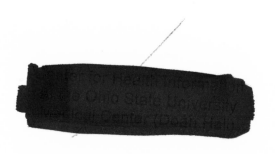
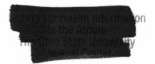

THE COLUMBIA UNIVERSITY SCHOOL OF DENTAL AND ORAL SURGERY'S GUIDE TO FAMILY DENTAL CARE

THE
COLUMBIA UNIVERSITY
SCHOOL OF DENTAL
AND ORAL SURGERY'S
GUIDE TO
FAMILY DENTAL CARE

by

REBECCA W. SMITH

and

The Columbia University School
of Dental and Oral Surgery

W · W · NORTON & COMPANY
New York   London

This book is intended for informational purposes only. It is not meant in any way to substitute for the advice and knowledge of your dentist or physician. If you have or suspect you have any dental or medical problems or disorders, you should consult a dentist and/or physician.

Copyright © 1997 by Rebecca W. Smith and the trustees of Columbia University in the City of New York through its School of Dental and Oral Surgery

For information about permission to reproduce selections from this book, write to Permissions, W. W. Norton & Company, Inc., 500 Fifth Avenue, New York, NY 10110.

The text of this book is composed in Times Roman
with the display set in ITC Fenice Regular
Composition and manufacturing by
The Maple-Vail Book Manufacturing Group
Book design by Jacques Chazaud

Library of Congress Cataloging-in-Publication Data

Smith, Rebecca W.
The Columbia University School of Dental and Oral Surgery's guide to family
dental care / by Rebecca W. Smith and the Columbia University School of Dental and
Oral Surgery.
p.   cm.
Includes bibliographical references and index.
ISBN 0-393-04036-4
1. Dental care—Popular works.   2. Consumer education.
I. Columbia University.   School of Dental and Oral Surgery.   II. Title.
III. Title: Guide to family dental care.
RK61.S666   1997
617.6—DC20   96-27434
CIP

W. W. Norton & Company, Inc., 500 Fifth Avenue, New York, N.Y. 10110
http://www.wwnorton.com

W. W. Norton & Company Ltd., 10 Coptic Street, London WC1A 1PU

2 3 4 5 6 7 8 9 0

CONTENTS

LIST OF EDITORS
AND CONTRIBUTORS

EDITORS

ALLAN J. FORMICOLA, D.D.S., M.S.
Dean, Columbia University School of Dental and Oral Surgery. Dr. Formicola is a periodontist. A past president of the American Association of Dental Schools, he is internationally recognized as an authority in the field of dental education.

ENID A. NEIDLE, Ph.D.
Senior Consultant to the Dean; Professor Emeritus, Pharmacology, New York University. Dr. Neidle is a past president of the American Association of Dental Schools and was the Director of Scientific Affairs at the American Dental Association.

WRITER AND EDITORIAL DIRECTOR

REBECCA W. SMITH
Rebecca W. Smith is a writer and editor specializing in medical and personal health subjects.

CONTRIBUTORS

DAVID A. ALBERT, D.D.S., M.P.H.
Assistant Professor of Dentistry and Public Health. Dr. Albert practices general dentistry in an inner-city community and develops and directs Columbia off-site dental practices and public-school-based prevention programs.

ERIC ASHER, B.A., M.A.M.S.
Associate in Clinical Dentistry. He is a maxillofacial prosthetist, Division of Prosthodontics, who also holds an appointment at the Bronx Veterans Administration Medical Center. An experienced medical illustrator, he has created all the illustrations in this text.

JEFFREY R. BURKES, D.D.S.
Associate Clinical Professor of Dentistry. A prominent forensic odontologist, Dr. Burkes is Chief Dental Consultant for the Office of Chief Medical Examiner of New York City.

THOMAS J. CANGIALOSI, D.D.S.
Professor of Clinical Dentistry, Associate Dean for Postdoctoral Education, and Director, Division of Orthodontics. Dr. Cangialosi is a diplomate and a current director of the American Board of Orthodontics.

MARTIN J. DAVIS, D.D.S.
Professor of Clinical Dentistry, Assistant Dean for Student and Alumni Affairs, and Director of the Division of Pediatric Dentistry. Dr. Davis is a diplomate of the American Board of Pediatric Dentistry and a former president of the American Academy of Pediatric Dentistry.

ROBERT GOTTSEGEN, D.D.S.
Professor Emeritus of Dentistry and former Director of the Division of Periodontics. Dr. Gottsegen is an internationally known periodontist, diplomate of the American Board of Periodontology, and past president of the American Academy of Periodontology.

FARHAD HADAVI, D.M.D., M.S.
Professor of Clinical Dentistry, Dr. Hadavi is Director of Preclinical Operative Dentistry and an expert in dental materials.

GUNNAR HASSELGREN, D.D.S., Ph.D.
Professor of Clinical Dentistry and Director of the Division of Endodontics. Dr. Hasselgren is internationally recognized for his scholarship in endodontics.

DAVID I. HENDELL, D.D.S.
Assistant Clinical Professor of Dentistry. A respected general dentist, Dr. Hendell lectures widely on the subject of cosmetic dentistry.

SIDNEY L. HOROWITZ, D.D.S.
Professor Emeritus of Dentistry and former Associate Dean for Academic Affairs. Dr. Horowitz is a distinguished orthodontist and is internationally recognized for his work on growth and development of the orofacial complex. He is a diplomate of the American Association of Orthodontists.

HOWARD A. ISRAEL, D.D.S.
Associate Professor of Clinical Dentistry. Dr. Israel is a diplomate of the American Board of Oral and Maxillofacial Surgery. In addition to his active surgical practice, he has expertise in the diagnosis and treatment of temporomandibular disorders.

IRA B. LAMSTER, D.D.S., M.M.Sc.
Associate Professor of Dentistry and Director of the Division of Periodontics. A leading researcher in the field of new diagnostic strategies for periodontal disease, he is a diplomate of the American Board of Periodontology.

RICHARD LICHTENTHAL, D.D.S.
Associate Professor of Clinical Dentistry. Dr. Lichtenthal is the Director of
Restorative Dentistry at Columbia and a distinguished dental educator.

IRWIN D. MANDEL, D.D.S.
Professor Emeritus of Dentistry. Dr. Mandel is an internationally recognized
researcher in the field of preventive dentistry, caries, and saliva. He was the first
recipient of the American Dental Association's Gold Medal Award for Excellence
in Dental Research.

LOUIS MANDEL, D.D.S.
Clinical Professor of Dentistry and Assistant Dean for Extramural Hospital Programs. Dr. Mandel is a diplomate of the American Board of Oral and Maxillofacial Surgery and Director of the Salivary Gland Center.

STEPHEN E. MARSHALL, D.D.S., M.P.H.
Assistant Professor of Dentistry and Public Health. Dr. Marshall is an expert in
the financing and organization of dental care plans.

MONA E. McALARNEY, M.S., D.Eng.
Assistant Professor of Dentistry. Dr. McAlarney is a researcher in dental materials and bioengineering.

JOHN L. McCABE, D.D.S., M.D.
Assistant Professor of Clinical Dentistry. A diplomate of the American Board of
Oral and Maxillofacial Surgery, he directs courses in pain control, anesthesia,
and sedation.

MARC W. MICHALOWICZ, D.D.S., M.Sc.
Assistant Professor of Clinical Dentistry. Dr. Michalowicz is a Diplomate of the
American Dental Board of Anesthesiology and is Chief, Dental and Oral Surgery
Service at the Helen Hayes Hospital.

LETTY MOSS-SALENTIJN, D.D.S., Ph.D.
Professor of Dentistry (in Anatomy and Cell Biology) and Associate Dean for
Academic Affairs. She is an international expert on the embryology and histology
of the orofacial region.

RONNIE MYERS, D.D.S.
Associate Professor of Clinical Dentistry. Dr. Myers is Assistant Dean for Patient
Care Activities and maintains an active general practice.

ZOILA E. NOGUEROLE, B.S.
Executive Assistant to the dean and the faculty of dentistry at the School of
Dental and Oral Surgery. She has been the coordinator for this project.

STEVEN M. ROSER, D.M.D., M.D.
Professor of Clinical Dentistry (in Surgery and Otolaryngology), Dr. Roser is a diplomate of the American Board of Oral and Maxillofacial Surgery, Director of Oral and Maxillofacial Surgery at the Presbyterian Hospital, and Director of the Division of OMFS at the dental school. He is an expert in reconstructive oral and maxillofacial surgery.

ANDREA SCHREIBER, D.M.D.
Assistant Professor of Clinical Dentistry. Dr. Schreiber is a diplomate of the American Board of Oral and Maxillofacial Surgery, has a busy surgical practice, and directs, among other courses, the course on medical emergencies.

NEILL SERMAN, B.D.S., M.S. (RAD), D.D.S.
Professor of Clinical Dentistry. He is Head of the Division of Oral Radiology and maintains an active general practice.

STEVEN B. SYROP, D.D.S.
Associate Clinical Professor of Dentistry. He is a general practitioner whose practice focuses on patients with temporomandibular disorders and facial pain. Dr. Syrop is a diplomate of the American Board of Orofacial Pain and co-director of the TMD program at Columbia's School of Dental and Oral Surgery.

KENNETH TROUTMAN, D.D.S., M.P.H.
Professor of Clinical Dentistry. Dr. Troutman is a diplomate of the American Board of Pediatric Dentistry, a past president of the American Academy of Pediatric Dentistry, and an expert in the hospital treatment of children with special healthcare needs.

ROBERT F. WRIGHT, D.D.S.
Associate Professor of Clinical Dentistry and Director, Division of Prosthodontics. He is an expert in the field of prosthetic reconstruction of maxillofacial defects and prosthodontics.

DAVID J. ZEGARELLI, D.D.S.
Professor of Dentistry (in Pathology), Dr. Zegarelli is a diplomate of the American Board of Oral Pathology and the American Board of Oral Medicine. He is internationally recognized on the subject of lesions of the oral cavity.

JOHN L. ZIMMERMAN, D.D.S.
Associate Professor of Clinical Dentistry and Assistant Dean for Information Resources. He is in the practice of general dentistry and is one of the few internationally recognized dentists in the field of dental informatics.

ACKNOWLEDGMENTS

Rebecca W. Smith wishes to thank her husband, Dana Gumb, for the unfair share of baby-sitting and other sundry tasks he performed to allow her to complete this book. She also thanks her children, Tyler and Derek, who were patient and understanding throughout the writing of this book; her agent, Judith Riven; and her editors at W. W. Norton, Mary Cunnane and Patricia Chui. Finally, she extends her profound appreciation to the members of the faculty of the Columbia University School of Dental and Oral Surgery for the considerable time, energy, and medical expertise they devoted to this project.

The Columbia University School of Dental and Oral Surgery's Guide to Family Dental Care represents the fruitful collaboration of faculty and staff from the School of Dental and Oral Surgery and a scientific writer, Rebecca Smith, who quickly absorbed the principles and problems of dentistry and transformed them into a highly readable and valuable book. We owe thanks to the dentists on the Columbia faculty, who patiently read parts of the book, made invaluable suggestions, and brought to the finished product an unassailable accuracy and unmistakable authority. To the staff who participated in this process in myriad ways, we offer our appreciation. We are particularly indebted to Zoila E. Noguerole who managed the complicated interactions between the writer, the publisher, the faculty, and the staff. And we commend Rebecca Smith for her willingness to venture into new territory with such felicitous results.

Allan J. Formicola, D.D.S.
Enid A. Neidle, Ph.D.
co-editors

ABOUT THIS BOOK

If you're like most Americans, you like and trust your dentist. In Gallup polls during the past 20 years dentists have placed consistently within the top 6 of approximately 25 occupations in traits of honesty and ethical standards. In a 1994 Gallup poll, for example, dentists were ranked third in these traits, behind pharmacists and clergy, but ahead of college professors, medical doctors, bankers, and lawyers. This is not surprising.

The relationship most people have with their dentist is the most enduring they have with any healthcare provider. It is not unusual for individuals who remain in the same community to have the same dentist provide care from cradle to grave, not only for themselves but for their children and parents as well. This continuum of care reveals the trust we have in our dentists to provide us with high-quality care, to deliver it painlessly, and to make our smile more attractive.

Dentists can do this because of the incredible progress modern dentistry has made in improving dental health and appearance. Within the last 50 years, the major dental problems—dental caries (tooth decay), periodontal disease, and tooth loss—which have plagued humans for centuries, have been subdued. And with the state-of-the-art dental care available currently, it is now possible for most people to achieve the age-old dental ideal of even, straight, white teeth. "You look different, better, younger," someone might compliment us, not knowing that a dental treatment was responsible for the subtle yet profound changes in our looks.

The advances in prevention, diagnosis, materials, and treatment that have revolutionized dental care within the last two decades also have made it more complex. As a savvy healthcare consumer, you realize it is no longer enough to care for your teeth by brushing them haphazardly and relying on your dentist to "choose" from the one option or material available. Yet the choices you are offered and the vigilance required in oral hygiene to keep dental diseases at bay (which, at times, feels Sisyphean) can be overwhelming. It seems as if an orientation course is needed just to steer through the dizzying array of dental care products at the drug store!

And even though you may be pleased with the care you receive from your dentist, you probably have questions about the exciting new technologies that you've heard or read about. These include bone-integrated implants; bacterial tests (DNA probes, enzyme assays), guided tissue regeneration, and subtraction radiography for periodontal disease; home teeth-bleaching kits; computerized imaging; the use of resin materials for bonding and restorations; and orthodontic treatment for adults. Since many of these are elective and many, especially cosmetic procedures, are not covered by insurance, deciding which treatment to have or restorative material to choose requires that you evaluate many factors, among them, how it looks, how long it will last, and how much it will cost. To make appropriate decisions, you need to consider the choices, weigh the pros and cons of each alternative, and determine how much you can afford. But given the current complexity of care and the options available, to do all this requires more information, knowledge, and time than your dentist will be able to give you during the period allotted for an office visit.

With this in mind, we have written this reference guide to help you maneuver through the new and ever-changing terrain of modern dental care. Our book answers both the practical and medical questions you have about preventive care at home and in the office and about proposed treatments. We explain the rigorous training and education your dentist has undergone to be highly qualified to treat you and describe to you what standards of care you have a right to expect from your dentist. These include screenings for oral cancer, periodontal disease, and dental caries; treatment planning; control of pain; informed consent; and infection control. Our book supplies you with the information you need to educate yourself at your own pace and in your own home, so you can determine what is best for the dental health, aesthetic preferences, and pocket book of you and your family.

As teachers at the Columbia University School of Dental and Oral Surgery we are well qualified to write this current, complete dental guide for you. We not only educate our students to become dentists on the forefront of clinical practice and research, we also teach the patients we treat in our clinics, who come from a wide range of ethnic backgrounds and have diverse dental problems, how to take care of their oral health. In the process we are able often to introduce them to new diagnostic, preventive, restorative, and surgical therapies before dentists in private practice are aware of them. And since our students take their basic science courses with the medical students at the Columbia University College of Physicians and Surgeons, we are especially attuned to the important interrelationships of both common and unusual medical and dental problems.

Our book is divided into seven parts. Throughout it we try to use the correct dental terms instead of the more common ones. For example, we use the term "gingiva" when referring to the gums. We do so because we respect your ability and desire to gain a more accurate understanding of the subject.

Part 1 describes the anatomy, as well as the normal and abnormal development, of the teeth, gingiva (gums), and supporting structures. The chronology of dental eruption is illustrated to provide an instructive reference for parents.

Part 2 answers questions you have about dentists' education and training. We explain the various types of dental insurance and give authoritative advice on how to choose a dentist and dental specialist and how to pay for dental care. The important issues of informed consent and treatment planning also are discussed.

In Part 3, all aspects of the two most prevalent and potentially destructive dental diseases, dental caries (tooth decay) and periodontal disease, are fully covered: their causes, mechanisms of action, treatments (different kinds of fillings, surgeries), and the preventive therapies performed at home and in the dental office (sealants, dietary modification, topical and systemic fluorides). We guide you through the maze of dental products and devices, show you the correct ways to brush and floss your teeth, and list foods to eat and to avoid.

In Part 4 you learn about the dental concerns you may have at different stages of your life: from birth to adolescence, the adult years, and after 65. The chapter for women elaborates on the problems specific to them, and the chapter for the medically compromised and physically challenged, the problems specific to them.

The largest section of our book is Part 5, which discusses specific problems and treatments, many of them requiring the services of a dental specialist. The chapters in this section cover cosmetic dentistry for improving the aesthetics of the smile; prosthodontics for ways of replacing missing teeth, including implants; orthodontics for "straightening" the teeth and correcting problems of occlusion, that is, how the teeth come together; endodontics (root canal therapy); and oral surgery, including a discussion on the removal of the wisdom teeth, or third molars. A chapter devoted to temporomandibular disorders provides a rational discussion of this all-too-common and frequently misunderstood problem.

Part 6 deals with many topical controversies and concerns, among them pain and the anxiety about it, dental emergencies, the transmission of infectious diseases, radiographs (x-rays), fluoridation of water, and mercury and gallium fillings.

In Part 7, you find out what advances in dental care you can look forward to in the near and not-so-near future.

In the back of the book are two handy references. A chart identifies dental symptoms, their possible causes, treatments, when to call the dentist, and what to do while awaiting professional help. A glossary provides definitions of common dental terms.

The appendices list the addresses of dental schools, associations, and organizations from which to obtain more information about specific procedures and state dental societies from which to ask for referrals of dentists.

As dentists, our role has been and will continue to be that of helping our patients keep their teeth and smile healthy and attractive throughout their life. It is a mission we cannot accomplish alone. We know that informed patients will take better care of their own oral health and that of their families.

PART I

ORAL
ANATOMY

CHAPTER 1

Dental Structure

T his chapter describes the anatomy of the teeth and their supporting structures and how different dental tissues function. This knowledge may not be critical for you to make appropriate choices about your dental care, but it will deepen your understanding of how and why dental diseases develop and the extent of damage they can cause. (Use Illustration 1.1 to help you identify the parts of a tooth and its surrounding tissues.)

I N S I D E   T H E   M O U T H

The teeth and the structures that support and supply nutrients to them (the gingival tissues, the dentogingival junction, periodontal ligament, and the alveolar bone) are composed of different types of tissues. Tissues are groups of more-or-less similar cells and their products that act in a characteristic manner to perform a particular function.

Oral Mucosa

When you open your mouth and peer inside, the soft pink-red lining that you see covering everything but your teeth is oral mucosa. Oral mucosa has two main functions: it protects the underlying connective tissues from trauma and bacteria, and it receives and transmits sensory information, such as temperature and pressure, from the external environment to the central nervous system.

There are three types of oral mucosa: *lining mucosa,* which covers the cheeks, lips, soft palate, and area under the tongue; *masticatory mucosa,* which lines the attached gingiva and hard palate; and *specialized,* or *gustatory, mucosa,* which lines the top surface of the tongue. The distinctions between them play an important role in the placement of dentures and other dental prostheses. For these to be secure, they must be

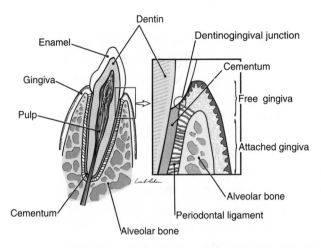

ILLUSTRATION 1.1. **PARTS OF A TOOTH AND SUPPORTING STRUCTURES.**

placed on the stable surfaces of the masticatory mucosa and not on the soft and movable surfaces of the lining mucosa.

Oral mucosa consists of two layers of tissues. The top layer is epithelium, a tissue that is in contact with the outer world and is found on other surfaces of the body, such as the skin and the lining of the digestive tract. It shields the underlying connective tissues from trauma and bacteria and loss of fluids. One way it does this is by keratinization. The process of keratinization changes the chemistry in the most superficial layers of the epithelium and renders them horny and impermeable to any water-soluble substances. The epithelial cells in these layers become filled with keratin, a fibrous protein also found in nails and hair and in a reptile's scales and a bird's feathers. Although not all layers of epithelium in the oral mucosa become keratinized, keratinization is especially prominent in the epithelium of the masticatory mucosa.

The basal (base) layer of oral epithelium contains melanocytes, cells that produce the pigment melanin. How brown an individual's oral mucosa is depends on the amount of melanin that is stored in his or her epithelial cells. The color of someone's oral mucosa does not always correspond to the amount of melanin in his or her skin.

Underneath the epithelium is a layer of dense connective tissue containing blood vessels and nerves. Its density provides mechanical support for the oral mucosa.

The gingiva is a special region of the oral mucosa. *Alveolar mucosa* covers the alveolar processes (the part of the jaw into which the teeth sink); *gingival mucosa* covers the roots of the teeth. Both help support and protect the teeth and make the mouth more attractive.

Gingival tissue (gums) is a specialized form of masticatory mucosa. It is bound firmly to the cervix (necks) of the teeth and the alveolar processes by collagen fibers. This firm attachment gives the gingiva a texture like an orange peel and protects the periodontal ligament beneath from invasion by bacteria. In healthy gums, the gingival tissues between the teeth are wedge shaped and fill the area. In most persons the gingival tissues are well keratinized; this makes them resistant to bacteria, chemicals, heat, and injuries.

The margins of the gums follow the contour of the neck of the tooth. However, from abrasion, most often caused by overzealous brushing, and, to a lesser extent, with age, they may recede and expose more of the cementum on the roots of the tooth. This makes the tooth appear larger and gives rise to the expression "long in the tooth."

If plaque, bacteria, and the food particles they feed on get trapped at the dentogingival junction (where the surfaces of the teeth and gingiva meet) and are not removed, the gums can become irritated and inflamed. This sets the stage for the development of periodontal disease. One of the diagnostic tests for periodontal disease involves inserting a probe to measure the depth of the gingival sulcus, a small space or crevice between the attached and free gingiva. *Attached gingival tissues* lie directly over the bone of the jaw and are so strongly bound to the underlying tissue that they cannot be moved. The *free gingiva* is the small strip (about 1.5 millimeters) along the margin of the gingiva.

THE TEETH

Teeth are composed of four dental tissues. Cementum, dentin, and enamel are hard or calcified. Pulp is soft or noncalcified.

Enamel

The visible part of the tooth is the crown. It is covered with enamel, the hardest substance the body produces.

When the tooth erupts or becomes visible in the mouth, the ameloblasts, the cells that form enamel, die. Because it contains no living
cells, enamel can neither repair nor replenish itself. As a result, any
defects that occurred during the prenatal formation of the tooth's enamel
(see Chapter 2) or damage that happens later will remain. Once formed,
it will not increase in thickness, nor is it able to repair damage from caries
or wear.

Although the teeth are often described as white, they are not. Enamel
has a gray or bluish tint to it that is only noticeable at the biting edges of
the incisors. The rest of the crown appears yellowish white, because
enamel is semitransparent and reveals the color of the dentin underneath.
When bonding or laminating teeth, the semitranslucent quality of enamel
needs to be replicated to retain a natural look. In older persons enamel
looks darker. When there is attrition, a natural wearing away of the
enamel surface with age, the dentin underneath may be revealed. Dentin
is a highly porous, slightly yellow tissue that can become stained by food
and appear orange, brown, or black.

Before birth, when the enamel is forming, the ameloblasts in the
grooves between the cusps of the molars are crowded, so areas that do
not calcify completely and are especially vulnerable to caries (or decay)
are created. Compounding the problem, these grooves are often so narrow
that a toothbrush or dental pick cannot easily fit between them, so food
particles and bacteria become trapped and the stage is set for the development of caries. Sealing these pits and grooves with an epoxy plastic that
forms a protective barrier against bacteria is a very effective method for
preventing this.

The enamel is composed of millions of microscopic and brittle
calcified structures called enamel prisms. Between them are spaces filled
with water and a minimal amount of protein. The enamel prisms run the
thickness of the enamel from the dentinoenamel junction to the outer
enamel surface. Their properties and arrangements play a crucial role in
a number of dental problems and the ways in which they are resolved.
For example, when dentists cut the enamel during the preparation of a
filling, they need to leave the prisms with enough support from the underlying dentin to prevent them from breaking. If the prisms are cut improperly, the margin of a filling can leak and weaken, and this can make the
teeth vulnerable to secondary caries at that spot.

Before bonding laminates or resins onto teeth, the inherently smooth surface of the enamel needs to be etched or roughened so that the materials can adhere to it. Whether a tooth's enamel takes the etching depends on the nature of its enamel prisms. In as many as 70 percent of permanent teeth, the outside layer of enamel lacks the prisms and the plastics may not adhere well.

Dentin and Pulp—The Essence of the Tooth

At the core of the tooth are the dentin and the pulp. Dentin (ivory) is a bonelike tissue that makes up the largest portion of the tooth. It is pale yellow and highly calcified. It is harder than cementum but not as durable or brittle as enamel. Dentin surrounds the pulp, except at the apical foramen, the opening at the root canals of the tooth, where blood vessels and nerves enter.

The shape of the pulp cavity conforms to the outline of the tooth (the root and crown). The space within the crown is called the pulp chamber, and the space inside the roots, the root canals. On the crown of the tooth, dentin is covered by enamel; on the root, it is surrounded by cementum.

Dentin is formed in the dental pulp by the odontoblast cells. During its production, the odontoblasts secrete dentin around long cell processes that are left behind to create dentinal tubules. The tubules wind in S-curved shapes through the width of the dentin in the crown. How dentinal tubules are involved in transmitting pain is explained in Chapter 13.

The pulp is composed of noncalcified loose connective tissue. Its blood vessels supply the oxygen- and nutrient-rich blood that nourishes the odontoblasts that maintain the dentin. If dentin is not maintained, the tooth will die. Dentin is manufactured continually throughout the life of a vital, or living, tooth. Its growth, however, is inward, so that, with age, it grows thicker by reducing the pulp inside. The pulp also contains a network of nerves that enter through the apical foramen and control the blood flow to the capillaries in the pulp. These are responsible for the perception of pain when the pulp is inflamed from caries or trauma.

THE TEETH'S ANCHORS

The root is the part of the tooth beneath the gums that is not visible. A tooth may have one or multiple roots, which are firmly anchored into sockets in the alveolar process. These vary in width depending on the shape of the tooth they hold.

Cementum and the Periodontal Ligament

The roots of the teeth are covered with cementum, a thin, pale-yellow layer of calcified connective tissue similar to bone but without the blood vessels and nerves. It forms very slowly throughout life. Cementum is attached to collagen fibers of the periodontal ligament, a tendonlike tissue surrounding the root. The periodontal ligament serves as a padding between the rigid bone and cementum to reduce stress on the alveolar bone during use.

Cementum, the alveolar bone, and the periodontal ligament anchor the teeth to the jaws. These three tissues can be compared to the parts of a suspension bridge. The cementum and alveolar bone serve as the towers; the periodontal ligament acts as the cables. When any of these tissues is compromised or missing, the teeth will loosen and eventually fall out. For example, the primary teeth fall out when the cementum and dentin in the roots, and sometimes some enamel, resorbs (dissolves). Teeth (usually permanent ones) will also loosen and fall out when bacteria from periodontal disease break down the periodontal tissue or destroy the alveolar bone.

Normally, cementum is not exposed. But with age and wear, the gums may recede and reveal the cementum where it meets the enamel. The line between the tissues can be readily seen on molars or other permanent teeth that have been extracted. Because cementum is softer than enamel and thinner at this line, it is more susceptible to caries. If your gums have receded, you need to be particularly vigilant in cleaning this area.

The Jaws and Temporomandibular Joint

The lower jaw, called the mandible, is the largest and strongest of the facial bones. It begins during development as two bones and then, around birth, fuses into a single bone, similar in shape to a horseshoe. The mandible is suspended under the upper jaw, the maxilla, by muscles, ligaments, fascia (a fiberlike connective tissue), and skin. Like those of other mammals, the teeth of humans are arranged equally between the two dental arches in the curves of the maxillae and the mandible. The temporomandibular joint (described in Chapter 17) allows the mandible to move.

SALIVARY GLANDS

There are three pairs of major salivary glands: the parotid, submandibular, and the sublingual. The parotid glands are largest. They are located in front of and below each ear and are the ones involved in the viral disease infectious parotitis, commonly referred to as mumps. Their main duct opens into the mouth on the wall of either cheek opposite the upper second molars. The submandibular glands are the size of walnuts. They are situated beneath the back of the tongue. The almond-sized sublingual glands are in the mucosa of the floor of the mouth. The spurts of saliva that sometimes erupt from the openings underneath the tongue and on the cheek near the upper molars can help you locate the glands.

In addition to the three pairs of major glands, minor salivary glands are distributed in the submucosa of the lips, cheeks, soft palate, and parts of the hard palate. The teeth opposite the ducts of the salivary glands develop more tartar. If not removed, it can irritate the gums and cause periodontal disease.

The salivary glands secrete two types of saliva: a thin, watery serous secretion, which helps clear away food and dead epithelial cells from the oral mucosa, and a mucous secretion, one of the functions of which is to help keep food together so it can be swallowed. The minor glands secrete the mucous solution, the parotid glands secrete the serous, and the submandibular and sublingual glands secrete both. Both minor and major glands produce saliva all the time, although the flow can be compromised by medical conditions and treatments. The amount that is secreted will vary between individuals, but on average, it is about 3 pints of liquid a day. (See Chapter 6 for a discussion of the important functions that saliva performs in maintaining oral health.)

DIFFERENT TEETH

Like other parts of our bodies, the purpose the teeth serve directs how they are shaped and what they are made of. Our teeth begin the process of digestion by breaking the food our bodies need into smaller pieces. Because we are omnivorous, our teeth need to be able to chew a variety of plant and animal foods that have different textures. To accomplish the daily chopping and grinding of our food, the enamel covering our teeth is made of strong tissue. And to remain intact after years of daily wear, our teeth are firmly anchored in the jaw.

Unlike many animals, we chew up and down (with only slight lateral, or side-to-side, motions made possible by the configuration of our skull bones and the temporomandibular joint). Although the structures of the different permanent teeth are similar, their shapes and surfaces vary, depending on the different kinds of chewing they do.

The cone-shaped canines, commonly referred to as cuspids or eye teeth, are the most stable. They are the only teeth with a single cusp, which is adapted for piercing food. Their roots are extra long and large, making them the longest teeth in our mouths. If they were not, they would be torn out of their sockets by the tearing movements they perform. Their shape, smooth with a single rounded cusp, tends to make them self-cleaning. As a result, the canines are some of the most resistant teeth to caries. This, combined with their secure anchorage, makes them among the last teeth to be lost to age. Canines also serve an important cosmetic purpose. Situated at the corners of the mouth, they give our smiles an aesthetic symmetry.

Incisors have been aptly named for their ability to cut. They are flat or chisel shaped; this makes them efficient for shearing and cutting food in preparation for grinding.

The first and second premolars (sometimes referred to as bicuspids for their two main cusps) are an intermediary type tooth, containing traits of both the canines and molars. With sharp cusps for piercing food and modified top surfaces for grinding, they effectively crush and tear food.

Molars have the largest grinding surfaces, with three to five main cusps. The lower molars usually have two roots, whereas the upper molars usually have three. Their roots are strong to secure the tooth for the grinding movements they make. The third molars, known to most as the wisdom teeth, can vary in size, shape, and position.

CHAPTER 2

Dental Development

NORMAL DEVELOPMENT

Like most other mammals, humans have two sets of teeth: the primary and permanent. Our primary teeth begin their development about the seventh week of prenatal life. After they are partially formed, secondary tooth buds start developing to form the permanent teeth. They continue developing through adolescence. The face develops between the fourth and twelfth weeks, whereas the hard and soft palates are formed between the fifth and twelfth weeks of prenatal life.

The Developmental Process

For either a primary or permanent tooth to form, two events, morphodifferentiation and cytodifferentiation, must take place. During morphodifferentiation, the shape of a tooth is formed; during cytodifferentiation, an undifferentiated cell type is transformed into a cell with a specific function.

Even though babies seldom have teeth showing when they are born, all the primary teeth, as well as the permanent first molars, are present. They are concealed beneath the gums, in various stages of enamel and dentin formation within the jaws. Slowly, in the early months of an infant's life, the tooth moves within the jaw toward the surface of the gums, until it erupts.

A tooth erupts over a span of time, during which its roots are forming. To form the roots, the epithelium on the enamel grows downward. (Epithelial tissue and embryonic connective tissue are the two types of tissues from which both primary and permanent teeth develop.) The cementoblast cells produce cementum, and the odontoblast cells undergo cytodifferentiation to produce dentin. When the tooth is fully erupted, the roots are only about two-thirds formed. The rest of the root, its apical foramen, the periodontal ligament, cementum, and alveolar bone are not completed until as long as four years after the tooth first appears in the mouth.

The Primary Teeth

The significance of our first set of teeth extends beyond their lifetime. Because they are not retained, many people believe that the primary teeth (also referred to as baby, deciduous, temporary, or milk, for their milk-white color, teeth) are not very important. To the contrary, while they remain in the mouth, which can be anywhere from 5 to 6 years for the front ones and 10 to 12 years for the back ones, primary teeth serve some of the same purposes as permanent teeth: they are needed for chewing food, making the face more attractive, and developing speech. In addition, they have independent functions: they maintain space to help the permanent teeth to emerge in proper alignment and to grow and develop normally.

In toto, there are 20 primary teeth, 10 in each jaw. They include 4 incisors, 2 canines, and 4 molars in each dental arch. Typically, they emerge in the mouth in a similar pattern: first come the lower central incisors, then the upper central incisors, the upper lateral incisors, the lower lateral incisors, the upper first molars, the lower first molars, the lower canines, the upper canines, the lower second molars, and finally the upper second molars. (See Illustration 2.1 for their average eruption times.)

Sometime between a child's second and third birthdays, his or her complete set of primary teeth should be fully erupted and visible. By the age of three, the roots are entirely formed. A year later the jaw often grows to such an extent that gaps form between the teeth. (The eruption schedule for primary teeth varies widely among individuals and among ethnic groups. Since most of the studies have been conducted on European whites, less is known about when the teeth of nonwhite, non-Europeans emerge.)

Primary teeth are lost after their roots resorb and the crown of the tooth loses its support. Thus, all that is left for the tooth fairy is the visible portion of the tooth. Parents who hold their child's tooth after it has fallen out will notice it ends in a jagged line a little beneath the cementoenamel junction. (Refer to Illustration 1.1 to locate the parts of the tooth.)

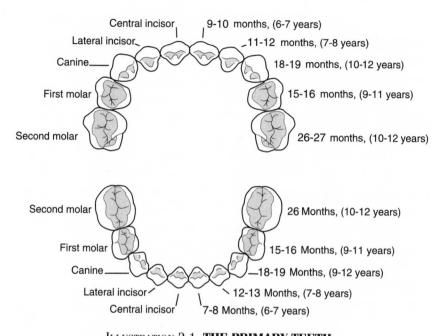

ILLUSTRATION 2.1. **THE PRIMARY TEETH.**
The average ages when the teeth erupt are shown.
The ages in parentheses are the average ages when they fall out.

Maintaining the health of primary teeth is very important. If they are lost prematurely, malocclusions (irregularities in the way the upper and lower teeth bite together) that may require orthodontic treatment can develop. Retaining primary teeth until they are ready to exfoliate (fall out) increases the odds of the permanent teeth erupting in normal alignment. If injured, the primary teeth can become discolored or disfigured. And if decayed, the disease may spread quickly to the permanent successors.

The Permanent Teeth

Most of us use our permanent teeth for 90 percent or more of our lives. Even though they are not visible in the mouth until a child is between four and six years old, on average, some of them begin calcifying (developing enamel and dentin) in infancy, as early as three or four months after birth.

Almost always before any of the primary teeth are lost, the first permanent molars, dubbed the six-year-old molars because they usually erupt by that time, emerge behind the primary second molars. The permanent central incisors in the lower jaw soon follow. (See Illustration 2.2 for the eruption schedule of the permanent teeth.)

The timetable a child's teeth follow in emerging is largely determined by heredity. Because many processes are underway simultaneously, such as the formation of the roots, growth of the jaw, and pressures from muscular action, researchers find it difficult to determine which process is most instrumental in provoking the teeth to erupt. Although there is no medical significance attached to the time when a child's teeth come in, teeth that are very retarded in their eruption may indicate a systemic disorder and frequently are seen in persons with Down syndrome, cretinism, and growth hormone deficiency.

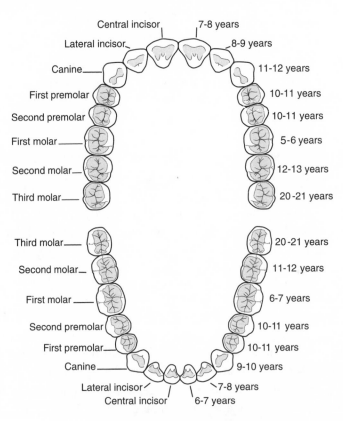

ILLUSTRATION 2.2. **THE PERMANENT TEETH.**
The average ages when they erupt are shown.

A full set of permanent teeth totals 32. By the age of 13, most children have 28 of their permanent teeth (4 central and 4 lateral incisors, 8 premolars, 4 canines, and 8 molars). The last four to arrive, the third molars, usually come in somewhere between the ages of 17 and 21.

PRENATAL INFLUENCES

For the most part, unless a woman has severe nutritional deficiencies, which are rare in the United States, her diet will be adequate in the nutrients the teeth of her fetus need to develop normally. There are, however, an array of influences on a woman other than her nutritional status during pregnancy that more often adversely affect her baby's teeth and other oral and facial structures. These include certain medications and substances she takes, illnesses she contracts, and chemicals or other environmental hazards to which she is exposed, especially during the crucial time when her baby's teeth, face, and jaw are forming. For example, high and prolonged fevers from infections and viruses, such as rubella or chicken pox, during gestation when the teeth are developing, can cause defects in the enamel and dentin, which can compromise both the aesthetics and integrity of the tooth.

ABNORMAL DEVELOPMENT

A host of conditions are associated with a range of oral and facial defects. Some of the more common dental abnormalities described here may be associated with systemic disorders but can also occur in the absence of them. Most are a consequence of hereditary factors or of problems for which the reason is unknown. In general, more defects affect the permanent teeth than the primary ones and more occur in the teeth of the upper jaw than in those of the lower jaw.

Defects of the Teeth Caused by Genetics

Anodontia. Occasionally, all or some of the teeth are missing because they never formed. This condition appears more often in the permanent teeth than in the primary ones.

When the anodontia is complete, all the permanent teeth are missing.

This rarely happens, but when it does, it is associated most frequently with a genetic defect that also affects the hair, nails, and sweat and salivary glands. Partial anodontia (hypodontia), in which one or more but not all of the teeth are missing, is not uncommon. It affects between 5 and 8 percent of the population in the United States and appears more frequently when there is a family history of it. The teeth missing most often are the lower second premolars, the upper lateral incisors, and the third molars. When a primary tooth comes in peg shaped, it is frequently an indication that the succeeding permanent tooth is missing. Treatment options for people missing permanent teeth involve different types of restorations.

Supernumerary. Some people develop too many teeth—a tendency that also runs in families. Most extra teeth appear in the upper jaw, in both primary and permanent sets.

Most commonly, only one extra tooth, usually a fourth molar, develops. It is most often discovered by radiographs (x-rays). When there are multiple supernumerary teeth, it may indicate Gardner's syndrome, an inherited disease characterized by extra bony growths in the jaws or face or long bones. Most supernumerary teeth are extracted, especially primary ones that might interfere with the eruption of permanent teeth, cause a malocclusion, or predispose the individual to caries and periodontal disease.

Microdontia and Macrodontia. The size of teeth is largely determined by heredity. Although there are substantial variations in size, when teeth are abnormally small, it is referred to as microdontia; when they are uncharacteristically large, it is called macrodontia. This abnormality can affect one, several, or all of the teeth. No treatment is performed for macrodontia. Microdontic teeth that are impacted are removed; others are restored to resemble normally sized teeth.

Amelogenesis Imperfecta. This is a catchall term for a number of rare genetic defects (they afflict 1 in 14,000 children) that affect the texture and color of the enamel of both the primary and permanent teeth. Often the teeth are also highly susceptible to caries. In general, the condition causes at least three different types of imperfections in the enamel. It may develop localized chalky white spots and variations in color from white to brown, flake off the teeth, or be pitted. Depending on the type and extent of the imperfection, treatments can include bonding, crowns, implants, and fixed partial dentures (bridges).

Enamel Projections. Sometimes during the formation of the enamel, extra cells stray and form a globule or projection, dubbed a talon's cusp. They form most frequently on the front or back of the upper incisor. Although rare, these enamel pearls may be unsightly and, if they project from the cementum at the gumline, may adversely affect periodontal health. Occasionally, they can interfere with the occlusion. If they are composed of enamel only, a dentist will be able to trim them easily. If they include part of the pulp or dentin, their removal will be more difficult because the pulp might be exposed, and this would threaten the vitality of the tooth.

Fusion. Occasionally during development, two adjacent teeth that have normal and separate teeth germs may crowd and fuse, or grow together, for reasons that are not clearly understood. When this happens, the crown is larger and usually appears joined, or "twinned," in much the same way Siamese twins are.

A number of variations on this theme can take place. The teeth may have separate or common roots and pulp chambers, one large crown, or two crowns fused together. This anomaly appears more frequently in primary teeth than it does in permanent teeth. Replacing the tooth is not always necessary but is warranted if it affects the occlusion or the individual finds it aesthetically unacceptable.

Gemination. The teeth may appear fused but share one root canal; this may require endodontic treatment before the tooth can be crowned. This anomaly is found most frequently in the primary teeth, in the incisors and canines.

Dentinogenesis Imperfecta. This disorder causes defects in the dentin, giving teeth an unattractive blue-gray to yellow color and an opalescent appearance. Radiographs will reveal a partial or total lack of pulp chambers and canals. A defect in the dentinoenamel junction prevents the enamel (though normal) from adhering properly to the dentin. As the enamel chips off, the dentin is exposed, and the teeth are quickly worn down. Treatment most frequently involves installing full crowns on all the teeth.

Hutchinson's Teeth. In this disorder, which results most often from prenatal syphilis, both primary and permanent teeth are shaped like a screwdriver and often have notches on the sides of their crowns. With antibiotic therapies widely available in developed countries, few teeth today are affected by this sexually transmitted disease. Similar-looking teeth can develop in individuals who have Down syndrome, even if they were never exposed to syphilis.

Taurodontism. Up to 5 percent of the population has this defect, in which the pulp chambers are larger and the roots are shorter than normal. Persons with Down and Klinefelter syndromes, as well as some other conditions, commonly have taurodont teeth. (Klinefelter syndrome results from a chromosomal abnormality in males that causes small, firm testicles; long legs; breasts; and infertility.) Because the roots are not nestled as deeply into the supporting structures as is normal, there is an increased risk of tooth loss when gum recession or periodontal disease are significant.

A Defect of the Teeth Caused by Trauma

Sometimes a tooth develops an abnormal curve or bend in its root or crown. Called *dilaceration,* this is believed to result from a trauma the tooth sustained during the development of its root. When this happens, the position of the calcified part of the tooth is altered and the rest of the tooth develops on an angle. The bend in either a permanent or primary tooth can occur anywhere along the root and is most frequently discovered by radiographs. No treatment is necessary. Radiographs should be taken before the tooth requires endodontic therapy or is extracted, as the defect may cause difficulties with these procedures.

Anomalies of the Jaw

Many malocclusions fall within a range that is acceptable aesthetically and physiologically. There are two facial abnormalities, mandibular retrognathism and mandibular prognathism, that lie at the extreme unacceptable ends of this spectrum. Both can cause disfigurement and problems with chewing. Sometimes these conditions can be corrected by long-term orthodontic treatment; more often a combined orthodontic-surgical approach is required. (For more information, see Chapter 18.)

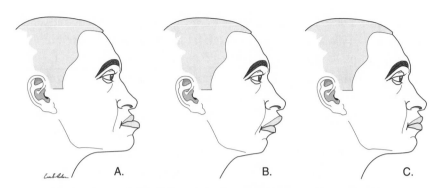

ILLUSTRATION 2.3. **SKELETAL ABNORMALITIES OF THE JAW.**
A. Mandibular prognathism. **B.** Mandibular retrognathism. **C.** Normal jaw.

Mandibular Retrognathism. In this skeletal deformity, the upper jaw appears large in comparison to the lower jaw, the chin appears receded, and there is a large overjet or protrusion (between 5 and 10 millimeters) of the upper teeth relative to the lower. The resulting profile gives rise to nicknames, such as buck teeth, overbite, and bird face.

Mandibular Prognathism. In this less common skeletal abnormality, the reverse occurs: the lower jaw juts forward and the chin is prominent. Names given to this condition include jut jaw, underbite, or Dick Tracy bite.

Cleft Lips and Palates

Each year in the United States, about 6,000 children are born with their lip or palate not completely closed. This causes functional, as well as cosmetic, problems and has attendant psychological repercussions. In addition to feeding disorders and difficulties with control of the muscles in their mouth that can affect speech, children with clefts have missing, misaligned, and malformed teeth.

Clefting is a common congenital malformation that comprises about 25 percent of all birth defects. The prevalence of the condition is higher with Asians, especially Japanese (about 1 in 400), than with Caucasians (about 1 in 700) or African Americans (about 1 in 1,500). The incidences of clefts have been increasing in recent years in the United States—a result of the greater numbers of pregnancies that involve the risk factors listed subsequently.

Girls experience isolated cleft of the palate more frequently. The cleft in the lip alone and in the lip and palate together are more common in boys. About 20 percent of facial clefts can be considered genetic.

Most clefts result from the interaction of environmental and genetic factors. They are associated with excessive maternal intake of alcohol, malnutrition (of calories and protein), illnesses, anticonvulsant and some other medications, and chemotherapy and radiation during the second and third months of pregnancy. Women who give birth after the age of 35 have an increased risk of delivering a baby with congenital malformations. This risk is intensified if the mother has diabetes and / or epilepsy.

Genetic testing can assist couples who have family histories of clefting in determining their risks of bearing a child with the malformation. Counseling can help women with other risk factors to evaluate their risks, whereas prenatal care can help improve a woman's nutritional status and warn her about the hazards of ingesting certain substances. The condition can be diagnosed using ultrasound between the sixteenth and twentieth weeks of gestation.

Rehabilitative therapy for children with clefts continues from birth until the age of around 20 years. Depending on the extent of the defect, dental therapies include orthodontics, prosthodontics, and surgery. Speech therapy and social and psychological support is often needed, as well (see also Chapter 18).

Defects Caused by Substances

(See Chapter 14 for treatments for these conditions.)

Fluorosis. When a child ingests high levels of the mineral fluoride during the years the teeth are forming, the enamel on the permanent teeth can become mottled, discolored, and pitted. This condition, called fluorosis, is usually caused by drinking water with a high level of fluoride (many times greater than the 1 part per million normally added to municipal water supplies) and sometimes by fluoride supplementation. Depending on the severity of the staining, bleaching, bonding, and sometimes crown restorations can be effective therapies. (For more information on fluorosis, see the sections on fluoride in Chapters 8 and 21.)

Tetracycline Stain. Tetracycline antibiotics, taken by a pregnant woman, infant, or child, may stain the developing dentin and cementum and very slightly, the enamel. The critical period seems to be between the fourth month *in utero* until the child is about eight years old.

The severity of the stain, which varies in color from yellow to gray-brown, depends on how much of the drug is taken and for how long. The front teeth are the ones most often discolored for two reasons. First, they develop during the critical exposure time, and second, they are most exposed to sunlight which, over time, turns the tetracycline-exposed teeth darker. (Tetracycline forms an orthocalcium phosphate complex with enamel and dentin that is oxidized by ultraviolet light. The pigments that result stain the hard tissues of the teeth.) The primary teeth usually have generalized staining, whereas the permanent teeth may or may not, depending on the age at which the antibiotics were prescribed. Tetracycline-stained teeth can be treated by bonding, veneering, and sometimes bleaching—cosmetic dental procedures that are covered in Chapter 14.

Problems with Eruption

A number of problems, some of which are listed here, are associated with the eruption of the teeth into the mouth.

Embedded and Impacted Teeth. At least 10 percent of the population have impacted teeth, teeth that do not erupt because of an obstruction. This usually happens because there is not enough room, a result of premature loss of a primary tooth, as well as the evolutionary diminution of the human jaw. (The jaws of primitive humans were larger.) Most impacted teeth are the third molars or the upper canines.

Canine teeth (lower and upper) are also problematical in other ways. Often they are the last teeth of the primary series to be replaced. Their permanent successors may emerge in peculiar places in the mouth; this necessitates orthodontic intervention to correct their position.

Embedded teeth are teeth that remain under the gums because there is not sufficient force to cause them to erupt. When this occurs, it may be a sign of a more-generalized systemic syndrome. When the entire set of the primary teeth are slow to fall out and when the permanent teeth include supernumerary ones, accompanied by a failure of the bones, especially the skull and clavicle, to develop, this indicates the hereditary condition cleidocranial dysostosis. Impacted and embedded teeth can be difficult to diagnose and, therefore, must be evaluated on a case-by-case basis.

Rotation. Teeth (most frequently the upper second premolars) that emerge twisted or rotated, sometimes as much as 180 percent out of their normal alignment, may require orthodontic correction.

Ankylosis. In this condition, teeth erupt only partially, so that they appear submerged beneath the gums. This can happen spontaneously, but it can also result from an infection or injury to the periodontal ligament. Frequently but not always this occurs in a primary tooth where the following permanent tooth is missing. When ankylosed teeth affect the occlusion, they may need to be extracted.

PART II

—

VISITING
THE DENTIST

CHAPTER 3

Your Dentist

WHO IS YOUR DENTIST?

If asked to explain who dentists are, most Americans would answer, "doctors for the teeth and gums." Yet the anatomy within the province of the dentist extends beyond this limited domain to encompass all the oral tissues. As doctors of the oral cavity and related structures, dentists detect oral diseases and diagnose and treat problems that also affect the tongue, lips, jaws, and other soft tissues of the oral mucosa. A dentist is often the first healthcare provider to identify diseases such as oral cancer or AIDS.

The dentist most patients routinely visit is a general dentist. When you require special procedures or therapies, among them braces, dentures, implants, periodontal treatments, and surgery, frequently you go to a dental specialist. What areas of expertise and treatments are within the realm of the various specialties, how general dentists and dental specialists are educated and trained, and what you need to know when deciding which dentist or dental specialist to choose are among the issues discussed in this chapter.

DENTAL TRAINING

Knowing what training a dentist has is one of the most important factors to consider when selecting a general dentist to provide routine care and when deciding whether to have complex procedures performed by a general dentist or a dental specialist. Many of the more recent innovative procedures being offered, such as osseointegrated implants, demand a level of knowledge and training you should be certain your dentist has before undergoing them.

Dental School

On successfully completing four years of dental school, a graduate is awarded a Doctor of Dental Surgery (D.D.S.) or a Doctor of Dental Medicine (D.M.D.) degree. The educational programs and accreditation requirements are the same for both degrees, and the regulatory and licensing agencies regard each the same. Despite this, they are often confusing to patients and leave many with the unspoken impression that holders of D.M.D.s may have more or different training or have degrees in both medicine and dentistry. They do not. The difference is one of semantics only.

Qualifications for Practice

To practice dentistry, the D.D.S. or D.M.D. must pass both a written national board and a state or regional examination. To become licensed to practice dentistry (after passing the boards), a dentist applies to the state board of dentistry in the state in which he or she intends to practice. The application process varies among states, but, in general, it is a means by which the board verifies an applicant's academic qualifications, moral character, and maintenance of professional standards (by checking with the National Practitioners Data Bank described in Chapter 4).

For most dentists, the educational requirements for licensure are fulfilled by graduation from an accredited dental school (all dental schools in the United States and Canada are accredited). Some states accept graduates from foreign dental schools that are recognized in the countries where they are located, other states accept foreign dental school graduates if they were licensed or admitted to practice in the countries in which they were educated, and still other states accept foreign dental school graduates if their educations meet established standards for curriculum (course content and clinical experience) and duration of education. As of this writing, 18 states accept foreign dental school graduates if they receive supplementary education given at some institutions within the state in lieu of a D.D.S. or D.M.D. degree. The majority of states, however, require foreign-trained dentists to receive a D.D.S. or D.M.D. degree before they can be considered for licensure. Regardless of how different states allow foreign-trained dentists to fulfill their educational requirements for licensure, all foreign-trained dentists who are licensed within the United States must pass the same national, and state or regional boards that are required of graduates of accredited dental schools.

Postgraduate Training

In 1993 a sizable portion of the graduating class of dentists (about 36 percent) went on for advanced training either in general dentistry or a specialty. Although postgraduate training is essential to become a dental specialist, it is not required to obtain or retain licensure.

For General Dentists. There are two types of postgraduate programs for general dentistry: a general practice residency (GPR) that is conducted in a hospital setting where the dentist gains experience managing hospitalized patients, as well as outpatients, and an advanced education in general dentistry (AEGD), that is typically provided at a dental school, to give dentists additional experience caring for all types of dental patients. Both offer one- to two-year programs, culminating in a certificate in General Dentistry from the university or hospital sponsoring the program. Dentists in these programs, like those for specialty training, are awarded a certificate and not a degree. To find out whether a dentist has this additional training, you need to ask.

For Specialists. To become a dental specialist requires a minimum of two years postgraduate training in a program sponsored by either a dental school or a hospital. It is each institution's prerogative to choose where the program takes place and whether the dentist pays for the training or receives a stipend. Paid residency programs in hospitals are usually offered for pediatric dentistry and oral surgery (as well as the general practice residency program for general dentists). Postgraduate programs in dental schools (for which tuition is required) are more common for the other specialties. (See Box 3.1 for a description of the different specialties.)

Other Additional Training

In recognition that lifelong learning helps to keep dentists current with the changes taking place in dentistry, more than half the states require dentists to take some type of continuing education. Continuing

BOX 3.1

DENTAL SPECIALISTS

The American Dental Association (ADA) recognizes the eight dental specialties described here. Currently, approximately 20 percent of dentists are specialists.

Dental specialists have the option of limiting their practices to their specialty or of practicing it in addition to general dentistry. Dentists who restrict their practices to a specialty, for example, orthodontics, are required by the ADA to have met the educational requirements and the standards set by the ADA for that specialty. (Although general dentists may practice orthodontics or one of the other specialities, they are not allowed to confine their practice to a specialty.) Unless otherwise indicated, all dental specialties require two or more academic years of post-doctoral training.

Endodontists. Diagnose and treat (with root canal therapy and other procedures) diseases and injuries to the dental pulp and the tissues surrounding the root of the tooth.

Oral and Maxillofacial Surgeons. Diagnose and surgically treat diseases, injuries, and abnormalities of the hard and soft tissues of the neck, face, head, and jaws. Using surgical procedures, among them implants, tissue and bone grafts, and extractions, they repair and restore oral tissues and supporting structures. Nearly half the programs that provide the requisite four years of full-time training also either offer or require an M.D. (Doctor of Medicine) degree in a five- or six-year combined program.

Oral Pathologists. Study and sometimes diagnose the causes, mechanisms, and effects of diseases of the mouth and surrounding regions. Most confine their work to examining tissue specimens through a microscope, but a small number diagnose and treat patients referred to them by other dentists. Oral pathology requires two or more years of full-time postgraduate training.

Orthodontists. Diagnose and treat problems of occlusion and malformations of the jaws by slowly repositioning the teeth and facial bones using different appliances to restore normal function and appearance.

Pediatric Dentists. Treat the dental needs of children from birth through adolescence. Some treat physically and mentally challenged adults.

Periodontists. Prevent, diagnose, and treat periodontal diseases and surgically place dental implants. Additional training of three years is required.

Prosthodontists. In complex cases, replace missing teeth with a variety of prostheses: fixed or removable complete and partial dentures and dental implants. Some prosthodontists (maxillofacial prosthodontists), working with oral surgeons, specialize in placing prostheses to replace lost parts of the face, such as eyes, noses, and ears. Postdoctoral training involves three years.

Public Health Dentists. Concentrate on the prevention and control of dental diseases. They generally work for public health agencies, federal, state and local government, universities, and hospitals. They plan, implement, and evaluate programs to improve oral health care. A specialist in dental public health has earned the M.P.H. and/or Ph.D. degree and completed a dental public health residency.

education is offered by a variety of organizations, schools, dental societies, manufacturers, and private entrepreneurs.

Specialty organizations may provide courses that include hands-on patient care in a specific treatment or procedure. The American Dental Association and the Academy of General Dentistry provide and encourage, respectively, continuing education for general dentists. In addition, there are groups of dentists who, on their own, organize local study groups, which host speakers. Continuing education from a recognized university and/or in conjunction with large, well-organized professional meetings is the usual way for dentists to keep abreast of new developments.

The short courses in specific procedures given by manufacturers of the equipment or devices used, which culminate in a certificate issued by the manufacturer, may or may not be helpful to the dentist. If you are considering having a general dentist perform a procedure that he or she learned at a manufacturer-sponsored seminar, especially inserting implants, you should question whether the dentist also undertook training in other formats to make sure a well-rounded educational program was taken.

CHOOSING A DENTIST

Ideally every family should identify a general dentist and perhaps a pediatric dentist to take care of its preventive and restorative dental needs. He or she will monitor your oral health, diagnose and treat most of your dental problems, and refer you to a dental specialist if and when you have a problem that requires more expertise. The general dentist who serves these functions may be the dentist for your entire family or for the adult members only (some general dentists do not treat children).

If you are choosing a dentist, the ideal time to make your selection is when you or the members of your family have no immediate dental concerns and before you experience a dental crisis. Since your dental care is individual, the choice you make should be tailored to your and your family's dental needs. To make an intelligent choice, call or visit the dental office and speak with a staff member or the dentist. If either the dentist or office staff is unwilling or uncomfortable responding, consider going elsewhere.

Selecting a dentist is a two-part process. The first step is to locate a practitioner whose office is convenient to your work or home and who accepts your insurance (if this is a consideration); the second is to check his or her qualifications, training, and other qualities we enumerate later.

Finding Dentists

The following are some ways of identifying (but not evaluating) a dentist.

Friends. Although friends or family members usually cannot evaluate the clinical expertise and knowledge of their dentists, they can give you subjective information, such as that the dentist is trusted and well liked, has a pleasant personality, is a good communicator, and performs services in a satisfactory manner.

Physician. Implicit in the recommendation of a dentist by a trusted family or primary-care physician *may* be an unspoken affirmation of his or her competent professional qualifications.

Previous Dentist. If you are moving, ask your present dentist to recommend a dentist in your new community.

The Local Dental Society. Patients who call their local dental society, which is a chapter of the American Dental Association (ADA), are given names only of dentists in their area who are ADA members. Membership in the ADA is voluntary and does not confer any degree, stature, or additional training or qualifications on the dentist. Rather, it is a professional organization to which most practicing dentists belong. Because the local dental society only lists and does not evaluate the professional qualifications of member dentists, this is simply a resource for consumers to find *a* member dentist in their area. Seeking a more personal recommendation from a friend, doctor, or another dentist is preferable.

To contact your local dental society, look in the white pages of the telephone directory under "Dental Society of (your state)," or look in Appendix 3 at the back of this book for your state chapter of the ADA.

The American Dental Directory. Many public and dental libraries have a copy of this compendium, published by the American Dental Association, which includes a geographical listing of *all* dentists (both members and nonmembers of the ADA) in the United States, including those living abroad. It supplies the following information: name, current mailing address, year of birth, membership status in the ADA, specialty, dental school from which graduated, year of graduation, and home or office telephone number. Dentists are also listed alphabetically and by specialty.

In general, the libraries of state-supported dental schools, where this directory and other information are available, are open to the public. Nonstudents are able to use the books, journals, and reference guides on the premises. Checkout privileges and the on-line computer reference services usually are available only to paying students, faculty, administrators, and some staff members. See Appendix 2 of this book for a listing of state dental schools.

Hospitals. A hospital in your area may have a hospital-based practice or be able to recommend a dentist. If it is not listed under "Dental Services" under the hospital's name in the telephone book, call the hospital's general number.

Dental Schools. Most if not all dental schools have dental clinics that are open to patients. (See Appendix 2 for a listing.)

Advertisements. Many dentists advertise in newspapers and local business fliers. Some also send newsletters to actual and potential patients. Most of these are purchased from a company that researches and writes them, with the dentist affixing his or her practice logo to the letterhead. Dental advertising and marketing are vehicles by which dentists promote their practices. Although the ADA, in its "Principles of Ethics and Professional Conduct Code," cautions dentists against printing false or misleading information, these guidelines are subject to some degree of interpretation and usually are not enforced; this leaves the consumer with little or no protection against unscrupulous dentists or deceptive advertising.

In looking for a dentist through an ad, you should be skeptical, especially about ads in which the dentist advertises fees, offers services free or for nominal fees as an inducement to visit, or promises to provide all services, no matter how invasive or recently introduced. Given the complexity of modern dental care, no dentist can be a "supergeneralist" and deliver a high standard of care for all services. Ads do not provide the information patients need to make an educated choice about a healthcare professional. Finding a dentist through advertising, the yellow pages, or the newspaper alone should never be the sole way to choose your dentist. Nevertheless, an advertisement can be an appropriate way to identify a practitioner who is conveniently located to you or to find out what hours and amenities the office offers. However, additional investigation is needed to verify professional qualifications and training.

Yellow Pages. The listings and advertisements under "Dentist" in the yellow pages of the telephone directory will not reveal the traits and qualifications of a competent dentist (training, whether they are prevention minded, practice good infection control, etc.), but they will disclose which ones are near your home or job and identify dental specialists. The same caveat as for advertisements applies here.

Considerations

Listed below are factors you should consider in selecting a competent dentist.

Location. Choosing a dentist who is conveniently located to your home or place of employment makes it easier for you to keep regular appointments and allows you to arrive at the office more relaxed.

Financial. The following may take priority when selecting a dentist:

INSURANCE PLANS. Assistance from dental insurance plans is limited. Most plans include an annual limit of $1,000, so the freedom to choose a dentist when major dental expense is recurring has little to do with what type of insurance plan you have. Most employers offer employees only a limited range of dental plans, some of which, such as HMOs, restrict an enrollee's choice of dentist (see Chapter 4). If you are picking a dentist on the basis of what you must pay out of pocket, you will want to know whether a dentist participates (accepts your insurance company's payment in full for the services) in an insurance plan you have or whether he or she accepts partial reimbursement from your insurance carrier. All insurance carriers should be able to provide you, on request, with a list of participating dentists in your area. If you know and trust a dentist on the list, you may decide to select that insurance plan; however, remember, if you continue to visit a dentist who does not participate in your insurance plan, you will be required to pay out of your own pocket; in some plans (PPO plans) compensation for out-of-plan dentists will be provided.

PRICE. To budget for dental expenses or comparison shop for other dentists, you may be interested in knowing beforehand what the fees for visits and procedures are. Although paying for dental services differs from buying a consumer item, such as a car or an appliance, in that you are buying the *services* of a professional, price is a factor, *after* professional qualifications are weighed, especially if you have no or minimal dental insurance coverage or are undergoing procedures not covered by insurance.

PAYMENT OPTIONS. What method of payment the dentist accepts

(checks, cash, and/or credit cards) or whether he or she will set up an individual payment schedule over weeks or months may be important to you.

Personal Rapport. The following traits will help you feel more comfortable with your dentist and may affect the quality of your care:

COMMUNICATION. You need to feel free to convey your dental needs to your dentist, and you need a dentist who listens to you and informs you thoroughly and accurately in language you can understand about dental problems you have, the different therapies available, their benefits and risks, their costs, and how long they last. Communication also encompasses both informed consent and treatment planning, issues described in Chapter 4.

TRUST. No matter how informed or knowledgeable you become, you ultimately must trust your dentist: to identify your dental problems accurately, to communicate them adequately to you, to use proper infection control, to perform appropriate procedures competently and safely, and to charge fairly for services. This element of trust, which is fundamental to your relationship with a dentist, is why, when you are making your selection, you ask people you already trust, such as friends, family, and physicians, for their recommendations. *Before* you "open wide," though, you need to be sure a dentist *earns* your trust by practicing or possessing the traits discussed here.

FEARS AND ANXIETIES. All dentists should provide appropriate measures to minimize the discomfort some dental procedures cause. If you are anxious or fearful about aspects of dental treatment or practice, you need a dentist with whom you feel comfortable discussing your apprehensions and who is able and willing to employ the numerous modalities, detailed in Chapter 19, to ease them.

RESPECT AND COURTESY. The dentist and staff should treat you with respect and courtesy. Except for extenuating circumstances, as when an emergency arises for another patient, you should not have to wait consistently more than 30 minutes in the waiting room for an appointment. Most dentists are very efficient with their time and hence very prompt. You, too, should return the courtesy and be on time for appointments.

Professional Qualities. The following are essential traits of a competent dentist:

INFECTION CONTROL. All dentists and their assistants should adhere to standard infection control procedures, which are detailed in Chapter 21. If a dentist is uncomfortable answering your questions regarding sterilization procedures and efforts to prevent cross-contamination or does not follow them, do not hesitate to seek another practitioner.

PREVENTIVE APPROACH. At the first or second visit and annually thereafter, a dentist should perform the following four preventive screenings: complete head and neck exam, including a screening for oral cancer; periodontal exam; temporomandibular joint evaluation; and an examination of the condition of your teeth (with radiographs, if indicated, depending on when the last set was taken).

TRAINING. Whether you are seeking a general dentist or dental specialist on your own or through a Preferred Provider Organization (PPO) or a Health Maintenance Organization (HMO), ask what kind of training and affiliations a dentist has (whether in hospitals and/or large academic medical centers). If you are having complex treatments, such as implants, ask how often he or she has performed the procedure. While not universally true, dentists with university and hospital affiliations are exposed to a broader range of dental problems and the techniques and procedures to treat them. Although they may not necessarily be more skilled practitioners, the fact that they have pursued and secured the affiliation reveals their motivation for and interest in staying current with developments in their field. Since universities often prohibit dentists from advertising their association with them, you should ask whether a dentist has one and to judge this adequately you need to find out about the range of treatment that the dentist does in the hospital setting.

DISCIPLINARY ACTION. The regulatory laws governing disciplinary action against licensed professionals and the agency responsible for disciplining them vary by state. The state board of dentistry located in the capital city of your state can either tell you whether individual dentists have had any disciplinary actions taken against them or direct you to the agency that can supply you with this information. (See Chapter 4 for a description of these agencies.)

EMERGENCY CARE. Because prompt treatment in a dental emergency may mean the difference between losing and saving a tooth, it is essential that *before* one arises, you ask the dentist (or a member of the office staff) how he or she or an associate handles emergencies, how quickly he or she responds, and who provides this care when the dentist is out of the office. It should not be routine policy for a dentist to tell patients to go to a hospital emergency room for a dental emergency. You should be able to contact a dentist or associate 24 hours a day, 365 days a year. Your calls should be answered directly, by an answering service, or by an answering machine that is regularly monitored or provides a beeper number. When the dentist is away from the office, coverage should be provided for dental emergencies.

REFERRALS. Check your dental insurance policy carefully, keeping in mind that for a dentist to be part of an insurance plan, most only have to be willing to accept a discounted fee, have a license, and have no disciplinary actions pending. Since some dental insurance plans—for example HMOs or PPOs—will reimburse enrollees only if they go to certain dentists or dental specialists, inquire whether the specialists to whom you are referred are accepted by your plan. HMOs reimburse only for specialists if you were evaluated first and referred by a general dentist. If you have made an appointment without the referral, you may have to pay the entire bill, but remember that to get the specialist of your choice, it may be well worth it. To find out what portion will be paid out of pocket in a fee-for-service plan, you need to ask at what percentage of the UCR (Usual, Customary, and Reasonable) or other schedule of allowances (see Chapter 4 for a definition) the plan covers for the fees of a specialist.

WHEN YOU NEED
A DENTAL SPECIALIST

Certain dental treatments, among them orthognathic surgery, bone grafts, and complex orthodontic care, require the skills and expertise only dentists specialized in that branch of dentistry can offer. Whether you need to see a dental specialist is an assessment the dentist who cares regularly for you should make; you should not diagnose yourself. There may be situations in which, even though a general dentist is willing and capable of performing a procedure, for example, inserting implants, you may be better off being treated by a specialist (e.g., an oral surgeon, periodontist, and/or prosthodontist). In these circumstances or when a general dentist cannot refer you to a specialist who participates in your dental plan, you may have to find a suitable specialist on your own. In doing so, follow the suggestions in the preceding section "Finding Dentists."

THE DENTAL HEALTH TEAM

Dental Hygienist

The dental hygienist is the member of the dental team responsible for making sure patients obtain regular preventive services. Hygienists frequently perform the most important preventive maintenance services, among them scaling and polishing teeth and applying topical fluorides and sealants. In addition, they take radiographs, record case histories, and chart dental conditions. In a number of states they are by law permitted additional duties which can include administering local anesthesia and preparing impression trays. In Colorado, dental hygienists can maintain an independent practice.

The minimal educational requirement to become a Registered Dental Hygienist (RDH) is two years of college in an accredited dental hygiene program for an associate degree. Dental hygiene education is also offered as part of bachelor's and master's degree programs. To be licensed by the state in which they will practice, hygienists need to pass a written national board and a clinical state or regional examination.

Dental Assistant

Assistants help dentists perform a wide range of administrative and secretarial duties. How they assist the dentist chairside (by helping during surgery or in preparing the teeth for bonding, for example) and what educational requirements they need to do so vary greatly from state to state and are determined by the dental regulations of each state.

TYPES OF DENTAL PRACTICES

Dentists work in different types of practices. Each has pros and cons depending on what you are looking for in your dental care. A fair question for patients to ask, for all types of practices, is what provision there is for emergency coverage.

Solo

In 1994, almost 80 percent of dentists operated as sole proprietors, that is, alone. Patients who want to see and establish a personal relationship with the same dentist most likely prefer a solo practitioner. The downside can include longer waits for appointments.

Group

In this type practice, two or more dentists share an office, staff, and patients. The patient, especially one with an unusual dental problem, benefits from the expertise and experience of all the dentists in the practice. Another benefit is that there is always coverage for emergencies. A group practice, however, may not provide you with the same personal contact that the solo dentist can.

Group practices come in a number of variations. Dentists can be partners who each have a financial interest in the practice. Some may be owned by a primary practitioner, most often a dentist who hires dentists as associates (employees) who are not partners in the practice. (The dental offices in malls and stores that were popular in the mid-1980s were often regional and national chains that operated in this fashion.) Dentists who belong to health maintenance organizations (described in Chapter 4) using the staff model only also are employees who are paid a salary by the plan.

Dental School Clinics

Clinics operated by dental schools offer a number of advantages to patients who live near them and have time. The ongoing dialogue between students and the faculty can allow you an opportunity to interact and participate in your care. In general, the care given is excellent and the cost is lower.

Routine care is provided by dental students and residents in training, under the supervision and approval of faculty, who are dentists. General dentists also practice at dental schools. For complicated and more recently developed procedures, such as osseointegrated implants, these clinics offer state-of-the-art care by dental specialists who are in the forefront of the research, technology, and techniques involved. Unlike the routine care given at these facilities, treatments using specialists whose practices are in the university or dental school facilities will be as expensive, if not slightly more, than those offered elsewhere in the community. Due to the restricted number of dental schools and the fact that most are located in large metropolitan areas, this type of practice is not an option for most Americans, especially those who live in rural areas.

Hospital-Based Clinics

Dental clinics, which may or may not have affiliations with dental schools, also can be located in private, public, or Veteran's Administration hospitals (at the latter only veterans of the armed services are eligible). These clinics offer services from attending dentists and residents under the supervision of attending faculty.

WHEN YOU SWITCH DENTISTS

If you move or change dentists for other reasons, you can avoid receiving unnecessary radiation and incurring additional and unnecessary charges by having copies of your dental radiographs sent to your new dentist. This will also provide your new dentist with a chronological visual record of your dental condition.

In most states the radiographs and dental records are the property of the dentist who created them. Some states require dentists to provide patients with copies of their radiographs and charts (often for a small fee to cover the costs of copying and handling) when the request is made in writing. Even in states in which dentists are not obligated to do so, many dentists voluntarily supply patients with copies of them. If your care has been complicated, you should try to have your chart and/or a summary of treatment transferred to your new dentist; otherwise, a copy of your radiographs should suffice.

CHAPTER 4

Paying for
Your Dental Care

I f you are like most consumers, you feel the pinch for dental services more than you do for medical care. The reason is that, on average, people pay for a much greater proportion of it directly out-of-pocket. Private dental insurance picks up approximately one-third the total cost of all dental care in the United States, and public assistance programs, such as Medicaid, pay for less than 4 percent of the total. You, the patient, pay the rest.

Because dental care is, for the most part, elective and the reasons for it life threatening only in very rare instances, it is one of the first services that many will reduce or forgo during times of economic hardship. Yet postponing preventive dental care can be very costly in the long run. Left untreated, dental problems almost always escalate and eventually require more extensive and expensive treatment than they would have had they been prevented or treated early. For example, a carious lesion that can be filled for less than $100 can end up costing $800 or more if the decay is allowed to continue to the point where root canal therapy and a crown are required. The smart consumer, as well as the good dental plan, emphasizes preventive care, routine visits to the dentist, and early treatment of dental disease to help prevent the high costs that may accrue from neglecting dental care.

DENTAL INSURANCE

Approximately 40 percent of employed Americans have some form of dental coverage. This leaves about 150 million Americans with no private third-party dental insurance coverage and limited coverage under public programs.

Most Americans who have private insurance are employed and between the ages of 25 and 54 or are the children or dependents of individuals with plans. A critical time for young persons is between the ages of 18 and 24 when many have lost the insurance coverage they had under their parents' plans and have not started working at jobs through which they have their own insurance. Older Americans also lack dental insurance; only 15 percent of people over 65 are covered.

Whether you have coverage through your job often depends on your income. The greater your salary, the greater the likelihood you have private dental insurance. Almost 60 percent of Americans with a yearly income of $35,000 or over are insured, compared with about 10 percent below the poverty level (about $13,000 for a family of four) who are.

Dental coverage varies from plan to plan, but, in general, its benefits are not as comprehensive as those provided by medical insurance, and it traditionally reimburses at lower levels for many procedures, especially the more expensive ones. Although medical plans typically pay 80 percent of the cost of major treatments, dental plans usually reimburse no more than 50 percent (of the cost of the treatments they do cover) after out-of-pocket co-payments and deductibles (see Box 4.1 for definitions) are subtracted. Furthermore, dental insurance does not insure its beneficiaries against the uncommon, high-cost extensive treatment, as medical insurance does with most hospitalizations. Instead, it generally covers the lower-cost preventive and restorative services and can exclude or limit some higher-cost treatments, such as cosmetic services (bleaching, veneer facings, crowns), temporomandibular joint-related procedures, and ortho-

---

BOX 4.1

DEFINITIONS OF SOME COMMON DENTAL INSURANCE TERMS

Beneficiary. The patient who is receiving benefits under a dental insurance contract. Also called the insured, subscriber, member, or enrollee.

Capitation. Dentists participating in this type dental program are paid on a per capita (or per patient/enrollee) basis for providing the dental services that are covered under the dental plan.

Co-insurance. The percentage or portion of the dentist's fee for a covered dental service that the beneficiary pays (after his or her deductible is met or paid). Typically, a dental plan pays 50 percent of the allowed benefit of the service that is covered and the beneficiary is responsible for the remainder. Also known as co-payment.

Co-payment. See co-insurance.

Deductible. The amount of payment for which an enrollee in a dental plan is responsible before the dental insurance plan will pay for any benefits. This may be a one-time or once-a-year charge and may be set on an individual or family basis.

Enrollee. See beneficiary.

Exclusion. Services not covered as benefits under the insurance plan.

Fee-for-Service. These dental plans pay the dentist on a service-by-service basis.

Limitation. A restriction on benefits in a plan. These may include age, waiting periods before coverage, duration of coverage, and the extent to or conditions under which some services are covered.

Premium. The cost to purchase benefits from a plan, for a specific time, usually a year.

Quality Assurance. A formal program that includes an assessment of the quality of care delivered by the plan and the requisite changes that may be necessary to maintain and improve the quality of care. These usually involve an assessment of the plan's cost, use, professional care delivered by dentists involved, program for prevention of dental disease, infection control, cleanliness of building, satisfaction of the participants, etc.

Usual, Customary, and Reasonable (UCR). A way of determining the reimbursement level for benefits based on dentists' charges and location. *Usual* refers to the fee the dentist normally charges to private, noninsured patients, *customary* refers to fees dentists with similar training and experience in the same geographic area charge for the same service, and *reasonable* refers to a payment that a dentist charges above his or her usual charge if the case is more involved than usual or there are extenuating circumstances, and therefore it is reasonable for the dentist to charge more. Some plans pay 90 percent of the UCR; this means they pay if the dentist's fee does not exceed 90 percent of the fee for the same service in the same area. Others pay only 50 percent or less.

dontics for persons over the age of 19. More expensive materials or treatments, such as implants, fixed partial dentures (bridges), gold fillings, and crowns, usually are not covered fully if there are less costly but professionally acceptable alternatives. In some plans, when a subscriber submits an insurance claim for these more expensive procedures, only the lower-cost alternative is covered; this leaves the enrollee responsible for paying the difference in cost.

Private Insurance

There are many private dental insurance plans, but most fall into three broad categories: capitation, preferred provider, and fee-for-service. Hybrids of the three, for example, point-of-service plans, are becoming much more common. Most dental insurance is offered through group plans and not to individuals. This protects the insurance industry from adverse selection (in which only individuals who feel they need a dental plan purchase one) and its disadvantageous economic consequences (of having to provide coverage primarily for persons who require more frequent and/or more expensive treatments).

The caveat "buyer beware" seems to have more relevance when choosing dental insurance than when selecting medical insurance. Since dental insurance consumes less than 11 percent of the total cost of healthcare plans, employers have less incentive to evaluate thoroughly the management and design of dental plans. As a result, corporate advisors on health plans are less knowledgeable generally about the specifics of dental plans and less able to give their employees advice about them. Bearing this in mind, you need to recognize that you must evaluate for yourself and your family the coverage that is best for the dental services you anticipate using.

As with all insurance, if you are offered a choice of plans, there are many considerations to make. For example, if your dental health and that of your family has been excellent, and the premium or the portion of it your employer requires you to pay for dental coverage is too high or the dental insurance eats up too many of your points or dollars in a flexible benefits plan, you may be better off not having dental care insurance coverage at all, and pay for preventive visits out of pocket or save your points for another benefit option.

To continue with a dentist you regularly visit and with whom you are satisfied, ask your dentist if he or she participates in any of the plans you are offered. If not, you must choose between loyalty to your dentist and the savings you will incur from visiting a dentist who does participate in a plan you are offered. The choice is personal. Individuals who desire or require extensive dental work may feel forced, for financial reasons, to establish a relationship with a new dentist.

The following are descriptions of the major types of dental plans available.

Fee-for-Service Dental Plans (also called Indemnity Plans). Traditionally, this type of insurance, in which patients are free to choose their dentist, has been the most common third-party method of paying for dental services. Their hold on the market has weakened due to the increased popularity of dental HMOs and PPOs in the 1980s and 1990s. In a fee-for-service plan, you are reimbursed by the commercial or nonprofit corporation that administers the plan for each service that is covered. There are usually deductibles, certain services that are limited and/or excluded, a maximum dollar amount of care the insurance company will pay for services and care per year or for your lifetime, and co-insurance. For example, if the plan covers 80 percent, you must pay the other 20 percent, after the deductible has been paid.

A simple fee-for-service plan, which is endorsed by the American Dental Association, is *direct reimbursement,* where you pay the dentist for dental care and submit the receipt to your employer for reimbursement. Sometimes referred to as bill payer, this simple type plan gives you the greatest amount of choice, allowing you the freedom to visit any dentist you desire and to be reimbursed up to the amount that the plan covers. There usually are no restrictions on what is covered. However, there are annual limits on the maximum the plan will pay, such as $1500 per person. Some direct reimbursement plans pay for a percentage of dental care received. It is up to you to decide whether to use your allowances for cosmetic dental services, preventive care, treatment of temporomandibular joint disorders, or any other dental service.

Capitation or Dental Health Maintenance Organizations (DHMOs). In a capitated arrangement, a dentist is paid a set amount per month for each patient enrolled in the plan, regardless of what and how many procedures or visits an individual requires. For employers DHMOs have become attractive alternatives to the traditional fee-for-service plans because they are easier to budget for and are usually less costly. DHMOs generally cover preventive and basic services, restorative work, and most dental specialty services.

The methods by which DHMO dental plans deliver services vary. In the *staff model* of delivery, dental plans operate a clinic or one or more dental offices, staffed by dentists who are paid a salary by the plan. The *Individual Practice Association (IPA)*, or *network, model* is the most common method of delivery; with it, dental services are provided in many dental offices. An IPA is a dental HMO without walls, in which dentists work in their own offices, under a capitated arrangement. Overtreatment is discouraged because the dentists receive the same monthly capitated amount regardless of the mix of services rendered. In both the staff and network models, you must visit a dentist who participates in the plan to receive benefits. If you seek care from a dentist outside the plan, you will not be covered under a traditional capitated plan. *Open-ended,* or *point-of-service,* plans combine features of the HMOs and conventional fee-for-service care by allowing enrollees to seek treatments by dentists outside the plan but at a reduced benefit.

As with all plans, capitated arrangements have advantages, as well as disadvantages. Their satisfaction depends, to a great extent, on how well they are managed. Well-managed dental HMOs provide close monitoring of the care they provide, with strict control of quality and review of utilization. They are designed to keep costs down by providing cost-effective preventive care and early treatment. Dental HMOs require little paperwork of their enrollees, though there often is a small co-payment for each visit.

When poorly managed, dental HMOs may discourage visits (by requiring long waits for appointments and separate visits for exams, radiographs, and cleanings) and provide minimal and sometimes only emergency care. In general, especially in staff model plans, there are fewer offices from which to choose; this potentially requires patients to travel longer distances.

Preferred Provider Organizations (PPOs). These plans are organized as a network of dentists who have agreed to discount their fees or to charge reduced set fees to PPO beneficiaries. Although individual PPOs can vary, most offer advantages, as well as restrictions.

Care is provided by the PPO dentists in their offices. Most dentists who belong are in private practice and a particular PPO is just one of a number of insurance plans in which they participate. When an enrollee seeks care outside the list of participating dentists, it is likely that the visits and treatments may be covered by the PPO, but the patient will usually have a larger out-of-pocket expense.

PPOs usually give subscribers a brochure detailing the services covered, the amount the plan pays for each, and the portion for which the subscriber is responsible. As with fee-for-service plans, there is a financial incentive for dentists to provide services as they are paid on the basis of services rendered. When fee allowances (the amount the plan reimburses the dentist) are too low, there may be insufficient numbers of dentists in the plan within an area to provide subscribers with conveniently located offices.

Cafeteria or Flexible Benefits Plan. A new movement in employee benefits is to allow employees to tailor the benefits they receive from their employer to fit their individual and family needs. It has been compared to a cafeteria line, from which the employee chooses from an array of options (in this case prescription drug benefits, extra sick leave, disability, and dental and health insurance instead of turkey, hamburgers, lasagna, etc.). Each benefit has either a dollar or point value ascribed to it and the employee has *x* number of benefit dollars to spend however he or she wants, usually on a fee-for-service, DHMO, or PPO plan.

If you have the option of a flexible benefits plan, you may or may not want to include dental insurance as one of your benefits. To determine whether it is worth it for you to use your benefit dollars for dental coverage, you need to evaluate your dental health and that of your family and calculate how much you have spent the last three or four years for it. You should find out what the plan covers and the amount the services you anticipate using will cost. To do so, you need to consider deductibles, co-payments, what services are covered, and what percentage of a dentist's fee is reimbursed. This often is based on the UCR value, which stands for usual, customary, and reasonable value. In fee-for-service plans, the insurance company frequently sets maximum fees for procedures that are a percentage of the UCR. When evaluating plans and deciding whether you will use your benefit dollars for dental care, you need to know at what percentage of the UCR the plan reimburses you. Lower-quality dental plans may only reimburse you 20 or 30 percent for every dollar on your dental bill. The higher the UCR schedule used for reimbursement by the plan, the less out-of-pocket expense you will have. This advice also applies when evaluating other dental plans.

Public Programs

Medicaid. As part of its coverage, this federally financed, state-run program provides low-income individuals and families in some states with dental services. Although each state determines who is eligible, what services are covered, and how much dentists are reimbursed, there is a minimum of some children's services that must be covered under the EPSDT (Early and Periodic Screening Diagnosis and Treatment) program. Of the $77 billion spent on Medicaid in 1991, less than 1 percent went for dental care; the majority went to children through the Aid to Families with Dependent Children Program. For the most part, the coverage for adults is very limited if it exists at all. Specific questions can be answered by a local social service agency or Social Security Administration office.

Medicare. This government health insurance program for persons over 65 and for those who are disabled, regardless of age, is calculated according to an individual's eligibility for Social Security and not his or her income. Dental care, with the exception of medically necessary dental work and surgery on the jaw that does not involve the teeth, is *not* covered. More information can be obtained from a local Social Security Administration office.

BEFORE TREATMENT

When extensive dental care is needed, there usually are a number of ways to restore oral health, each with practical and economic considerations. For example, missing teeth can be replaced with either a fixed or a removable denture. Ultimately, which option is selected depends on many factors, among them the particulars of your medical and dental history, the dentist's recommendation, and your aesthetic preferences and finances. Before deciding which treatment to have, you need to find out from your dentist what options and alternatives exist and what the costs, disadvantages, and advantages of each are. This is especially important if you have a dental plan that only covers the least-expensive, professionally acceptable treatment.

Treatment Planning

For very simple procedures, the treatment planning process is usually straightforward. But when your dental needs are complicated and perhaps expensive and when there are choices to be made, then you and your dentist should, ideally together, create a treatment plan. The best time for this is not in a few minutes after a visit or initial examination. Ideally, you should return for another visit, during which the dentist can spend time explaining the costs and other details of the different alternatives and show you radiographs, models, or mock-ups of a proposed restoration or prosthesis, or pictures of the treatment on other patients. You need to be sure you understand the advantages and disadvantages of the different treatment options for you personally, taking into consideration your priorities and finances. After this, you choose the treatment plan from the ones presented by the dentist; the dentist should not dictate the "only" option to you.

Pretreatment Estimates

Once you have decided on a treatment plan with your dentist and before beginning dental treatment, your dentist should give you a written estimate of the costs, as well as the amount of time the treatment will take to complete. Some insurance plans require a dentist to submit a pretreatment estimate if the costs are over a certain amount, often $200, or if specific procedures, such as prosthetics (dentures, crowns, and bridgework), temporomandibular joint therapy, root canal therapy, orthodontics, and extensive periodontal treatment, are involved. The insurance company may require that it approve the treatment before it begins.

Informed Consent

Before giving medications, performing procedures or surgery, or enlisting patients' participation in a study, dentists have a legal obligation to give their patients information about the known risks and benefits involved, any alternatives that are available and the risks and benefits of each, and the estimated length of time for recovery.

There are two types of informed consent in dental care: *consent to examination* and *consent to treatment.* At the initial dental visit, most dentists require that you fill in a detailed medical history form, which includes a paragraph that, when signed by you, gives your consent to a dental examination.

When a final treatment plan is developed (after it has been thoroughly discussed and agreed on by the dentist and patient), many dentists ask a patient to sign a form, giving *consent to treatment.* By signing this agreement, you are attesting that you:

- Have given permission for the treatment.
- Are giving your permission without coercion.
- Understand the information.
- Have been informed by the dentist about the reason for the proposed procedure, what the procedure does, its risks and benefits, any alternatives that exist, and their known risks and benefits.
- Are of sound mind and therefore are capable of giving consent. (Patients who are mentally or emotionally incompetent to understand what the treatment involves and therefore to give their informed consent must have it given by a designated surrogate, who is usually a family member. Similarly, persons under the age of 18 are not asked to sign consent forms: instead consent is given by parents or guardians.)

Signing a consent form does not absolve you from all responsibility. Implicit in a *consent-to-treatment* form is your agreement to follow the dentist's posttreatment instructions, such as performing oral hygiene at home, returning for follow-up visits, and paying for the treatment.

Consent is not required in emergencies when a patient is unconscious or otherwise unable to communicate, as while under anesthesia, during surgery when a serious or life-threatening complication arises, or when a guardian or the parents of a minor cannot be reached. In these instances, the law allows the dentist or physician to treat the patient without obtaining consent.

There are dentists who do not require patients to sign informed consent agreements, but, by submitting to the treatment, the consent is implied, on the assumption that the dentist has explained the treatment and the patient has understood the explanation. For the protection of both parties, *signed consent* is preferable to *implied consent.*

Before signing the form and certainly before proceeding with treatment, you should be sure all your questions regarding the procedure, medication, or treatment have been answered. If the form is not explicit, you may make additions in the margins for clarification before signing. Once signed, you have little leverage to claim you did not understand the proposed treatment, for the law assumes that as a competent adult who has signed such an agreement, you have both read and understood it.

PAYING FOR YOUR TREATMENT

You should expect to pay for your dental care as you do for any service, at the time it is rendered. Most dental offices make accommodations for the convenience of their patients. Many accept credit cards, and most help patients submit insurance claims and require payment only for the portion of the bill that the insurance does not cover. Some even allow for deferred billing: the dentist first files a claim with the insurance company and, after finding out what portion the insurance plan will pay, bills the patient for the balance.

WHEN YOU ARE NOT SATISFIED

Much of the time when patients are unhappy with the dental care they have received, it is either because they did not convey their expectations to the dentist accurately or the dentist did not explain thoroughly to them what could be expected realistically of the treatment, its costs, outcome, alternatives, and duration of recuperation involved. (Recognizing this, many dental schools now include in their curriculums courses on how dentists can improve their communication skills.) But when the communication between you and your dentist has been adequate and you are still dissatisfied with some aspect of dental treatment, what steps should you take?

Talk to the Dentist

If you are unhappy with your dental care, you should first speak with the dentist who performed it. Explain why you are dissatisfied and how you would like it corrected. The dentist may describe the remedies he or she can and is willing to make. If, after speaking with the dentist, you are still dissatisfied, the next step, depending on the nature and seriousness of the problem, might be to try the peer review process.

Peer Review

Each constituent dental society of the American Dental Association (ADA) operates peer review proceedings as alternatives to litigation. Their purpose is to air, review, and decide disputes between patients and dentists or among a patient, dentist, and a third-party payer (i.e., an insurance carrier).

Although the peer review process varies among the different constituent dental societies, each must function in accordance with state laws and should conform to the guidelines the ADA sets for it. To find out how the dental society for your area conducts its peer review, call your state (or constituent) dental society, listed in the white pages of your telephone directory under "Dental Society of (your state or region)" or call the ADA (see Appendix 1 for the telephone number).

The procedures described here are those followed by the Dental Society of the State of New York, which generally is regarded as a model for the process. Peer review, as practiced in New York, is not appropriate for cases involving malpractice to be determined in a court of law or where damages are sought. It is most suitable in cases where the quality of care or the appropriateness of treatment presumably has not met acceptable standards and the patient only wants to recover all or part of the fee paid. The most a patient can receive monetarily is the fee for the original treatment in question.

To be accepted for the process, a complaint in New York must meet the following criteria:

- The dental treatment must have been completed within the last two and a half years (the dental malpractice statute of limitations) and must be able to be seen and examined (it cannot be altered or removed).
- The dentist who performed the work must be a member of the ADA.
- The case cannot be in litigation or under review by the Office of

Professional Conduct of the New York State Department of Education.

- Both the consumer and the dentist must agree to abide by the ruling. With this agreement, the patient and dentist contractually relinquish the right to pursue future litigation.

First, a dentist mediator tries to resolve the dispute. If this mediation fails, a hearing takes place before a peer review committee, the chairperson, and, in some components (local dental societies), a lay observer. If the treatment was rendered by a specialist, the panel consists of dentists certified in the same specialty. The hearing includes a discussion with the patient and dentist, a review of the radiographs and records (and any documents from subsequent treating dentists), and a clinical exam. The panel discusses the findings and renders its judgment. Either the dentist or patient may appeal the decision within 30 days. If he or she meets certain qualifications, a rehearing may take place before a new panel.

Decisions rendered through the peer review process are private and are not given to any outside agency. If the judgment is in favor of the patient and the dentist makes a payment through an escrow account set up by the component dental society, nothing will be reported to the National Practitioners Data Bank (described later). If, however, the dentist requests that the payment be made through a liability carrier, the liability carrier is required to report the judgment to both the National Practitioners Data Bank and, in New York State, the Office of Professional Discipline of the Department of Education.

Filing a Formal Complaint

If you believe a dentist's conduct has been improper, you may report him or her to the agency in your state responsible for handling disciplinary actions against dentists. Although this varies from state to state, the state entity that oversees the licensing of dentists should be able, if it does not handle the complaints itself, to steer you to the right department. Because the state entities responsible for disciplining dentists do not have authorization to return a patient's money, patients who complain usually do so because they feel it is their public duty to prevent what they consider to be a lapse in professional conduct from happening to other patients. (If you want monetary restitution, you are better off pursuing peer review.)

Dentists can be disciplined if professional misconduct or unprofessional conduct, such as verbal or sexual abuse, negligent or incompetent dental treatment, or criminal conduct has taken place. The disciplinary actions meted out vary and include fines, probation (during which a dentist still practices but is monitored to be sure he or she is practicing in compliance with standards of practice), or revocation of the license to practice. Once the agency responsible for disciplining dentists determines that a complaint is credible, a process, which usually cannot be stopped, is set in motion. This can involve different levels of investigations and hearings before a professional conduct officer or consultations with members of state boards of dentistry.

Judgments resulting in disciplinary actions are reported to the National Practitioners Data Bank. The information in this data bank is used by state licensing boards, hospitals, and professional societies when hiring dentists and other healthcare providers.

Litigation

Litigation is an option a consumer can always exercise. Due to the costs involved and the seriousness of the process, it should be reserved for cases of negligence or irreparable or unacceptable damage. Most minor problems can be solved either by the patient's talking with the dentist or through the peer review process.

PART III

ROUTINE
CARE

CHAPTER 5

Preventive Care— In the Home and Office

Though the motivation for practicing good oral hygiene changes as we age. For the most part, children need to take care of their teeth to avoid or minimize dental caries (tooth decay). Although this risk does not disappear as we grow older (adults are especially susceptible to caries at the roots of their teeth), the problem is often superseded by a new concern, periodontal disease. Good preventive care that involves the control of plaque, dietary modification, and the use of fluorides and sealants help prevent or control one or both of these ubiquitous dental problems.

ASSURING SAFETY AND EFFECTIVENESS

All dental devices have to be safe and effective to be marketed. The criteria the Food and Drug Administration (FDA) uses to assess safety and efficacy varies depending on the degree of risk involved in the device or product. Before marketing a new dental device with what would be considered the highest degree of risk (most of these would be used in dental offices), a manufacturer must prove to the FDA through clinical and other studies that its product is safe (for instance, is not toxic, does not cause cancer, will not disrupt or change the genes) and that it is effective (does what it claims to do). A manufacturer of a product that is substantially equivalent to a legally marketed one does not need to conduct new clinical studies but instead submits an application to the FDA for approval.

At the present time, no regulation obligates manufacturers to do this with over-the-counter dental products. Most, through good faith and the fear of being held liable if they market an unsafe product, comply with the FDA recommendations (which are in the process of being made mandatory): the label lists all active and inactive ingredients, indicates how the product is to be used, and includes warnings and directions for use. If a claim is made for the product, such as it reduces plaque, there must be proof.

A dental product with the American Dental Association (ADA)'s Seal of Acceptance has been scientifically proven to be both safe and effective for the claims it makes. To receive the seal, manufacturers voluntarily submit data from laboratory and clinical tests that meet stringent guidelines to the ADA's Council on Scientific Affairs to demonstrate that the product is both safe and effective. Conversely, if a product does not have the seal, it can mean either that the manufacturer never applied for it or that it did and its submission was rejected. A provisional Seal of Acceptance may be granted for certain products at an intermediate stage when the evidence reasonably supports the product's value.

HOME PREVENTIVE CARE

Controlling Plaque

To prevent caries and periodontal disease, plaque, the transparent mat of bacteria and its toxic by-products that coat the teeth, needs to be regularly removed. At home, plaque removal can be accomplished mechanically, with brushing and flossing and the use of other aids to clean between the teeth, and, to a lesser extent, chemically, with some mouthrinses and toothpastes.

Toothbrushes. Brushing the teeth regularly removes plaque, cleanses the teeth, and stimulates the gums to help prevent periodontal disease. Combined with flossing, it is the single most important thing that you can do to maintain the health and vitality of your teeth and their supporting tissues.

Over the centuries, the design of toothbrushes, the materials from which they are made, and their method of use have changed as the knowledge about dental diseases has increased. The Chinese in 1000 AD are credited with inventing them. The well-to-do during the Victorian era put silver handles on theirs and made them part of their ornate toilet sets. In the early twentieth century it was not uncommon for members of the same household, boarding house, or college dormitory to share the same toothbrush. But the precursor of the dazzling variety available today was the inexpensive toothbrush with a plastic handle and nylon bristles that made its debut in the late 1930s.

Although it is hailed as one of the new kids on the dental care block, the electric toothbrush was initially introduced in 1938. The models vary in form and in the frequency their heads rotate per minute, with the most sophisticated resembling professional dental cleaning devices. In a number of short-term studies some of them have been shown to be more effective at removing plaque and reducing gingivitis than manual ones. And although they do seem to have the ability to clean between the teeth better than manual brushes, dental floss is still needed to remove the plaque on the sides of the teeth where they touch. But the statistical advantage electric brushes have in studies may evaporate over time in practice. Some owners object to the care required to maintain them. Others dislike their noise, feel, or weight. Electric toothbrushes may be of special use for individuals who are mentally impaired, wear braces, have arthritis, or otherwise lack the manual dexterity or steadiness of hand necessary to manipulate a manual toothbrush. If children are more excited using one, they may brush better and longer, at least initially.

A new twist is the electric sonic toothbrush that emits high-frequency sonic waves (the sounds can be heard by the ear) that help to propel away food and bacteria. The heads of these toothbrushes vibrate even more rapidly than the regular electric toothbrushes, at over 30,000 strokes each minute, 150 times faster than it is possible to brush manually. Studies on them have been promising, revealing a very effective rate of removal of plaque and certain stains from the teeth. Although they are designed to be used with regular toothpaste, many people prefer to use them with toothpaste in gel form. There is also an ADA (and FDA) accepted ultrasonic toothbrush (using frequencies unable to be heard by the ear) with some clinical support. All electric toothbrushes are relatively expensive, as are their brushes or heads.

Deciding which kind of toothbrush to use may involve trial and error and will depend on your dental problems, oral configurations, and personal preferences. Your dentist probably will be helpful in steering you to the right size and shape. Individuals with small mouths may find it easier to reach back teeth with a brush that has a small angled head. The left-handed may prefer a brush designed for lefties, and persons with teeth that are sensitive to temperature or pressure may choose a soft bristled brush with rounded nylon bristles. For others, the feel or grip of the handle may dictate how long they will continue brushing.

What is more important than the physical configuration of a toothbrush or whether it is manually or electrically powered, is whether it is thoroughly, consistently, and correctly used. The ADA's Council on Scientific Affairs does not recommend any one design or product for removing plaque. What it does recommend and what studies over the last 15 years have revealed is that plaque can be effectively removed with regular and proper brushing and flossing with any manual or electric toothbrush.

For instructions on how to properly brush your teeth, see Box 5.1. For tips on mouth care, see Box 5.2.

BOX 5.1

HOW TO BRUSH YOUR TEETH

Through the years, different methods have been suggested for brushing the teeth. An effective one is described and illustrated below. The minimum time recommended is two minutes.

1. Start on a section of the outside of your teeth. Hold your tooth brush at a 45-degree angle at your gumline. Gently brush from where the tooth and gum meet to the chewing surface in short (half-a-tooth-wide) strokes. Use the same motion to clean all outside surfaces of your teeth.

2. Use the same procedure to brush the inside surfaces of your teeth.

3. To clean the chewing surfaces, use short sweeping strokes, tipping the bristles into the pits and fissures.

4. To clean the inside surfaces of your top and bottom front teeth and gums, hold the brush almost vertical. With back and forth motions, bring the front part of the brush over the teeth and gums.

5. Using a forward sweeping motion, brush your tongue. Place the brush as far back on the tongue as you can comfortably without gagging.

6. To clean your palate, use a sweeping motion to pull your brush across the roof of your mouth.

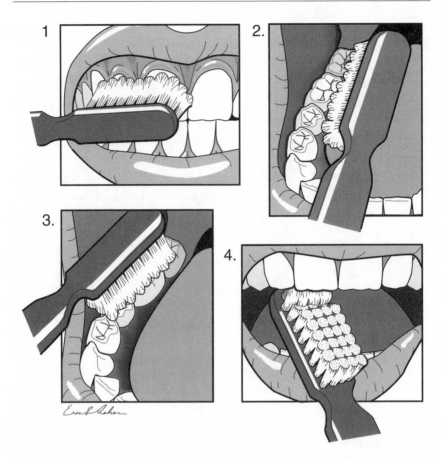

ILLUSTRATION 5.1. **HOW TO BRUSH YOUR TEETH.**

Toothpastes (and Gels, Liquids, and Powders). Toothpastes contain abrasives, detergents, and foaming agents. The addition of fluoride, the most common active ingredient, helps control dental caries. The claims made by manufacturers for their toothpastes are almost always based not on the power of the gel or paste alone but on its actions when combined with brushing. Most plaque removal takes place from the mechanical act of brushing. Although using a toothpaste may enhance this physical cleansing, a real value it has is that it motivates most people to brush longer because its pleasant taste freshens the breath and makes the mouth feel good.

Toothpastes can be marketed for specific purposes. Antitartar tooth-

BOX 5.2

MOUTH CARE TIPS

Use a brush that has soft nylon bristles with rounded or polished ends.

- Choose smaller toothbrushes for children.
- Brush your teeth at least twice a day with a toothpaste that contains fluoride. If you can, brush every time after eating.
- Children should use only a pea-sized amount of toothpaste to avoid swallowing too much fluoride.
- Floss your teeth at least once a day. The ADA recommends spending a minimum of ten minutes a day brushing and flossing.
- Replace your toothbrush every three months. If you need to do so more often, you may be brushing too hard and may damage your gums and the enamel on your teeth.
- Rotate toothbrushes. Have two or three different ones and use them consecutively, throwing the oldest one out as you introduce a new one.
- Never share a toothbrush with anyone.
- Supervise children under the age of six years when they use toothpaste.
- Follow the cautions on the packages for toothpastes designed for specific purposes, e.g., antitartar, sensitive teeth.
- Do not swallow toothpaste.
- Visit your dentist regularly.
- Have your teeth professionally cleaned on a regular basis.

pastes most commonly contain pyrophosphates or zinc salts, chemicals that interrupt the formation of mineral crystals. They will not remove tartar (hardened or calcified plaque) from the teeth (only a professional cleaning can do this), but they can slow its accumulation above the gums. They also will not influence its buildup below the gums, where it can irritate the soft tissues and encourage periodontal disease. Because they lack these therapeutic benefits, antitartar toothpastes receive the ADA Seal of Acceptance only for their caries-reducing properties because they contain effective levels of fluoride and not for their antitartar properties. The ADA does not approve any toothpaste that does not contain fluoride.

Approximately one in ten persons has a tendency to accumulate tartar very rapidly. Using antitartar toothpastes and mouthrinses and spending additional time brushing the teeth near the salivary glands (the inside of the lower front teeth and the outside of the upper back teeth) may retard but only modestly the development of new tartar.

If used regularly, toothpastes marketed for sensitive teeth can desensitize teeth to heat, cold, and pressure. The desensitizing agents are usually strontium chloride or potassium nitrate. Most also include fluoride, an important ingredient for persons whose gums have receded and exposed the more caries-susceptible cementum and dentin on the surfaces of the roots. They should not be used for more than four weeks, nor should they be used by children under the age of 12 years unless directed by a dentist. If you suffer from sensitive teeth, you should bring the condition to the attention of your dentist. It may indicate a more serious problem, such as dental caries or inflammation of the dental pulp (nerve).

No toothpaste can remove stains that are incorporated into the tooth structure itself, such as those from fluorosis, tetracycline, antiperiodontitis medications, or aging. Those targeted to remove external stains contain slightly abrasive granules and detergents to scrub off stains from food and beverages only.

In recent years, baking soda, a home remedy to clean and whiten teeth, has been added, in a less abrasive form to toothpastes, with the addition of fluoride and sometimes hydrogen peroxide. Despite the extensive advertising, no clinical studies have shown baking soda to have any special cleaning or whitening abilities or to reduce caries or periodontal problems more effectively than other cleaning agents.

The hydrogen-peroxide-containing pastes promoted to reduce stains can indeed bleach teeth and reduce intrinsic stain if the concentration is high enough. The ADA's Council on Scientific Affairs has some of the same questions regarding their safety as it does of the peroxide-containing bleaching products used with mouthguards to bleach teeth (described in Chapter 14). These are can they cause damage to the pulp, irritate the oral mucosa, result in irreversible cell changes, and/or enhance the effect of carcinogens, substances that cause the growth of cancer? To address these issues, the council has developed guidelines to be used in conjunction with its Provision of Acceptance that apply both to dentist-prescribed and over-the-counter peroxide-containing oral hygiene products to ensure their safety and effectiveness.

Flosses. Brushing the teeth will not remove the plaque and particles of food between the teeth, under the gumline, or under fixed prostheses. To clean these spaces, flossing is recommended. It will also polish the surfaces of your teeth and make your breath smell and feel fresher. Adults (including those with bridges, crowns, and fillings) and children over the age of 10 years should floss at least once a day, ideally spending five minutes at it. For instructions, see Box 5.3.

The type of floss to choose depends on the spaces between the teeth.

BOX 5.3

HOW TO FLOSS YOUR TEETH

1. Take about 18 inches of floss. (Some floss is sold in precut sections.) Lightly wrap most of one end around the middle finger on one of your hands. Wind most of the rest around the middle finger of your other hand, leaving a small section between both middle fingers.

2. Hold the floss taut between the thumb of one hand and the forefinger of the other, leaving about an inch between the two.

3. Carefully insert the floss between two teeth, using a back and forth or sawing motion. Gently bring the floss to the gumline but do not force it under the gums. Curve the floss around the edge of your tooth into the shape of the letter "C" and scrape it up and down the side. Reverse the curve of the floss and slide it along the edge of the other tooth. When cleaning your bottom teeth, you may find it easier to grasp the floss in your forefingers.

4. Repeat this procedure between the other teeth.

Although unwaxed floss is often recommended because it is thinner, can easily slide through small spaces, and the debris more readily adheres to its tiny filaments, a number of studies have shown no significant difference in the effectiveness of any of the different kinds of floss. Unwaxed floss may present difficulties because it has a tendency to fray and break when it catches on deposits of tartar, fillings, and other restorations and to become stuck between tightly spaced teeth. Waxed floss resists breakage, and bonded unwaxed floss prevents fraying but not tearing. Flat-sided, wider waxed tapes, often called ribbon floss, are often recommended when there is space between the teeth from gum recession and bone loss. Used alone, however, floss is not adequate to clean these spaces. Other interproximal devices, such as brushes, also need to be used.

Superfloss consists of a yarnlike section for cleaning under a bridge or braces and an unwaxed section for cleaning the normal spaces between teeth. Its stiff end makes it easier to thread through dental work and is especially useful on implants, related bridges, and dentures.

A new type of floss is made with polytetrafluoethylene, the material used in Gore-Tex the fabric for foul weather. It costs more, but it is claimed that it slides between the teeth more smoothly and does not shred. Fluoride has been added to some flosses, although a clinical benefit has not been demonstrated as yet.

Dislodging partially metabolized food particles during flossing can produce a bad taste in the mouth. The addition of flavoring, such as cinnamon, peppermint, wintergreen, and spearmint, makes flossing more pleasant tasting. Floss with the flavor of bubble gum may appeal to children.

Floss holders (usually Y-shaped) are especially recommended for persons who have physical or mental disabilities, lack manual dexterity, or have large hands or a small mouth. The floss is pulled tightly between the two prongs and then inserted between two teeth, where it is pulled forward and back, and up and down along the sides of the teeth. Studies show the holders to be as effective for removing plaque as finger-held floss. With any floss or floss holder, care should be taken not to snap the floss but instead to use a sawing motion to avoid injury to tissues.

For up to a week after starting to floss, your gums may be sore and bleed. These symptoms should abate when the bacteria have been removed and the plaque broken up. If the bleeding persists beyond this time, call your dentist.

Tongue Cleaners. Regular brushing of the palate (the roof of the mouth) and tongue will further reduce the accumulation of plaque and bacteria in the mouth. For most, this can be effectively accomplished with a very soft bristled manual toothbrush. Persons who smoke, have a coated or deeply fissured tongue, or have hairy tongue, a harmless condition caused by certain medications and characterized by a dark coating, may prefer a tongue-cleaning device. To use, the oblong cleaner is placed on top of the tongue as far back as it can comfortably go without stimulating the gag reflex and pulled forward using gentle pressure.

Other Ways to Clean Between Your Teeth

Long before the invention of dental floss, people (and other primates) fashioned implements out of twigs and bone splinters to remove bits of food trapped between their teeth. Today, there are other aids almost as effective as flossing and sometimes more suitable for individuals with specific dental problems and appliances or physical impairments.

Toothpicks. At one time, the toothpick was the main tool for cleaning the teeth. The wealthy had theirs fashioned of metal, carved wood, and ivory; the less affluent whittled sticks. In recent years their use has waned, although they are still offered at restaurants.

Toothpicks are not appropriate when there is little space between the teeth or when the gum tissue fills that space. Only gentle pressure should be applied on the gums with them. Before using, premoisten with water or saliva.

Wedge Stimulators. These implements should be used only when there is enough space between the teeth and the gums for them to easily slide back and forth, with the flat base placed on the gums. Although they do not entirely remove plaque from the surfaces of the sides of the teeth, they do reduce its accumulation and dislodge food particles.

The wooden wedges should be premoistened before using by sucking on them or placing them in water. To avoid injuring the gums, they should be discarded as soon as they splinter and after every use. The plastic wedges are reusable if thoroughly washed.

Tip stimulators. The conical-shaped rubber tip at the bottom of some toothbrushes can supplement floss in removing plaque and is effective for massaging the gums and dislodging food particles from between the teeth.

Interproximal Brushes and Swabs. Dental floss is ineffective if the spaces between teeth are wide. For large spaces, interproximal brushes with small, spiral bristles or swabs are usually the most effective.

The diameter of the brush should be a little larger than the space between the teeth being cleaned. To avoid damage to the gums, moisten the brush before inserting it and move it carefully in and out of the space. Because the brush bristles can scratch titanium, special interproximal brushes with plastic coverings on the wire portion or ones with swab tips are preferable for cleaning implant abutments.

Irrigation Devices. These deliver a steady or pulsing stream of water (and sometimes mouthrinses with antiplaque agents) to a specific area in the mouth to irrigate or flush out debris and toxic bacterial products, although they do not remove plaque. If used cautiously and correctly, these devices are appropriate for certain situations. They can help clean the spaces between the teeth and normal gum pockets and are useful to supplement but not replace brushing and flossing for persons with braces or complex restorations like crowns and fixed bridges.

For individuals susceptible to bacterial endocarditis (see Chapter 12) there is a risk of bacteria entering the bloodstream when excessive water pressure forces air, water, and bacteria into underlying tissues. Holding the nozzle at a right angle to the length of the tooth will circulate the water, yet help avoid forcing bacteria into tissues. It is a good idea to ask a dentist, before using an irrigator, to recommend a pressure setting (usually low to prevent trauma to the soft tissues) and to rule out reasons not to use them. When the gums are inflamed, a dentist always should be consulted before use and when gum inflammation is severe, irrigators never should be used.

Mouthrinses. In normal circumstances, mouthrinses are never substitutes for brushing and flossing. In special situations, however, they can supplement (and very occasionally substitute) for these staples of oral hygiene. Used in this way, mouthrinses are appropriate for persons with dental problems, for example, exposed roots or devices, such as bridges or braces that are difficult to clean by brushing and flossing alone, and those with physical impairments for whom grasping and manipulating a toothbrush is too challenging. Individuals who have medical conditions, such as Sjögren's syndrome, or take drugs that encourage decay or periodontal disease (e.g., phenytoin) also may need the additional therapeutic effects of these chemical agents. Of course, healthy persons who are not at any particular risk for developing dental diseases may use mouthrinses as an adjunct to brushing and flossing and to freshen their breath.

Mouthrinses can be either cosmetic or therapeutic or a combination of both. A cosmetic mouthrinse (mouthwash) will help rinse away debris and food particles, make the teeth feel cleaner and the mouth smell better for a while, and temporarily stop harmful bacteria from developing. Cosmetic mouthwashes available over the counter usually contain an active ingredient to inhibit the growth of bacteria, a flavoring, an astringent to impart a tingling feeling in the mouth, and water. They also contain ethyl alcohol in as much as 18 to 26 percent concentration, a potential hazard for young children. No mouthrinse is recommended for use by children under the age of six and all should be kept out of their reach.

Therapeutic mouthrinses bring about a medicinal effect, by reducing either caries or gingivitis. The caries-reducing mouthrinses contain fluoride and are discussed in "Fluorides" subsequently.

Two antimicrobial mouthrinses have plaque-fighting properties that have merited the ADA Seal of Acceptance. They are Listerine and its generic or brand-name equivalents, sold over the counter, and chlorhexidine gluconate, sold by prescription and marketed under the trade names Peridex and PerioGard.

Listerine, a combination of thymol, eucalyptol, menthol, and methylsalicylate oils, a phenolic-like antiseptic, in a water and alcohol solution, has been used safely for over a century. The phenol oils in Listerine reduce plaque by destroying its bacterial cell walls and inhibiting the bacterial enzymes. In studies it has been shown consistently to reduce both plaque and gingivitis by over 20 percent, when used in conjunction with regular oral hygiene. Rinsing with it two times a day is as effective in combating gingivitis as using it more often.

After using Listerine for a few days, the bitter taste and burning sensation some persons experience usually dissipate. In response to these complaints, a modified version, Cool Mint Listerine, which has a different taste and a lower alcohol content (22 instead of 26 percent), has been introduced.

Unlike Listerine, the broad-spectrum antimicrobial chlorhexidine gluconate is able to sustain its bacteria-killing ability over a period of time because it has substantivity, the ability to adhere to hard and soft tissues (the teeth and gums). Studies have shown chlorhexidine's abilities to reduce plaque and gingivitis to be significant, around 50 and 45 percent respectively, with no long-term (up to two years) ill health effects. When taken with red wine, tea, coffee, and other beverages, either brand can stain teeth and restorations brown. A professional cleaning can remove the staining, but it remains unattractive in the interim. Chlorhexidine's propensity to promote tartar, especially for individuals who have a tendency to develop it, may be troublesome. To reduce these side effects, the level of chlorhexidine gluconate would have to be lowered to a point where it no longer would be effective at reducing plaque and gingivitis.

Listerine, Peridex, and PerioGard all have shown promise when used with power irrigators. A recent study revealed that 0.06 percent of chlorhexidine (half its usual strength) delivered through a power irrigator is more effective in reducing plaque and gingivitis than rinsing with undiluted chlorhexidine or using the irrigator with only water. The reason is that the irrigating device can distribute the antiseptic 3 to 4 millimeters under the gum, whereas using it as a mouthrinse cannot. Similarly, a recent study showed Listerine used with an irrigator was both beneficial in controlling plaque and gingivitis in the three weeks following scaling and root planing therapies for periodontal disease and when used this way at home after in-office irrigation with it. Further research needs to be done to determine whether these preliminary findings will be substantiated.

Both these antimicrobial agents have uses for other dental problems. Studies have shown that chlorhexidine significantly reduced the incidence and severity of oral candidiasis, a fungal infection, and mucositis, a condition causing the soft tissues in the mouth to become sore, develop ulcers, and bleed easily. Mucositis frequently occurs in patients undergoing cancer chemotherapy and immunosuppressive therapy for organ transplants. A study showed Listerine, when used in conjunction with an antifungal denture cleanser, to be as effective for persons with oral candidiasis who wear full or partial dentures, as nystatin, a drug used to treat it.

Sanguinarine, an extract from a blood root plant *Sanguinaria canadensis,* promoted as an antiplaque and antigingivitis agent, is used in a mouthrinse, as well as a toothpaste. Studies have been equivocal over the use of a mouthrinse containing the herbal extract: some reported a significant reduction in plaque and gingivitis, whereas others reported little reduction.

The quaternary ammonium compounds, cetylpyridinium chloride, known as CPC; domiphen bromide; and benzethonium chloride are widely used in over-the-counter mouthrinses. Like chlorhexidine, quaternary ammonium compounds attach to the teeth and soft tissues; however, they are released much more quickly than and are not as effective as chlorhexidine. Quaternary ammonium compounds also produce side effects similar to those of chlorhexidine: a burning sensation in the mouth and a propensity to stain teeth and encourage tartar formation.

The results from a recent study revealed cetylpyridinium chloride's antibacterial properties in reducing plaque and gingivitis were about equivalent to a rinse containing a placebo (an inactive substance given as if it were a drug) with which it was compared. No mouthrinses with these compounds carry the ADA Seal of Acceptance.

Cleaning Dentures

The plastics of denture bases absorb fluids and sometimes metabolites, products resulting from the metabolism or breakdown of the foods and fluids they come into contact with in the mouth. When these by-products, along with the yeast organism *C. albicans,* are present on the denture base, they can inflame the soft tissues in the mouth covering the hard palate on which they rest; this results in reddened, shiny areas, often infected by candidiasis. This condition, called denture stomatitis, is estimated to occur in as many as two out of three denture wearers. Cleaning dentures removes the inorganic and organic deposits that cause denture stomatitis. It also removes stains before they become embedded in the denture base or teeth and prevents the appliance from acquiring an unpleasant odor.

Dentures traditionally have been cleaned with some kind of commercial or homemade cleansing agent. As many as half the people who wear dentures clean them with ingredients they have at home, such as mild dishwashing liquid or hand soap, both of which can be acceptable. How effective the substances or products are depends, to a great extent, on how thoroughly, carefully, and appropriately they are used.

Commercially available denture cleansers in paste or powder form contain mild abrasives, such as calcium carbonate powder. When they are applied properly and carefully with a brush adapted to the contours of the denture, abrasive cleaners can be effective in mechanically removing plaque and stains and sometimes the calcified deposits that develop on dentures. Too vigorous scrubbing can abrade the acrylic materials in dentures and/or bend the metal clasps of removable partial dentures.

Another method for cleaning dentures is to soak them in chemical cleansers, often tablets or powders of alkaline detergents and agents. When dissolved in water, they release bubbles of oxygen, which dislodge the plaque and other debris. The oxidizing agents remove stains and some bacteria. Soaking solutions can also contain enzymes that clean by breaking up the substance in which the cells of dental plaque are embedded.

The first chemical soaking solutions contained hypochlorites, which have antibacterial and antifungal properties. They are effective at bleaching stains and dissolving mucin, the sticky and main component of mucous, and other organic substances of plaque. Their corrosive effect on metals was later moderated by the addition of alkaline materials. Still, since prolonged soaking of dentures in a chlorine-containing commercial or homemade solution (such as one-half teaspoonful of commercial bleach to one-half glass of water) may corrode appliances made of cobalt-chromium alloy or other metals, no more than 15-minute soaks are recommended.

The metal components of prostheses (the framework and clasps of removable partial dentures and perhaps the pins used to anchor the porcelain denture teeth) also can be damaged by cleansing solutions containing acids (hydrochloric acid used alone or in combination with phosphoric acid); therefore these should never be used on dentures containing any type of metal. Acid solutions may be effective at removing the recalcitrant stains the peroxide and hypochlorites cannot. But due to their caustic nature and the care required to handle them, they almost always are used only by dental personnel and are not recommended for home cleaning.

At night dentures need to be immersed in water or a soaking solution to prevent them from drying out and losing their shape. Commercially available products are effective for this purpose, except for appliances with metal attachments that can be tarnished.

Sonic and Ultrasonic Devices. A more recent way to mechanically clean dentures is with a device using frequencies that are sonic (the sounds are audible) or ultrasonic (the frequency of the sound waves emit-

BOX 5.4

CLEANING AND CARING FOR YOUR DENTURES

Instructions for Using a Denture Cleaner

1. After removing the denture from your mouth, rinse with water to remove food particles.
2. Apply a denture cleaner approved by your dentist to a moistened denture or soft-bristled tooth brush.
3. Carefully but thoroughly scrub all surfaces of the denture.
4. Rinse the denture thoroughly with water.

- Keep all denture cleaning agents out of the reach of children.
- Have the denture cleaned at least once a year by a dentist.
- Clean the denture daily.
- Only use a cleaning agent approved by a dentist.
- Be careful not to scrub too vigorously.

Instructions for Using an Ultrasonic Denture Cleaning Device

1. Rinse the denture with water to remove food particles before placing it in the ultrasonic device.
2. Follow the manufacturer's instructions carefully. Leave the denture in an activated ultrasonic device no longer than recommended.
3. After removing the denture from the solution, rinse thoroughly with water.

- Supplement ultrasonic cleaning of the denture with hand brushing.
- Have the denture cleaned by a dentist when calcified deposits or stains accumulate on it.
- Use only the cleaning agent recommended by the manufacturer. Do not substitute harsh alkaline or caustic solutions that can damage and discolor the denture and ruin its fit.

ted are above the normal hearing range). Ultrasonic devices take the electrical energy available from ordinary household current and convert it into mechanical energy at ultrasonic frequencies to move or agitate the cleaning solution.

Cleaning dentures in an ultrasonic device that uses a commercially prepared cleansing soaking solution has been shown to be more effective than cleaning the appliances with either a sonic device or by soaking them in a cleansing solution alone. Tests by the ADA's scientific laboratories have shown that the devices will not remove all stains and debris without some hand brushing. Neither the sonic nor the ultrasonic devices will prevent the eventual staining or, in some cases, the calcified deposits from developing on dentures. Damage to the denture may occur if it is left for an extended period of time in either of these types of devices.

Persons who are handicapped or have difficulty grasping or manipulating objects may find it easier to use the ultrasonic devices or the soaking solutions than to clean their dentures with a paste or powder cleanser. For instructions on cleaning dentures, see Box 5.4.

Assessing Your Cleaning

Most studies show that the average American devotes less than one minute to brushing his or her teeth, time inadequate to remove plaque effectively. Disclosing tablets or liquids, made from harmless vegetable dyes and available from either a drugstore or dentist, enable you to evaluate the effectiveness of your oral hygiene efforts by temporarily staining the plaque above the gumline.

After brushing and flossing, chew the tablets or paint the solution on your teeth and rinse your mouth with water. Next, look in a mirror to identify the stained areas on your teeth you missed. Further brushing and flossing will remove any of the remaining colored plaque.

PREVENTION IN THE OFFICE

Professional Cleaning (Prophylaxis)

A professional cleaning accomplishes a number of things. It removes the stains caused by food, beverages, and tobacco and the tartar above the gumline that brushing and flossing cannot. Below the gums, it forestalls or prevents periodontal disease because it removes both the plaque and tartar that initiate and accentuate the disease process. Finally, it polishes the teeth to make it easier for the dentist to visually examine them and more difficult for new plaque to accumulate.

The process takes between one-half and one hour, depending on the condition of your teeth. First, the tartar is scraped off with a scaler. Scaling can be done manually, with a handheld instrument or with ultrasonic and sonic instruments. Studies have revealed all to be equally effective at removing tartar, though the ultrasonic ones make removal easier and quicker. Ultrasonic and sonic instruments, however, should not be used on persons with certain types of heart pacemakers or on composite resin or porcelain restorations. Next, the surface is smoothed with a motorized instrument and a polishing paste, often containing fluoride, to remove stains and any plaque that remains.

Because the rate at which adults and children accumulate tartar and develop stains varies, it is not possible to make a blanket recommendation on how frequently teeth should be professionally cleaned, although every six months may be the average. Your dentist will tell you the appropriate schedule for cleaning your teeth. Oral prophylaxis is usually performed by a hygienist and then checked by the dentist.

Sealants

Coating the biting surface of back teeth with plastic resin to prevent the bacteria from attacking the enamel has been shown to be highly effective in preventing caries in children. When combined with fluoride mouthrinses in children, their effectiveness in preventing caries increases. Sealants also have been shown effective in the very early stages of caries by trapping the bacteria and depriving them of the energy they need to multiply.

Sealants work best on first and second molars with pits and grooves on the biting surfaces so narrow that the bristles of a toothbrush cannot reach between to remove food debris and plaque. If premolars and third molars are also grooved, sealants can be applied to them.

The best time to apply sealants is soon after the teeth have fully erupted, when the immature enamel is especially vulnerable to destruction by acids. For the primary teeth, this is usually between the ages of 3 and

4 years, and for the permanent ones, between the ages of 6 and 7 years for the first permanent molar and between 11 and 13 years for the second permanent molars and the premolars.

It has been suspected that sealants can also be helpful for adults, especially during times when their teeth are more susceptible to caries, such as during orthodontic treatment, when the wires and appliances trap more food and bacteria, there are dry mouth conditions, or the consumption of sugary foods has increased, as may occur when hard candies are substituted for cigarettes in an effort to quit smoking. There are, however, no clinical studies on sealant use in adults.

Sealants are not appropriate for use on caries around old, leaking fillings or open, carious lesions. To be effective, there must be enough enamel to which the resin can adhere and the pits and fissures must be deep.

Application is painless and quick. The teeth are cleaned, air dried, and isolated. The enamel is etched briefly with acid, after which the teeth are rinsed with water and dried. The sealant is then painted on. The tint chosen (clear, white, yellow-orange, pale or bright pink) depends on the color of the enamel and personal preference. Depending on the type used, it will cure itself (a chemical catalyst is in the sealant) or require a special light to harden.

Sealants should be checked by a dentist or hygienist about every six months to be sure they have not worn off. If so, additional material can be added. Over the years, as sealants wear off, their effectiveness in preventing caries decreases. However, studies have shown that even when teeth lose much of their sealant, the rate of caries remains lower, possibly because some of the material remains embedded in the deep crevices.

There is debate whether it is cost effective to take this prophylactic measure. When the long-term costs of restoring decayed teeth are considered, studies reveal sealants are 25 percent less expensive than not using them. Economics, though, should not be the only consideration. There is a cosmetic and psychological value of having a mouth with no or few fillings versus one with multiple ones. Their use also may help shape a generation's attitude toward dental treatment. Fear is a learned behavior. Many adults who are anxious about dental treatment have had their impressions formed during childhood when what they remember of dental visits was drilling and filling. Children who grow up cavity-free or nearly so may be less apt to associate dental treatment with pain and, as a result, less likely to avoid it.

Costs vary according to the geographic region, but generally run between $30 and $50 per tooth. Dental insurance programs are increasingly including some reimbursement for sealants.

Caries Activity Tests

If you have recurrent caries, your dentist may measure the levels in your mouth of *Streptococcus mutans* and *Lactobacilli,* species of bacteria associated with the disease, with a simple in-office test. Although the threshold for the numbers of bacteria individuals tolerate before developing caries varies, in general higher levels have been found to correlate with more caries and higher susceptibility.

Dentists use caries activity tests for a variety of purposes, most often as incentives for patients to follow the regimen recommended for reducing their susceptibility to caries. This involves practicing good oral hygiene, eating a low- or noncariogenic diet, using antimicrobial mouthrinses, and monitoring the number of decay-causing bacteria. The test also can be valuable when used before and after restorative treatment. Some dentists may test a patient's *S. mutans* levels before placing extensive and expensive restorations to make sure the levels are low enough so that is it is unlikely that caries will develop around the edges of fillings or crowns, which would necessitate their removal. Other dentists may employ the test to determine whether a patient needs better or more dental counseling or whether reinfection has occurred and retreatment is needed.

FLUORIDES

The mineral fluoride is important for the teeth throughout our lives. It acts systemically during their development by incorporation into the enamel to increase their resistance to demineralization from bacterial acids produced in plaque. Once teeth have erupted, fluoride ions are present in saliva, where they help prevent demineralization and enhance remineralization.

In its various forms, it is the single factor most responsible for the decreasing incidence in caries. Fluoride can be present naturally in drinking water and in some foods. It also is added to drinking water, toothpastes, and mouthrinses and is available in lozenges, chewable pills, drops, and topical gels.

Fluoride is most effective on the smooth surfaces of teeth and is especially beneficial at the difficult-to-clean points where teeth are in contact with each other. It is not as effective on the pits and fissures of the molars; this is why they need the protection of a plastic sealant.

In Water

Over 60 percent of Americans are drinking fluoridated water (from supplementation of the municipal water supply or from the supply at schools). In the first years (1940s) after fluoride was introduced into water supplies (usually in the ratio of 1 part per million), water was one of the very few vehicles for it. A dramatic reduction (between 50 and 60 percent) in the incidence of dental caries was attributed to it.

We now receive fluoride from so many other sources that there are virtually no areas in the United States free of it. In addition to fluoridated toothpastes (used by over 90 percent of the population), one significant source is processed drinks and soda, which make up 50 percent of the liquid children consume and may be made from fluoridated water. Because of the presence of fluoride in so many products, the impact *water* fluoridation has on reducing dental caries has dropped and is now estimated to be between 17 and 38 percent. Even so, it remains an effective method of reducing caries for both children and adults. (For adults it is of great benefit in reducing the incidence of root caries.) If the water where you live is not fluoridated, your dentist may recommend one of the forms of supplementation listed below.

Toothpastes

All persons (unless discouraged by their dentist or physician) should use a toothpaste with fluoride. Use one approved by the ADA to ensure that it meets appropriate standards.

Mouthrinses

When used as a supplement to proper oral hygiene, fluoride mouthrinses, available over the counter (in a 0.05 percent sodium fluoride solution) and by prescription (with 0.2 percent sodium fluoride content), can reduce caries by as much as 40 percent. The additional protection provided by fluoride mouthrinses is especially useful for people who have receding gums, xerostomia (dry mouth) caused by an array of medications (see Chapter 10 for a listing), or disease (most frequently the autoimmune disorder Sjögren's syndrome, covered in Chapter 11), who are undergoing cancer chemotherapy, or who have recently had caries. All mouthrinses need to be expectorated, not swallowed. When children (only over the age of six years and only under a dentist's advice) are using them, the rinsing should be supervised to make sure none is swallowed.

Topical Office Application

Fluoride can be applied topically to the teeth via gel, solution, or varnish in the dental office by a dentist or hygienist. This is done routinely on children by some dentists when home applications of fluoride are not sufficient or on adults who are susceptible to caries (especially at the roots of the teeth) or have medical problems predisposing them to caries.

The teeth are first cleaned of tartar, isolated, and dried. The dentist or hygienist applies the fluoride by painting the solution on the teeth or placing the gel in a disposable or sterilizable tray and then inserting it over an arch of teeth, where it remains for four minutes before it is wiped off. A prop can be used for persons who are unable to hold their mouth open for the duration of the treatment. After the procedure, it is important to spit several times to avoid swallowing the fluoride and to refrain from eating or drinking for 30 minutes.

The varnish (which has only recently been introduced into the United States) needs to remain on the teeth for four hours before brushing, during which it forms a yellow film that hardens on contact with saliva. Because of its longer duration on the teeth, more of the fluoride is absorbed and more is retained than with the other forms. Since less is applied, accidental ingestion also is lower with the varnish than with the gels.

Topical Home Application

Fluoride can be applied at home using gel or drops of prescription fluoride that are loaded into a custom-made polyvinyl or disposable tray following a dentist's or hygienist's instructions. A gel form (such as Gel-Kam or PreviDent) also can be applied with a toothbrush. Home fluoride applications are recommended for persons who have dry mouth from a variety of causes, are undergoing radiation therapy, have severe caries or hypersensitivity on the surfaces of their roots, or need to prevent caries under an overdenture.

As with other topical fluoride preparations, the solution should not be swallowed. You may find it most convenient to apply it before going to bed, as you should not eat or drink for 30 minutes afterward. Since stannous fluoride, one of the preparations used, may stain teeth or porcelain and composite restorations, ask your dentist to choose the appropriate one for your particular dental condition and health.

CHAPTER 6

Dental Caries

Almost half the children in the United States between the ages of 5 and 17 are now free of dental caries (tooth decay). Despite these heartening trends and despite what many think, caries is not only a childhood disease. It can and does attack at any age. By the time children reach the age of 17, only 16 percent are free of the disease. For adults between the ages of 35 and 65, caries has not decreased, and for persons over 55, root caries is on the rise. In total, more than 95 percent of the adults in our country are afflicted. Its ubiquity makes dental caries, after the common cold, the world's most widespread ailment. Combined with periodontal disease, the two are so pervasive that virtually every adult has one or both in varying degrees.

Teeth infected with caries may no longer jeopardize life as they did before antibiotics were introduced, but they compromise its quality. Left untreated, caries can cause excruciating pain and result in the loss of teeth. This affects how we look and feel about ourselves, our ability to chew and speak, and, occasionally, even how well nourished we are. Restoring the damage it causes may mar the appearance of our smile. It is also expensive. Treating caries and its consequences (with restorations, crowns, bridges, dentures, root canal therapy, and implants) consumes a substantial percentage of the personal expenditures that are spent on dental services (which were almost $41 billion in 1994). Thus, the prevention and early treatment of this prevalent health problem remains a challenge throughout our lives and becomes even more important as more of us grow older and keep our teeth longer.

WHAT IS DENTAL CARIES?

Many people erroneously believe caries and cavities are the same. They are not. The word "caries" is Latin for "rot" or "decay." It is similar to the Greek word *Ker* for "death," which is appropriate, since a carious lesion is decaying tissue. Caries is a destructive infectious disease instigated by bacteria. A cavity or hole occurs later in the disease process, after the caries has destroyed the enamel and penetrated the tooth's dentin.

WHAT CAUSES IT?

For caries to develop, three things have to be present: specific bacteria, fermentable carbohydrates for them to feed on, and a tooth surface that is susceptible to the products that bacteria form.

The most cariogenic (caries-producing) bacterial species, *Streptococcus mutans,* which feeds on the sugars in foods, is the primary organism involved. It releases lactic, formic, and other acids, some of which are capable of dissolving the enamel on the teeth, beginning the disease process. Other organisms play lesser roles: *Lactobacilli* are associated with caries of the pits and fissures on the biting surfaces and *Actinomyces* with root caries.

In susceptible people, *S. mutans* forms a significant portion of *supragingival* plaque, the sticky substance that adheres to teeth and dental restorations (crowns, bridges, fillings, dentures, and implants) above the gumline. Supragingival plaque can be removed mechanically, but it will begin to reform within hours after the teeth have been brushed.

The plaque that is found in the crevices below the gumline is called *subgingival.* Although it contains some *S. mutans,* it also contains many other species, especially anaerobic bacteria that thrive without oxygen and are responsible for periodontal disease.

Plaque has a life cycle. First, pellicle, a thin film from saliva, covers the teeth. Bacteria quickly attach to it and start multiplying. If not removed, plaque, especially in areas opposite the salivary glands, can form hard deposits of calculus (tartar) on the teeth. If tartar is not removed (possible only by a professional cleaning), it attracts more bacteria, one of the factors in the development of periodontal disease.

Caries is the symptom of an infectious disease, spread by specific strains of bacteria from one person to another by saliva. Newborns who have no teeth do not have the bacteria responsible for caries, but they acquire them as the teeth erupt. By age five, more than half of children have been infected with the specific type of organisms their mothers have in their mouths. Most children infected with *S. mutans* acquire the infection between 19 and 28 months of age; 83 percent are infected by the age of four years. Sufficient quantities of the bacteria to cause infection are transmitted when a spoon is shared. Blowing on food and kissing are other common activities that may be capable of transferring the bacteria from an infected person to a young child.

THE DECAY PROCESS

The first visual sign of caries is a white or brown spot on the enamel. These occur in areas where plaque accumulates, such as in the pits and fissures of the molars and premolars, between the teeth, and at the gumline. This is not a cavity. Rather, it is an indication that demineralization has occurred below the tooth surface. If it is detected early (it is *not* noticeable to the untrained eye) and oral hygiene, topical fluorides, and plaque removal are begun, it is possible that the enamel can remineralize and the caries be arrested (see the subsequent section "Arrest of Precavitated Lesions"). But, once a cavity forms, remineralization cannot fill it up. If not treated, a cavity will continue until the entire crown (or root surface) is destroyed.

The disease can progress from the enamel to the dentin, and eventually attack the pulp and cause an infection called pulpitis. Since the dentin surrounding the pulp is a hard tissue, when the blood vessels within the pulp become inflamed, they cannot expand. The pulp dies after its blood supply becomes severed. This process may result in severe, stabbing pain. The pain may be difficult to locate, because nerve pathways can refer it to other teeth and even the other jaw.

In the worst-case scenario, after pulpitis has caused the death of the pulp, the infection can spread to the root and tissues surrounding it and create a periapical abscess. This usually causes a continuous pain exacerbated by pressure. If not treated with antibiotics, cellulitis, an inflammation of the skin, can ensue. Cellulitis causes the face to swell and a fever to develop, with the possibility that the infection may spread to the bones and soft tissues. The treatments for pulpitis and periapical abscesses most often involve either root canal therapy (endodontics) or extraction of the tooth.

THE ROLE OF SUGAR

The ingestion of sugar is the culprit in the development of caries. Carbohydrates (sugars and, to a lesser degree, starches) enhance the colonization and growth of bacteria in dental plaque. Sucrose is the most cariogenic sugar, with glucose (found in honey, fruits, and vegetables), fructose (in honey and fruits), and maltose (in grains) close behind. Fermented sugars quickly produce acids that can overcome the rate at which saliva neutralizes them to destroy the enamel of the tooth. Although sucrose is most often identified as refined white and brown sugar, it also occurs naturally (though in far less damaging form) in a variety of fruits and vegetables, including beets, bananas, peaches, melons, and sweet potatoes. When starches accumulate on teeth, the enzyme amylase in saliva can convert them to sugars, which produce the acids that initiate decay.

Through the Millennium

How much caries a society has tends to be proportional to the level of its technology, which, in turn, is associated with its consumption of sugar. Prehistoric man had very little caries: only 2 to 4 percent of the teeth examined from the remains of humans before the Iron Age revealed decay. Our early ancestors' diet was not conducive to caries. It consisted of fibrous foods, which require a lot of chewing and stimulate the production of saliva which helps wash away bacteria and food debris. The grains they ate were coarse ground and contained calcium and several phosphates, substances that assist in remineralizing enamel after an acid attack. The milling and refining processes of flours today remove these nutrients. Although the fruits primitive man ate contained sucrose, glucose, and fructose, their total content was modest. In contrast, the prepackaged foods and beverages we consume frequently and in great quantities in our present diets contain high concentrations of sucrose, glucose, and high fructose corn syrup.

Through the Roman, Anglo-Saxon, and Medieval periods, the incidence of caries hovered at about 10 percent. The rate remained constant until the end of the seventeenth century when, with the development and distribution of sugar cane, it began its steady rise. Queen Elizabeth I's infected teeth, which eventually led to her death, were a result of her fondness for sweets and her ability to obtain them, given her position and wealth. But most of the world's population could not develop a sweet tooth to satisfy because sugar remained prohibitively expensive until slavery provided a way of cheaply harvesting this labor-intensive crop.

When slavery furnished the "free" labor, the British supplied the ships, and the congregation of people in cities afforded easy access to markets, sugar became widely available. By 1850 sugar was eaten by most of the population, and the incidence of caries mushroomed. Both the consumption of sugar and the rate of caries continued to rise until the 1950s and 1960s. At this time, fluoride was added to municipal and school water supplies and toothpastes and the rate of caries began to decline. An exception to the increase in caries occurred in Europe during World War II when sugar was restricted because of naval blockade.

What to Eat When

When a great deal of sugar is consumed, as is the norm in our society, when and how often it is eaten may be more significant than how much is eaten. Usually there is a correlation between the two; the more sugar that is available, the more and more frequently it is eaten.

About ten minutes after eating food that contains sugar, the pH (a scale used to show the level of acid or alkaline in a solution) of the plaque that adheres to the tooth drops, often below the threshold (a pH of 5.5 and below) at which enamel begins to demineralize. (A pH of 7.0 is neutral. Below 7.0 is acid; above 7.0 is alkaline.) Depending on the type of food eaten, its sugar content, and the ability of an individual's saliva to neutralize the acids, the plaque will remain acidic for up to an hour. After this, components in the saliva neutralize the acids, and the destruction of the enamel starts to reverse. When sugary foods are eaten at frequent intervals throughout the day, the enamel is constantly exposed to acids with little opportunity for demineralization to reverse. To enhance remineralization, many researchers advocate a three-hour hiatus between eating foods with sugar.

In general, food containing over 15 to 20 percent sugar is highly cariogenic (caries producing). Despite this, how cariogenic a specific food is cannot be evaluated by its sugar content alone. Other factors are important, among them a food's ability to stimulate the flow of saliva, its particle size and shape, its ability to cling to the teeth, and how long it remains in the mouth.

Some foods assumed to be highly cariogenic are not as detrimental to the teeth as are others and vice versa. For example, some people substitute molasses, honey, or corn syrup for refined sugar, believing they are less harmful to the teeth. These "natural" sweeteners contain fructose, glucose, sucrose, and other sugars which, because they are sticky and linger on the teeth, may be worse for them. Hard candies, cough drops, and breath mints are especially damaging because they dissolve slowly in the mouth, and so allow the teeth to be bathed longer in acid.

Sugary or starchy foods eaten with a meal are less harmful to the teeth, possibly because the production of saliva, which washes away the sugar and bacteria, is increased. Conversely, sugary foods eaten before bed are potentially very damaging (especially if the teeth are not cleaned), as saliva production is reduced during sleep.

Sugar can be present naturally in food or added by the cook, consumer, or manufacturer. Most naturally occurring sugar is present in the form of lactose in milk and fructose in fruit. Although fructose can produce caries, whole fruits have little cariogenicity, due, in part, to their high water content. Although lactose alone is moderately cariogenic, milk products with it contain casein, a phosphoprotein, which may prevent bacteria from adhering to the tooth. Studies have revealed that older persons who had no root caries reported a high intake of milk and cheese.

Eating starchy foods alone is usually not enough to produce caries. Raw or unrefined cereal grains are low on the cariogenic scale. When starchy foods, like rice, potatoes, and bread, are cooked, they increase somewhat in cariogenicity. But when combined with even small amounts of sugar, they can become very cariogenic. Potent caries-producing foods are sweet baked goods, like cakes and cookies, which contain sugars and starches and remain on the teeth for a long time.

Eating fibrous foods may not prevent plaque from forming per se, but it does help stimulate saliva production. Saliva that has been stimulated from chewing is slightly alkaline; it does not have the acidity of unstimulated saliva. Fibrous foods, such as carrots, celery, and apples, also stimulate the periodontium; this increases the blood circulation, which bring nutrients that will help maintain the health of the area.

Aged cheddar cheese (and to a lesser extent peanuts) are two foods with the ability to keep the pH higher to counteract the acid released by bacteria. When cheese dissolves in saliva, calcium and phosphates are released and stored in the plaque, where they help slow the acidic breakdown of enamel. For this reason, some people have recommended ending a meal with either of these foods or with sugarless gum (especially ones containing xylitol), but there are other health reasons for avoiding cheese (e.g., its high fat content). For specific recommendations and warnings about what to eat and when, see Boxes 6.1 and 6.2.

BOX 6.1

EATING TIPS

• Eat carbohydrates (sugars and starches) with a meal.
• Don't eat sugary foods alone or between meals.
• If you don't brush your teeth after eating, rinse your mouth with water or chew sugarless gum.
• If you snack, substitute sweet or starchy foods with "safe" ones listed in Box 6.2.
• Take good care of your teeth and gums by following the recommendations in Chapter 5.
• Drink sugared beverages, such as fruit or soft drinks, and carbonated beverages through a straw.

The Attraction to Sugar

The fondness for sweets is innate. Babies prefer sweet foods over other taste sensations. When rats who have been made dependent on alcohol are offered a choice, they select sweets over alcohol. Some researchers have gone so far as to suggest that for some individuals, the preference and consumption of sweets is like an addiction and one not restricted to our own age. During the crusades, there were reports of Christian soldiers "abandoning their holy mission to languish in the land of the infidels in happy pursuit of Saracen sugar."

BOX 6.2

WISE SNACKING

If you snack, choose foods that are less cariogenic and therefore better for your teeth, such as:

Cheese	Meats	Sugarless gum or
Coffee or tea without	Milk	candy
sugar	Nuts	Tofu
Dill pickles	Olives	Vegetables, raw
Eggs	Peanut butter	Whole grains,
Fruits (e.g., apples,	(without sugar)	legumes
oranges, plums,	Popcorn	Yogurt, plain
cantaloupe,	Seeds	
watermelon)		

Some of these foods are high in fat, caffeine, or salt. If your physician has recommended that you avoid any of them, follow his or her advice.

Avoid eating foods such as these by themselves:

Cakes	Crackers	Popsicles
Candies	Dates	Raisins
Chips	Gelatin desserts	
Cookies	(jello)	
Cough drops		

For most people to successfully reduce their consumption of sugars, their emotional and psychological desire for it needs to be addressed. To change ingrained and pleasurable behavior, it is seldom enough to simply say, "stop." Instead of cutting sweets out completely, it is more realistic to follow the guidelines in Box 6.1 to choose when and how to eat them to minimize their potential to cause decay. To prevent children from developing an emotional response to sweets, they should not be given as rewards nor should their removal be used as punishment. Adults who are especially fond of sugary foods may find behavior modification, support groups, and other therapies helpful in establishing good eating habits.

INHERENT RESISTANCE TO CARIES

To what extent an individual's teeth are resistant to caries depends on a number of factors, especially the resistance of the enamel, the presence of fluoride, and the function and composition of the saliva and plaque. Genetic factors and the body's immune defenses also may play a role.

Resistance of Enamel

The strength of the enamel is influenced by what happens while teeth are developing within the jaw and what happens after they erupt. Although the crowns are formed before they erupt, the surface of the enamel does not fully mature for some time; this makes newly erupted teeth particularly vulnerable to the harmful pathogens. For this reason, the years between the ages of 5 and 8 and between the ages of 11 and 14, when most new teeth are emerging, are times when the teeth are especially susceptible to caries. Phosphorus, magnesium, fluoride, calcium, and other trace minerals present in saliva and supplemented, as with fluoride, in the form of toothpastes, water, rinses, and topical applications help the enamel mature. Most people in the United States receive adequate levels of these minerals. It is the intake of sugar and starches *after* teeth have erupted that has more of an impact on whether we develop caries than our nutritional status during their development and maturation does.

Still, despite a high standard of nutrition, similar oral hygiene habits and intakes of sugars, some individuals are prone to developing caries whereas others are caries-free. To find out why, some researchers have studied the small proportion (1 in 750) of adults whose teeth developed without benefit of fluoridated water and remained free of caries. The group without caries had about twice as many males as females, and the members' close relatives were 30 times as likely to have no caries. No relationship was found between a person's susceptibility or resistance to caries and a tooth's size, hardness, or degree of mineralization. However, subtle differences in the crystalline structure of the enamel may be related to caries resistance.

Subsequent studies have supported the evidence that genetic factors are in some way involved. With the emerging capabilities of molecular biology, it may be possible in the future to discover a specific gene or genes responsible for a resistance to caries.

The Role of Saliva

Saliva is instrumental in keeping caries at bay by washing away food particles and bacteria (also cancer-causing components in tobacco smoke) and by neutralizing acids generated from fermentable carbohydrates to maintain a near-neutral pH. In addition, saliva is supersaturated with phosphate, hydroxyl ions, and calcium, all ingredients of tooth mineral that play a role in reversing early carious lesions by remineralizing the enamel. Perhaps the strongest testament to the extent to which saliva helps prevent caries is what happens when its flow is substantially decreased.

Xerostomia (Dry Mouth). Also referred to as hyposalivation, this condition is characterized by dry mouth, which encourages the growth of bacteria and causes mouth soreness and difficulty in eating, swallowing, and speaking, as well as high susceptibility to decay. Xerostomia can be caused by radiation of oral cancers, tumors of the salivary glands, Sjögren's syndrome, and prolonged illnesses, such as lupus. It is most frequently found as a side effect of hundreds of medications (see Chapter 10 for a partial list). Unless measures are taken (such as artificial salivas, fluoride mouthrinses, fluoride varnishes, topical applications of fluoride, dietary modification to reduce the amount of sugary foods and beverages between meals, and thorough oral hygiene), rampant caries will ensue as early as three months after the xerostomia begins.

Chewing gum is a simple, effective, albeit temporary, treatment to increase salivation as long as there are functioning salivary glands.

BOX 6.3

ARTIFICIAL AND ALTERNATIVE SWEETENERS

The following are artificial and alternative sweeteners that will cause either no or little caries.

Artificial Sweeteners

These popular synthetic sweeteners have highly concentrated sweetening powers but do not contain calories (or contain so few as to be insignificant).

Acesulfame K has 200 times the sweetness of sucrose. It tolerates high temperatures and is considered safe.

Aspartame is a sweetener, as a well as a flavor extender, which lengthens, by five to seven times, the period chewing gums taste sweet. Unlike saccharin, it leaves no aftertaste. Among its approved uses are as a substitute for table sugar and in cold cereals, drink mixes, instant tea and coffee, puddings, toppings, chewable multivitamin food supplements, and gelatins.

Saccharin is between 300 to 500 times sweeter than sucrose and is included in processed foods and carbonated drinks. A major drawback is its bitter aftertaste. Because of conflicting research regarding its safety in food, all items containing it that are sold in the United States must contain the warning, "Use of this product may be hazardous to your health. This product contains saccharin, which has been determined to cause cancer in laboratory animals." Many scientists advise against its excessive use by anyone, heavy use by women of childbearing age, and any use by pregnant women or children who are not diabetic.

Alternative Sweeteners

Due to their chemical structure, these sweeteners are technically not sugars but sugar alcohols. They are described as sugar free but have about the same caloric content as sucrose. Because mannitol and sorbitol are about half as sweet as sucrose, if used as a sugar substitute, there may be a tendency to increase the amount used and hence the caloric content in order to equal the sweetening power of sucrose.

Mannitol occurs naturally in seaweed but can also be derived from the sugar mannose by chemical means. It is most often used in toothpastes and mouthrinses. It does not cause caries.

Sorbitol is used most often in chewing gum, toothpaste, and in some candy. It should not contribute to caries.

Xylitol, which has the same sweetening power as sucrose, is made from birch trees, corn cobs, oats, bananas, and some mushrooms. Not only does it not promote caries, but research has shown it can prevent new carious lesions from developing and, in some instances, cause a hardening of existing ones. Because sugar alcohols can cause diarrhea when used in excess, its use is restricted to small amounts, as in chewing gum or lozenges.

NOTE: All three can cause flatulence and diarrhea when above 50 grams per day are used.

Recently, the addition of sweeteners that do not ferment, especially xylitol (see Box 6.3), to gum has been found to reduce caries for people with this problem. Sugar-free lozenges also can be helpful for people who object to chewing gum.

Many people with xerostomia find artificial salivas unsatisfactory in overcoming oral dryness. One study found water to be as effective in relieving symptoms of dry mouth as either carboxymethylcellulose or mucin, the lubricating ingredients in artificial salivas.

If an individual is still able to produce some saliva, pilocarpine hydrochloride, a drug that stimulates the salivary gland to produce more saliva, can be used to improve the symptoms associated with Sjögren's syndrome and post-irradiation xerostomia (it has not been tested for drug-induced xerostomia), including dryness of the mouth, oral discomfort, and difficulty in speaking. Some patients experience minor side effects, most often sweating.

DETECTING CARIES

Early signs of caries are easy to see on the visible surfaces of the teeth, but they are more difficult to see in the pits and fissures or between the teeth. For a dentist to conduct an examination, the teeth should be dry and clean and free of heavy deposits of plaque or tartar. A hand instrument, an explorer, is used to examine teeth and locate caries. When it is inserted into the chewing surfaces of the teeth and there is early caries, it either sticks in decay or is difficult to remove and the area around the spot may be soft or stained. Questions have been raised over whether its sharp point may cause a cavity in the demineralized area and force bacteria into it. This has been of particular concern in recent years when many carious lesions have been progressing more slowly due to the use of fluoride and other preventive interventions.

The use of bitewing radiographs (which reveal the crowns of several upper and lower teeth on one film) remains the best way to discover caries between the teeth. However, fiber-optic transillumination using light is an alternative to radiographs to detect caries in the dentin between the teeth and sometimes on the biting surfaces. (See Chapter 21 for information on radiographs.)

There are newer high-tech methods to detect caries, some of which are still being investigated and others of which are beginning to be employed routinely in clinical practice. The use of staining dye has been explored at dental schools. It has proved helpful in detecting caries under amalgam fillings where it is frequently missed. Laboratory studies of an electronic caries detector with a battery-generated current that is applied through a probe for a digital readout of the degree of demineralization in a fissure have shown the device to be effective in discovering decay on the chewing surfaces, but it is not widely used because of its expense. With video technology, photographs (which eliminate radiation) and radiographs of the teeth can be taken and magnified 100 times or more onto a television screen. Subtraction radiography (explained in Chapter 7) for caries detection is still being evaluated.

Because carious lesions can reverse spontaneously and arrest in the early stages and because they have been slower to progress in recent years, the approach to diagnosing and treating decay is changing. The new philosophy holds that observation over time is required to diagnose all but the cavitated lesions that penetrate the dentin. An individual's risk for developing caries, based on past history, diet, use of fluorides, and microbiological factors, needs to be considered when making the diagnosis. A more conservative approach to repairing and replacing defective restorations also is being embraced (see Chapter 9).

TREATMENTS

If, despite preventive interventions, caries develops or actively recurs at the site of a previous restoration, it needs to be treated in some way. What treatment is undertaken depends on the stage of the carious lesion.

Arrest of Precavitated Lesions

Once a white spot lesion has developed and decalcification of the tooth has begun, measures are taken to increase remineralization and prevent demineralization of the enamel. Carious lesions that have not penetrated through the enamel may be treated with instruction in oral hygiene and fluoride mouthrinses, varnishes, and other topical fluoride treatments (covered in Chapter 5) for a finite period of time, often six months, in the hopes that the enamel crystal structure will stabilize and the damaged crystals will recalcify. Because caries does not always follow a steady path of destruction but instead may progress with periods of destruction sometimes interrupted by periods of arrest and even repair during its early stages, these treatments can sometimes work.

Fillings

If a cavity occurs, the tooth needs to be restored. *Restoration* in dentistry refers to any tooth filling, crown, denture, or other dental device that restores or replaces lost or infected (decayed) tooth structure and function. Fillings are most often used to replace carious tissue when enough sound tooth structure remains to mechanically support them. Teeth in which the caries has invaded the pulp need to be treated with root canal therapy or other endodontic treatment (see Chapter 13).

What material is used to fill an infected tooth depends on a number of factors, among them the location of the tooth, the size of the carious lesion, the strength of the material and how much biting force will be exerted on it, its costs, and the individual's personal preference, which often includes aesthetic concerns. Although some materials can last a long time, none should be considered permanent. The different materials, how they are used, and their advantages and disadvantages are discussed here and summarized in Box 6.4.

Procedure. For all filling materials, decayed tooth structure must be removed and a cavity prepared. This is usually accomplished with a variety of hand instruments and high- and low-speed rotary instruments with burs that use water and air for coolants. Lasers have been developed, but at the present time they have FDA approval only for penetration of the soft tissues in the mouth; they are under research for use in cutting the hard tissues of the tooth. A new air-abrasive device based on an older technology blasts a stream of microscopically fine powder of purified aluminum oxide (alpha alumina), a nontoxic material used in some medicine, foods, and whitening toothpastes, at the teeth. The device creates less heat, vibration, and noise, and therefore causes less pain, its proponents assert, than do rotary drills; this frequently reduces the need for anesthesia. The new device may be better suited, however, for preparing enamel for resin materials in lieu of acid etching than for removing decay. Whether this technology (which is much more costly than rotary drills) will be embraced more extensively by dentists remains to be seen.

Cavities can be simple, which means a carious lesion is confined to only one tooth surface; compound, which means lesions are on two surfaces of the same tooth; or complex, which means the carious lesions are present on more than two surfaces of the same tooth.

After the cavity is prepared, its walls are finished to provide a tight seal between the restoration and tooth structure to prevent microleakage and the development of staining, sensitivity, and recurrent caries. The cavity may or may not be lined with a varnish of natural or synthetic resins. Deep cavities may be lined with calcium hydroxide, glass ionomer cement, zinc phosphate, or other materials. This seals the dentinal tubules and potentially the pulp from reaction to heat and cold, chemicals, galvanic shock, corrosive and hazardous materials, and bacteria. In addition, a cement base may provide support for the restorative material.

With the rapid pace of progress in the field, each year different filling materials come on the market, most of them only slight variations of already available materials. They are usually modified to make their

BOX 6.4

DIFFERENT TYPES OF FILLING MATERIALS

Type	Reasons to Use	Not Recommended for	Advantages
Amalgam	Small, moderate, and some large decay	Teeth that have had root canal work, very large lesions	Strong, long lasting, good seal at margins
Composite resins	Aesthetics, small fillings	Very large fillings	Blends in with tooth
Cast gold inlays, onlays, and crowns	Large amounts of decay, for extra strength, to change bite	Adolescents	Long lasting, may improve strength of tooth for crowns

Type	Disadvantages	Longevity	Costs
Amalgam	Stains, silver color, can leak at margins.	Long lasting	$50+, prices vary with size.
Composite resins	Do not last long.	About 6 years	$60+, prices vary with size.
Cast gold inlays, onlays	Expensive, appearance, time required to place.	Long lasting	$400+, prices vary with type of metal and treatments.

application easier and improve their physical properties. A dentist will work most successfully with materials with which he or she feels comfortable and has the most experience.

Amalgam. This is the most commonly used filling material. Although it is often referred to as silver, as this metal is its major ingredient, it is an alloy of different metals, among them silver and tin, with lesser amounts of copper, indium, zinc, mercury, gold, and palladium. In response to the reputed problems and anxieties over mercury (see Chapter 21), a mercury-free metallic filling is under development. At the present time, though, its mechanical and chemical properties are not advanced enough to make it an equivalent or acceptable substitute for the mercury-containing amalgam.

Amalgams have many advantages: they are long lasting and strong, are easy to insert, retain their form, and are the most reasonably priced filling material. They are best used on the back teeth, which sustain most of the chewing and grinding movements. For cosmetic reasons, they are not used on front teeth because of their dark color.

Amalgam must be worked quickly since it begins to harden within three to seven minutes. Because amalgam conducts heat and cold, a base material is usually put down first to protect the pulp in deep cavities. Next, the amalgam is added a little at a time and packed down until the cavity is overfilled. Finally, the surface is carved out to conform to the contours of the tooth and polished to produce a smooth surface and to prevent the amalgam from fracturing at its margins.

Composite Resin. The filled or composite resins in use today are composed of different sizes of particles of hard inorganic material or filler, usually quartz silica or glass, which are bound to an acrylic BisGMA (Bisphenol A-Glycidyl Methacrylate) using a coupling agent. The addition of inorganic fillers has increased the material's resistance to wear, decreased the amount it expands and contracts with temperature fluctuations, and increased stiffness.

To prevent microleakage and improve retention, the cavity is etched briefly with phosphoric acid to develop micro irregularities so the material can bond with the tooth in a manner similar to Velcro. Before placing the composite resin (and depending on how deep the cavity is), the cavity is lined with glass ionomer or calcium hydroxide. The composite resin is added in layers, which are cured, or hardened, by light, and then smoothed and shaped. Fluoride is sometimes incorporated into the resin, but since it is unable to leach out in sufficient quantities, it does not provide significant protection against caries.

Composite resins are not without their drawbacks. The success of the filling depends on the technique used by the dentist. When the proper technique is not followed, problems can occur with the seal at the margin of the filling and with recurrent caries. Allergic reactions also have been reported. Because of these disadvantages and composite resins' limitations in longevity, wear resistance, and strength under the stress of chewing, it is widely recommended that they be limited to areas where aesthetic concern is paramount.

In general, it costs more to fill a tooth with composite resin than it does with amalgam because it takes the dentist longer to place it. When the cost of refilling the tooth is factored in (they do not last nearly as long), composite resins become much more expensive than amalgams.

Glass Ionomer Cement. This material is used most often for filling root caries, because it retains fluoride and releases it to the tooth. Some dentists use it to fill cavities on the front or back sides of a tooth near the gums and the biting surfaces of primary teeth. It also is used as a base under restorations to protect the pulp.

Sealants. Normally applied as a preventive measure, sealants (which are usually BisGMA resins or lightly filled composites, sometimes with slow-release fluoride added) also can be used effectively to treat

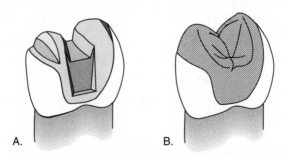

ILLUSTRATION 6.1. **ONLAY.**
A. Preparation of tooth for onlay. **B.** Tooth with onlay.

caries that has not invaded the dentin. Using them over more-advanced caries that has penetrated the dentin is not advocated.

Gold Foil (Cohesive or Direct Gold). Due to its longevity, gold foil, in the hands of an experienced clinician, is still considered by some the "gold standard" for filling small carious lesions. It is rarely used anymore, however, because the time and technique required to apply it makes it much more expensive than other filling materials. To apply it, small pieces of 24 karat gold are cold welded together with pressure to form a strong and extremely long-lasting restoration.

Inlays and Onlays

An *inlay* fits within a prepared cavity. An *onlay* covers the entire biting surface and most of the cusps (the peaks of the tooth), as well as fitting within the prepared cavity. This more extensive coverage protects a tooth that has little tooth structure left. If an onlay is placed over a tooth that has had root canal therapy or a previous filling, its edges will be placed on the tooth to protect it from further fracture. In a *pinlay,* pins are placed through the dentin, near the gumline to help anchor the thin cast restoration. Very little of the tooth needs to be removed to prepare it for this type of onlay.

Ideally, onlays and inlays are made from an alloy of metals—gold, silver, copper, platinum, palladium, zinc—and some additives. Onlays that extend onto the front portion of the teeth can have the visible portion filled with a tooth-colored resin or porcelain.

These restorations usually require two to three visits. During the first visit, the dentist prepares the tooth by removing the caries, preparing a cavity, and making an impression (a negative reproduction) of it. From this, a die (a positive reproduction of the tooth) of a hard material is made. Next, a waxed pattern is carved from which the molten gold alloy is cast. A temporary filling, usually made of acrylic resin, protects the tooth until the second visit, when it is removed and the restoration is permanently placed using a dental cement.

Crowns are discussed in Chapter 16.

CHAPTER 7

Periodontal Disease

WHAT IS PERIODONTAL DISEASE?

"Periodontal disease" is a broad term to describe a group of diseases that affect the hard and soft supporting structures of the teeth that together are called the *periodontium:* the soft tissue around the teeth (the gingiva or the gums), the alveolar process or part of the jaw bone into which the roots of the teeth are anchored, the cementum, and the periodontal ligament. The word is derived from Greek: *peri,* meaning "around," and *odont,* "tooth."

Like dental caries, periodontal disease does not follow a linear progression. Instead, there usually are episodes of disease activity followed by periods of remission. If left untreated, periodontal disease can damage the structures that support the teeth and cause the teeth to loosen and fall out. Although it may take years for the disease to progress to this point (and not all do), once it has advanced so far, there is a point of no return where tooth loss is inevitable. Fortunately, there are traditional and innovative methods of intervening to halt its progression.

Because periodontal diseases are often painless in their earlier, reversible stages, some patients have difficulty understanding why they need to undergo expensive and time-consuming treatments. But, these are necessary to retain the teeth.

WHO SUFFERS FROM IT?

At some time during his or her life, every adult has gingivitis (described subsequently). At the other extreme, between 10 and 15 percent of adults have moderate to advanced periodontitis requiring extensive treatment. The incidence of periodontal disease and the severity of its symptoms escalate as we grow older. For adults, periodontal diseases remain a major cause of tooth loss. Researchers believe women are not as severely affected as men because they practice better oral hygiene.

WHAT CAUSES
PERIODONTAL DISEASE?

For nearly 30 years, the accumulation of plaque has been implicated in the progression of periodontal disease. About 20 of the 300 or so different types of bacteria that have been found in the mouth are associated with specific types of periodontal disease. The consensus among researchers is that the diseases are infections caused by one or more of these bacteria. Most of the bacteria associated with periodontal diseases are anaerobic, meaning they survive without oxygen. These microorganisms are most frequently found in the crevice of the gum, a potential space immediately beneath the gumline, where they thrive and multiply.

Whether disease develops depends on more than the presence of harmful organisms. How virulent the strain is, its presence below the gumline, whether it has invaded the tissue, and how numerous it is are contributing factors. And finally, whether someone develops disease depends on his or her reaction to the destructive pathogens: the environment in the mouth must be conducive to the growth of the disease-causing bacteria and their numbers must exceed an individual's threshold for them. Much of the research being conducted is focusing on this host, or individual, response to the bacteria, in an attempt to answer why, with the same bacteria in the same numbers, some people develop active disease and others do not.

Genetic factors that reduce the function of white blood cells (leukocytes) may be involved in some less common types of periodontitis that occur in young persons and tend to run in families. The types of periodontal disease seen in adults usually do not have obvious family patterns.

ITS PROGRESSION

Gingivitis, the first stage of the disease, begins as the plaque below and above the gumline builds up and the toxins released by the bacteria lead to gum inflammation. As the inflammation continues, the area below the gumline is colonized by bacteria, and the destructive types proliferate. Some of the collagen (the bundles of tiny fibers of protein) that forms the connective tissues at the margin of the gum is destroyed; this causes the gum to retract from the tooth surface and to lose its attachment to the

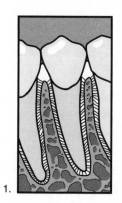 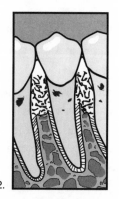 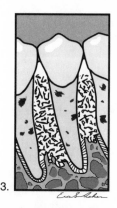

ILLUSTRATION 7.1. **PROGRESSION OF PERIODONTAL DISEASE.**
1. Healthy, normal. **2.** Plaque and calculus accumulate and cause the gums to
inflame. Harmful bacteria cause the destruction of the connective tissue and
bone. The gums begin to pull away from the tooth. The space between the tooth
and gum widens and deepens. **3.** Advanced disease. Disease has dissolved major
amounts of the bone and periodontal ligament and invaded the cementum, all the
structures that help anchor the tooth in its socket.

tooth. The space between the tooth and the gingiva widens and deepens.
This creates a pocket that allows the bacteria access to the periodontal
ligament, which anchors the tooth and cushions it from pressure, and to
the cementum, which covers the outside of the roots of the tooth.

When the inflammation involves the hard tissues and begins destroying the alveolar bone, the disease is called *periodontitis*. As the bone
dissolves, the tooth it encases loosens and either falls out or needs to be
extracted.

TYPES OF DISEASE

Different forms and stages of periodontal disease cause varying degrees
of damage to the different tissues of the periodontium. Not all teeth have
the same amount of disease around them and its location varies with individuals. It is most commonly found around the molars, situated in the
back of the mouth where plaque is difficult to remove, and, less commonly, on the front teeth, which are easier to clean and, because they are
more visible, are brushed and flossed more often.

Gingivitis

This is the most common form of periodontal disease in the United States and, fortunately, the mildest. It remains confined to the gums and does not involve the underlying bone and ligament. When plaque is removed and good oral hygiene habits are established, the gums usually return to their healthy state.

In its acute form, the gums swell, redden, bleed, and sometimes cause discomfort. Gingivitis usually starts at the gum margin and can extend to the attached gum tissue (the portion of the gingiva that is anchored to the underlying structures). Occasionally the swelling results in the formation of pseudopockets ("false" pockets). When acute flare-ups of gingivitis become chronic, the symptoms are less intense.

Gingivitis is almost always caused by an accumulation of plaque, which, in normal, healthy individuals, is usually due to lax oral hygiene. It also can be a response to chronic irritation from partial dentures; orthodontic bands and appliances; overhanging margins of fillings, crowns, and other restorations; or certain medications (e.g., some antiepileptic drugs) or can result from the eruption of a tooth. Even the habit of breathing through the mouth can contribute to the problem.

Other types of gingivitis, some of which are listed here, are influenced by secondary factors and are classified by the appearance of the gingiva. If left untreated, any of these forms may develop into periodontitis, although not all untreated cases will.

Acute Necrotizing Ulcerative Gingivitis (ANUG). In World War I, this noncontagious gingival disease was dubbed trench mouth because of its ubiquity in the trenches. It also is referred to as Vincent's infection for the person who first described it. It takes its proper name from the symptoms it causes: destruction of and sores on the gum tissues. The gums are inflamed and bleed easily and sometimes copiously upon pressure, and there may be a foul odor and taste in the mouth. The gingival papillae (the zpointed parts of the gums between the teeth) become eroded and destroyed, and a grayish-white layer of decomposing gum tissue may form over this area. The condition develops rapidly and causes such great discomfort that most persons who have it seek professional help promptly.

The disorder is usually confined to the gums surrounding the front teeth. It most often occurs in adolescents and young adults under the age of 30, though occasionally it is seen in adults who are weakened by other diseases. As with other periodontal diseases, bacteria are the culprits. However, stress, poor eating and oral hygiene habits, smoking, not enough rest, and overconsumption of alcohol can predispose some individuals to ANUG. It often recurs and may develop into *necrotizing ulcerative periodontitis,* a chronic condition associated with bone loss in the affected area. ANUG is occasionally seen in patients with HIV infection.

Gingivitis Associated with Systemic Disease. Certain systemic conditions and diseases, nutritional deficiencies, bacterial and viral infections, and medications can increase an individual's susceptibility to gingivitis. The medications phenytoin and other drugs to control epileptic seizures, and cyclosporin, given to recipients of organ transplants, can cause an overgrowth of gum tissue in some individuals. The reaction starts as beadlike swellings of the gum margin and the papillae and enlarges to form pseudopockets in the gums. Some medications for hypertension and cardiovascular disease can cause a similar response. Gingivitis is also associated with the hormonal fluctuations during puberty and pregnancy (see Chapter 11). Elevated levels of steroid hormones enhance the subgingival growth of some of the bacteria implicated in periodontal disease. Scurvy, though now a rare nutritional disorder caused by a deficiency of vitamin C, also can cause the gums to bleed and become ulcerated and the teeth to loosen.

Desquamative Gingivitis. This is a term for a group of relatively rare and painful disorders. The gingival epithelium (the outer layer of the gums) desquamates, or peels away, and the underlying connective tissues can become damaged. Postmenopausal women are most commonly afflicted, but older men also develop it. A number of types of desquamative gingivitis are autoimmune diseases. Because this type of gingivitis most often represents an oral manifestation of a serious skin disorder, such as pemphigus or bullous pemphigoid, it is essential that an accurate and quick diagnosis, which usually involves a biopsy, is made. These lesions can also result from allergic reactions.

Periodontitis

In this more-advanced stage of periodontal disease, the damage involves the cementum, periodontal ligament, and, finally, the alveolar bone. Unlike gingivitis, treatment for periodontitis may halt and repair the destruction, but, at present, complete regeneration is not possible. (See the following sections "Bone Grafts" and "Guided Tissue Regeneration.")

Periodontitis is associated with some of the same symptoms as gingivitis (see Box 7.1). The pocket formed in the gum crevice is deeper (sometimes with pus), and the gums detach further from the teeth. The teeth loosen as the inflammation extends deeply to involve and destroy the fibers of the periodontal ligament and dissolve the alveolar bone. Even though the damage is more severe, the symptoms of the early stages of periodontitis may not be any more bothersome than those of gingivitis.

BOX 7.1

SYMPTOMS OF PERIODONTAL DISEASE

If you experience any of the symptoms listed below, see your dentist.

- Gums that bleed when you brush your teeth
- Gums that are tender, swollen, or red
- Persistent bad breath
- Gums that no longer adhere to the teeth
- Pus in the crevice between your teeth and gums
- Teeth that are loose or pulling apart
- A change in your bite, or the way the teeth of your lower jaws contact those in your upper jaw
- A change in how your partial dentures fit

Because it is possible not to have any of these signs and still have periodontal disease, you should have regular visits with your dentist that include periodic periodontal exams.

When pockets form in the gingiva, they usually do not cause pain.

There are varying degrees of severity of periodontitis. During the early stage, the gum inflammation advances to the crests or peaks of the alveolar bone between the teeth, beginning the loss of alveolar bone, and the gum pockets are of moderate depth. Moderate disease is characterized by a deepening of the crevice about the tooth to between 4 and 6 millimeters. As bone loss progresses, the pocket often deepens and the teeth become mobile. When most of the bone surrounding the teeth is lost, frequent abscesses occur, and the teeth drift, the disease has entered the advanced stage.

Periodontitis usually progresses in bursts with brief episodes of active disease and longer periods of quiescence. (Some uncommon forms explained below proceed more quickly.) As with gingivitis, the damage can be localized and does not have to affect all teeth.

Listed below are the four major forms of periodontitis, all of which are associated with specific strains of bacteria, plus the newer designation of refractory disease.

Chronic Adult Periodontitis. Although it may begin during adolescence, both men and women over the age of 35 are most susceptible to this common type of slowly progressing periodontitis, which increases in severity with age. The amount of destruction (loss of attachment of the gingiva to the tooth surface and the loss of bone) is usually found on areas with plaque and tartar and is directly related to the amount of its accumulation. It is not related, as are some other forms of periodontitis, to an impairment in the functioning of neutrophils or lymphocytes (white blood cells that are instrumental in fighting infections). Faulty, large, or numerous restorations (fillings, crowns, and fixed dentures) and teeth that are missing or out of alignment contribute to the retention of plaque and can make an adult more prone to developing this form of periodontitis.

Prepubertal Periodontitis. Fewer than 1 percent of children develop this early and rapidly progressing form which can result in the premature loss of both primary and permanent teeth. It effects a number of teeth and can be seen in children who have a history of middle ear and upper respiratory infections, a white blood cell defect, or a systemic disease, especially a reduction in the numbers or functioning of the leukocytes (white blood cells).

Juvenile Periodontitis. This swiftly destructive but fortunately uncommon form can also result in tooth loss at a young age. As its name indicates, it strikes children (girls more often than boys), in their late childhood and early teen years, usually between the ages of 11 and 13. It is most associated with the bacteria *Actinobacillus actinomycetemcomi-*

BOX 7.2

FACTORS THAT CONTRIBUTE TO PERIODONTAL DISEASES

Most periodontal diseases are caused by plaque. Other factors, although they are not causes, can raise the risk, increase the severity, and hasten the speed with which diseases develop. They are:

- Increasing age
- Smoking or chewing tobacco
- Existing periodontal disease
- A family history of periodontal disease
- Ill-fitting bridges
- Impacted teeth
- Tooth mobility
- Tooth root length and form
- Caries
- Teeth with treated or untreated endodontic problems
- Oral cysts and other pathological conditions
- Systemic diseases, such as uncontrolled diabetes or AIDS
- Use of some medications, among them some antiepilepsy drugs, some calcium channel blockers, and cyclosporin
- Malocclusions
- Habitual clenching or grinding of the teeth
- Defective fillings
- Poor nutrition

---

tans and occurs more commonly in persons who have a family history of it (it may be inherited as an X-linked dominant trait or an autosomal recessive trait). The ability of the neutrophils and phagocytes (blood cells that digest bacteria) to function is depressed in individuals afflicted with this form of periodontitis.

In its early stages, the gums are not obviously inflamed nor do they exhibit the usual changes in color or texture. As the bone loss progresses, the teeth may drift or stick out. Often there is little or no pain. In the localized and more usual form, the deep pockets and rapid loss of bone are found on the first permanent molars and permanent incisors. In the less typical, generalized form, the problem is more evenly distributed throughout the mouth.

Rapidly Progressive Periodontitis. This rapid and destructive rare type of early onset periodontitis usually affects individuals during their twenties or later. Its severity is equally distributed among most of the teeth, and its tendency to occur in persons whose family members have it is not as strong as it is with juvenile periodontitis. *Porphyromonas gingivalis* and *Bacteroides forsythus* are among the pathogens associated with this disorder.

Refractory Periodontitis. This category includes periodontitis that is unresponsive to conventional treatment, no matter how thoroughly and frequently it is given (approximately 5 percent of treated patients do not benefit from it), and disease that recurs at a few or numerous sites throughout the mouth. Certain strains of bacteria are present in individuals with refractory disease, and the presumption is that the pathogens, for unknown reasons, continue to infect.

WHO TREATS PERIODONTAL DISEASE?

Early periodontal disease should be treated by a general dentist who, as part of regular visits, routinely examines the gingiva for signs of periodontal disease. When your dentist determines that the condition has advanced to the point where you would be better cared for by a periodontist, he or she will refer you to one. During the time you are undergoing care from the periodontist, you should continue to visit your general dentist. The two will work together and with other dental specialists, if necessary, or your physician if there are complicating medical conditions, such as diabetes or HIV disease, to coordinate your care.

HOW TO DETECT
PERIODONTAL DISEASE

Looking for Physical Changes

Until recently, detection concentrated on assessing the damage done during the active phases of the disease. These methods, the assessment of probing depth and radiographic bone loss, provide an historical record, revealing what physical changes or damage has already occurred. This is called *disease severity.* To determine *disease activity,* or how the disease will behave in the future (whether it will progress), dentists need to take at least two sets of tests that evaluate the disease severity at a specific interval ranging from weeks to months and then compare them. The tests include measuring the loss of attachment, pocket depth, tooth mobility, bleeding when probed, and destruction of the bone.

The traditional way of detecting periodontal disease is to insert a manual probe between the gum and the root surface of the tooth to determine whether the gum is losing its attachment to the tooth. If attachment has been lost, the depth of the pocket increases. The dentist then checks whether and how much the tooth can be moved, whether the gums bleed when they are probed, and whether the gum margin has receded. The occlusion of the teeth also may be noted. In some individuals, an incorrect bite may contribute to periodontal disease, but it is not as significant a factor as once believed. Finally, radiographs are made to determine whether the disease has affected the bone.

The manual probe is subject to a degree of error because it depends on the pressure each dentist applies when inserting it. Neither the manual probe nor radiographs can determine whether the disease is still in an active phase or whether the destruction has already occurred. A number of recent innovations have sought to overcome the problems inherent with these methods of detection. (See section on Automated Devices.)

Pocket (Probing) Depth

The gingiva is not entirely connected to the teeth. Between the margin of the gum and its attachment to the tooth surface there is a crevice, or sulcus. It is the depth in millimeters of the sulcus (or pocket that is created) that a dentist measures with a periodontal probe to help determine the status of periodontal health. In general, the measurements of pocket depth listed correlate with the following periodontal conditions:

Healthy gums	1 to 3 millimeters
Gingivitis	2 to 4 millimeters
Mild periodontitis	3 to 5 millimeters
Moderate periodontitis	4 to 6 millimeters
Advanced periodontitis	7+ millimeters

These categories only apply to gingiva that has not been treated. Patients with periodontitis who have been treated surgically may not have deep pockets but instead have recession associated with surgery. In addition, gingival swelling can create false pockets. These can usually be reduced by a periodontal cleaning.

Automated Devices

In seeking to standardize diagnostic assessments, the following automated devices have been developed.

Electronic Probes. Automated probes use a uniform force and angle to accurately measure the gum pockets. The data is then stored on a computer or memory card and can be retrieved in future visits to determine whether the pocket is increasing or decreasing.

Temperature Probe. This device measures the temperature at the bottom of the gum pocket and, using a mathematical equation, compares it to the temperature of healthy or uninflamed gingiva. A relationship between an elevated crevicular temperature and gingival inflammation has been established. This test has been most effective when the depths of the pockets are less than 4 millimeters.

Automated Tooth Mobility Device. This device overcomes the variation in force that individual dentists use to test how loose a tooth is. It exerts a uniform push against the tooth and automatically measures the time it takes the tooth to return to its starting position. Using a scale, the extent of tooth mobility is determined. Although a mobile tooth is *not* a sign of healthy gums, the relationship between how much a tooth moves and how far disease has advanced has not been determined.

Radiographs (X-rays)

Radiographs, commonly used to determine the amount of bone loss or gain, provide a valuable record of bone changes over time. However, they have limitations in determining bone loss over short periods of time. At least 30 percent of the mineral in the alveolar bone must be lost before it will register on a radiograph and the amount of destruction that is reflected will almost always be less severe than what exists. Furthermore, the quality of the image produced is influenced by how the radiograph is developed.

A new technique, *subtraction radiography,* addresses these drawbacks. In this method, two radiographs are made at different times. They are placed on top of each other and one is subtracted by computer to determine what structures have *not* changed (whether or not there has been bone loss) since the last radiograph. Subtraction radiographs can detect as little as 5 percent mineral loss in the alveolar bone and can identify changes as small as 0.5 millimeter versus conventional techniques which are not accurate until bone loss exceeds 1.5 millimeters. Subtraction radiography is currently a research tool, available at some university dental clinics, but not commonly used in private dental practices.

Alternate Methods to Detect Disease

The problem with the techniques described so far is that they all measure the disease after it has started. In the last decade, researchers have focused on determining who is at risk for periodontal disease *before* it develops in the hopes that intervention can begin and the disease can be either averted entirely or prevented from escalating. As a result, detection and diagnosis of periodontal disease are on the cusp of great change.

Some of the tests described here are available on a limited or experimental level.

Bacterial Tests. These diagnostic tests identify the bacteria in the subgingival plaque in different types of periodontal disease. Some of the tests (listed here) identify specific bacteria; others look for the enzymes (or proteins) that the bacteria produce.

CULTURE AND SENSITIVITY TESTS. Both identify some of the organisms associated with the active stage of the disease and determine their antibiotic sensitivity; this makes possible the use of a specific antibiotic rather than a scattershot approach. The test requires a laboratory specially equipped to grow the anaerobic bacteria and is available at some dental schools.

DNA PROBES. These tests identify the unique sequences of bases that form the DNA and RNA of bacteria implicated in periodontal disease. They can detect organisms even when their concentration in the samples is small. They can also identify organisms that are difficult to culture. For such tests, samples are taken in the dental office and sent to a lab. Unfortunately, no information about antibiotic sensitivity is available from this test.

ENZYME EVALUATIONS. These in-office tests identify enzymes produced by certain bacteria in subgingival plaque. They can identify existing disease sites. At the present time, none of these tests is commercially available.

Host Response Tests. Other new tests (all or most of these are not on the market yet) are based on detecting the disease by looking for responses to the bacteria that show up in saliva, blood, or gingival fluid.

GINGIVAL FLUID SAMPLES. Gingival crevicular fluid is released through the vessels of the gum tissues into the base of the gum pocket. When the gums are inflamed, more fluid is released in a response believed to be part of the body's defense mechanism to fight the infection. As it passes through the infected tissues, the fluid picks up enzymes and antibodies and other by-products of cells and tissues involved in the disease process. Active disease can be identified by testing a filter paper soaked with gingival fluid.

BLOOD TESTS. Using a drop of blood obtained from a finger prick, antibodies to bacteria in plaque can be identified. Although still in development, this test holds the promise of identifying persons at risk for getting periodontal disease by detecting the body's immune response to it before symptoms appear.

PREVENTION

Your best chance of preventing periodontal disease is by visiting your dentist regularly and conscientiously removing plaque by brushing and flossing your teeth. (For the most effective ways to brush and floss, see Chapter 5.)

TREATMENTS

There is no definitive way to treat periodontal disease. The available therapies range in their approach from conservative to radical; the appropriate treatment is probably a combination of the two. The goals of therapy are reducing the microbes that cause the disease, reducing gingival inflammation in the mouth by controlling plaque, and preparing the teeth and gingiva (by recontouring restorations and reducing excessive gum pockets) so that the patient can cleanse them efficiently.

Treatment involves four stages: (1) examination and diagnosis, (2) cleansing (debridement), (3) surgery, and (4) maintenance. Which stages each person progresses through and whether someone needs to complete all, varies and depends on many factors, not all of which are known. Some patients may spend six months in stages 1 through 3 and the rest of their lives in stage 4.

Examination and Diagnosis

To verify a diagnosis, you should be shown radiographs and the results of other evaluations. For you to understand why you need treatment, the periodontist should give you a clear explanation of your condition and, if possible, show you an illustration or radiograph comparing the condition of your mouth to a normal one.

Cleansing (Debridement)

Patients whose diseases are mild to moderate may be able to be treated conservatively, with instruction in oral hygiene, scaling, root planing, and orthodontic adjustment to correct a malocclusion (*if* it contributes to the problem). For some, these measures, combined with meticulous home hygiene and regular periodontal exams, may suffice. Persons with moderate to advanced disease may need surgery. If surgery has been advised or if you are not satisfied or comfortable with the explanation you have been given and the treatment recommended to you, you should seek a second opinion from another periodontist.

Scaling and Root Planing. Sometimes scaling (described in Chapter 5), which removes the plaque and tartar on the tooth surfaces below the gumline where the pockets have formed, will be sufficient. When it is not, the surfaces of the tooth roots may be planed with curettes (handheld, elongated scraping instruments) until they are smooth, to rid them of any irritants. A topical and sometimes a local anesthetic is used to lessen the discomfort. Creating a smooth surface enables the gums to reattach to the tooth and helps the pocket shrink.

How the tissues respond to scaling and root planing varies. In general, the smaller the pocket, the better the response. Pockets that are less than 4 millimeters have a better chance of shrinking and reattaching to the surface of the tooth than pockets of greater depth do.

Surgery

Surgery may be indicated for patients whose gums continue to bleed, exude pus, have pockets greater than 5 millimeters, or do not shrink after scaling and root planing. The purpose of surgery is to gain access to the roots so they can be cleaned thoroughly and to eliminate or reduce the pockets. Surgery will permanently expose tooth surfaces so that plaque can be removed at home daily by the individual. Surgery is also needed for regenerative procedures.

The type of surgery recommended depends on the kind and extent of damage to the bone and soft tissues and the position and configuration of the pockets. Not every one is a candidate for surgery. Surgery is not recommended:

If scaling and home hygiene can control the problem

For patients who are of an age that their teeth may last without it

If certain systemic conditions are present, among them severe cardiovascular disease, cancer, kidney and liver diseases, bleeding disorders, or uncontrolled diabetes (unless the physician and periodontist determine otherwise)

For individuals who either will not or cannot practice proper hygiene

If it will result in a very poor postoperative appearance

If tooth loss is inevitable

In general, the results of surgery are usually good for persons who are conscientious about practicing home prevention and seeking routine professional care.

Periodontal surgery sometimes has aesthetic and dental consequences. It may alter the line of the gums and reveal more of the tooth's surface. In the back teeth, this change is not apparent, but when done on the front teeth, the alteration may make the recipient appear "long in the tooth." Periodontal surgery also may cause further recession of the gums. As a result, the teeth may be more vulnerable to root caries and, if the pulp is still vital (living), may be more sensitive to extreme temperatures. Although this sensitivity is usually temporary, it may persist.

Surgery is usually done in segments on different portions of the mouth under local anesthesia. When the entire mouth is operated on at once, general anesthesia or conscious sedation is usually administered.

The following are the older, conventional surgical procedures.

Gingivectomy. The upper portion of the gum is cut off to reduce pocket depth. The exposed root surfaces are scraped of tartar and contaminants, and then dressed with an antibacterial gauze or bathed in a disinfectant solution. This procedure results in the reduction in the depth of the pocket, but it also exposes more of the root of the tooth, and thus enlarges the crown. Flap surgery has, for the most part, replaced this method.

Flap surgery. There are a number of different techniques depending on the configuration of the incision or flap, but the essential elements are the same. The periodontist makes an incision in the gums, lifts them, cleans out the infected tissue and scales and planes the root surfaces that

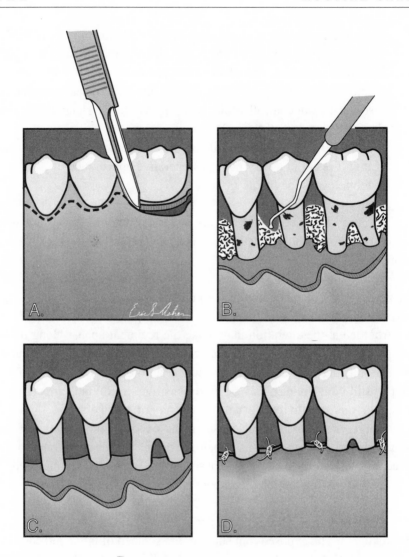

ILLUSTRATION 7.2. **THE PROCEDURE FOR FLAP SURGERY.**
A. An incision is made into the gums. **B.** Gum tissue is separated from underlying structures (flap) to remove diseased tissue and to clean calculus from the roots. **C.** The surface of the tooth below the gumline is then cleaned of infected tissue. **D.** The flap is sewn back in place. The surgery eliminates the gum pockets but leaves more of the root surface exposed.

are inaccessible without the surgery, and sews the flap back into place. The result is elimination of the gum pocket. During the procedure, bone also may be removed to improve its architecture or shape.

Modified flap surgery has the esthetic advantage of leaving less of the root surface exposed, although it does not always eliminate the gum pockets nor will the seal between the gum and the root surface be as stable. If postoperative oral hygiene and maintenance are not excellent and consistent, the pockets could reform.

Gum Grafts (Mucogingival Surgery). When a great deal of the root has been exposed from disease or gum recession, pieces of gum can be taken from other areas of the patient's mouth (usually the roof) and grafted onto the gum above the exposed root. This procedure is referred to as periodontal plastic surgery because it improves the appearance of the smile.

As with detection, there are innovative therapies that have been developed in response to some of the problems with the older surgical procedures. These new methods are geared toward regeneration or rebuilding of the bone. They include:

Bone Grafts. Bone, either taken from the patient (for example, from a different area of the jaw) or from a bone bank, which stores bone that has been harvested from a donor and freeze dried, is grafted onto the affected area. The grafting is done in conjunction with the flap procedure. The grafted bones stimulate the body to generate new bone cells to fill in the areas that were dissolved from disease.

Guided Tissue Regeneration. After flap surgery, the outer layer of gum tissue or epithelium grows down along the root surface of the tooth; this prevents the bone from regenerating. To solve this problem and to increase the gum's attachment to the bone, a membrane is put between the alveolar bone and the bone graft or replacement. Membranes made of teflon must be retrieved after six weeks; this involves another incision. Biodegradable membranes are available and do not require a second surgical procedure.

Growth factors are covered in Chapter 22.

Nonsurgical Treatments

Systemic antibiotics, either singly or in combination, are frequently prescribed during advanced periodontal treatment. In certain circumstances, systemic antibiotics are used for actively progressing periodontitis or for recalcitrant infections (those that return after other therapies have been tried). They also are frequently used during tissue regeneration surgery. This therapy is not recommended for routine or long-term use, nor should it be used to treat gingivitis or periodontitis that is not progressing. To select the appropriate antibiotic, the patient can be tested to determine which drug is appropriate for the pathogens that are present.

An alternative to surgery that was recently introduced involves implanting antibiotics in the infected pocket. At the present time, the placement of tetracycline-containing fibers in the infected pocket and their removal after ten days is the only method approved by the FDA. Other systems are in various stages of development. The antibiotic-impregnated fibers may have particular value for persons who have recurrences after surgery or who are medically compromised, elderly, or otherwise not good candidates for surgery.

Maintenance

After either conservative or surgical therapy, the teeth must be kept as free from plaque as possible or the disease will recur. The possibility of recurrence is also minimized by keeping all appointments with dentists and periodontists and following their instructions. Following treatment of periodontitis, it is quite common for oral prophylaxis to be required every three months.

Antimicrobial mouthrinses can be an important adjunct to brushing and flossing or other methods of cleaning between the teeth. Although Listerine can be effective, chlorhexidine is best (see Chapter 5). Flushing the teeth (at home or in the dental office) with a syringe irrigator and a diluted solution of peroxide or chlorhexidine may also help.

OTHER PERIODONTAL PROBLEMS

Periodontal Abscess

When the opening at the top of a (usually deep) gum pocket becomes blocked, the white blood cells, which normally marshal their forces to fight off bacteria, die. Pus forms, and an abscess, capable of destroying both hard and soft tissues, is created. When acute, the infection is localized and results in a swelling resembling a reddened bubble in the gum. This can cause the tooth nearby to become loose and painful. If the infection is severe, there may be fever or swelling of nearby lymph nodes.

Gingival pockets that are deep and narrow are prone to recurrent abscesses. Because the configuration of the periodontal pocket allows for the release of pressure, the symptoms of a periodontal abscess are not as severe nor do they cause as much pain as those normally associated with an endodontic abscess (these occur within the closed space of a root canal). Over time, recurrent abscesses can severely weaken the support for the tooth.

Periodontal abscesses are most often associated with deposits of tartar, but they can also occur when food becomes impacted in the pockets. They also occur more frequently in persons with diabetes.

Treatment depends on the severity of the abscess, how much bone has been destroyed, and whether the pulp of the tooth is involved. In its beginning stages, the infection may be controlled by cleaning out the pocket or with antibiotics. An incision, done under local anesthesia, may be required to drain the abscess. If bone loss is significant, the tooth may need to be extracted. In some cases, when the tooth can be retained, flap surgery, with or without a bone graft, can be done to excise and/or repair the defect the abscess has caused in the bone.

Periodontal Recession

As people age, their gums may recede. This condition is also seen in younger people. It has a number of causes, including using too much pressure when brushing teeth, tartar, braces, and teeth that are malpositioned in the jaw. The recession exposes cementum, the softer tissue on the tooth's root; this increases the risk of root caries. When the gums recede, the alveolar bone in that area dissolves, too. Although less likely, children can experience gum recession as a result of problems with the eruption of their teeth, trauma, and improper brushing.

Trauma

To maintain the healthy functioning of the periodontium, the teeth need activity. Although the supporting structures of the teeth will compensate for fairly heavy intermittent pressure, sustained heavy pressure can cause damage. Habitual grinding or clenching of the teeth can cause injury to the periodontal ligament and may contribute to bone loss.

PART IV

DENTAL CARE THROUGHOUT YOUR LIFE

CHAPTER 8

Birth Through Adolescence

Personal Cleaning
Professional Cleaning
Fluoride
Sealants
Lip Habits (Licking, Pulling, Sucking, and Biting)
Iron Stain
Malocclusions

THE TEEN YEARS

Dental Caries
Periodontal Problems
Sports Injuries
Removal of the Third Molars (Wisdom Teeth)
Sexually Transmitted Diseases
Chewing Tobacco and Snuff

BOX 8.5 SOME COMMON ORAL PROBLEMS CAUSED BY SOME SEXUALLY
TRANSMITTED DISEASES

F rom birth through adolescence a significant amount of dental development and growth occurs. During this time, many children develop dietary and dental hygiene habits they will practice the rest of their lives. The following pages discuss some of the dental concerns that commonly arise during these formative years. For more detail about some of the dental procedures that are performed, such as sealants, orthodontics, and extractions of third molars, you need to consult other chapters.

INFANCY AND THE PRESCHOOL YEARS

For most parents, the most notable and anticipated of the dental events of the early years of a child's life is the emergence of the primary teeth.

Because they set the stage for the health of their successors, primary teeth require the same amount of care and attention as do permanent teeth.

Natal Teeth

Although most babies are born with no teeth showing, in rare instances (between 1 in 700 and 1 in 6,000 births), teeth are present. Most often, they are normal lower incisors; however, fewer than 10 percent are supernumerary, or extra, improperly formed, teeth. Radiographs may need to be made to determine whether these extra teeth are normal.

These early erupted teeth seldom cause problems if they do not cause trauma. If they cut the bottom of the infant's tongue or the mother's breast during nursing, their sharp edges may need to be smoothed by a dentist. Supernumerary teeth or teeth that are very loose and in danger of being aspirated may need to be extracted.

Oral Growths

Babies can have a number of oral growths, most of which are benign, disappear in several weeks or months, and require no treatment. In about 75 percent of infants, small white spots, or keratin cysts, appear on the roof of the mouth or on the dental ridges.

Congenital epulis is a rare pink and firm tumor that forms on an infant's gum pads. It is more common in females, usually occurs in the upper jaw, and should be removed by a surgeon.

In rare instances, oral growths in newborns can have medical consequences or be associated with congenital conditions. To prevent any potential complications, you should show any unusual dental growth or swelling your baby has to your dentist who will determine whether the tissue must be removed.

Dental Injuries

By exercising proper precautions, parents and caregivers can prevent many of the dental injuries to which young children are especially prone. Since injury to or loss of the primary teeth can damage the buds or interfere with the eruption of the developing permanent teeth, all injuries to the primary teeth resulting in bleeding, chipping, loss, or loosening of a tooth or teeth, even those that appear to cause little damage, should be brought to the immediate attention of a dentist. Children who complain of pain or tenderness when eating or have a mobile tooth should not eat with that tooth until they have been seen by a dentist.

Falls. Many infants fall and injure their newly emerging teeth when they are learning to crawl and walk. Infants and toddlers fall frequently over coffee tables and other furniture and, when inappropriately restrained, from high chairs, shopping carts, and strollers. The primary teeth most commonly injured in these mishaps are the upper central incisors. When they protrude, they are two to three times more likely to be injured than when they are normally positioned. These risks can be minimized if adults pad the sharp edges of furniture, move objects from the center of rooms, and carefully watch young children at all times. The dental trauma that children with seizure disorders are prone to can be reduced by having them wear protective headgear and custom-made mouthguards.

Automobiles. In a collision or when a car stops suddenly, children who are not restrained by either infant or booster seats or who are not wearing seat belts can be hurled forward. Their teeth can be damaged if they hit the dashboard, windshield, or floor. You can reduce significantly the risks of these kinds of injuries by obeying the law and properly restraining your children every time they ride in a car or other vehicle.

Child Abuse. By far the most preventable cause of childhood dental injuries is physical abuse. Up to 50 percent of abused children sustain injuries to their head and neck, including dental trauma and fractures. Forcing a child to bottle feed can cause damage to the labial frenum (the skin that extends between the upper lip and the upper central incisors). Although laws vary in different states, most require dentists to report to the appropriate authorities cases of suspected child abuse. Penalties range from fines to jail sentences if they fail to do so.

Teething

Although there is no way to determine when your baby's first tooth will appear, the complete set of primary teeth (20) usually will be showing by his or her third birthday. Although the average age for a child's first tooth to erupt is six months, it is normal and not unusual for parents to have to wait up to 18 months for the event.

For years, parents have told countless tales of the tribulations they and their babies have endured during this infant rite of passage. Teething can make a baby's gums swell and redden and may cause drooling and fussiness, loss of appetite, a change in eating habits, and have been related to difficulty sleeping. Contrary to what many parents believe, teething has *not* been shown to cause diarrhea, fever, rashes, vomiting, or even pain. If your infant or young child has these or other medical symptoms or complains of pain in the area of the jaws, a pediatrician should evaluate the child to rule out ear infections or digestive problems.

Giving your child a teething ring (preferably cold), pacifier, or wet washcloth to suck on may relieve the fussiness that sometimes accompanies the process, but you should avoid giving them over-the-counter topical anesthetics that are rubbed onto the gums. Their most common active ingredient, benzocaine, may be acceptable in low-concentration (5 to 7.5 percent) infant preparations if used occasionally. In the highest strength (20 percent), it is too potent for infants and should never be used because it can cause serious illness and even death from drug overdose.

Eruption Cysts. A bluish, soft, round swelling sometimes forms over emerging primary molars or permanent incisors. The cyst should not be cut or punctured. If it is left alone, it will disintegrate spontaneously as the tooth erupts through it. If it is cut, a scar will form and may further delay the tooth's eruption.

Mamelons. The three little bumps that may develop on the biting edges of the permanent incisors are normal and will wear away usually within six months. If they develop on primary incisors, a dentist may need to smooth their edges to prevent irritation to the underside of the tongue.

Ankyloglossia, or Tongue-tie

At birth, the tongue is anchored to the floor of the mouth by a strip of skin called a frenum. In some children, the frenum prevents the tongue from extending across the lower incisors and out of the mouth to remove food particles stuck on the teeth.

A simple surgical procedure, called a lingual frenectomy, will correct this condition. It is performed most frequently by a pediatric dentist or oral surgeon when the child is between two and three years old. It should be done only if a dentist or speech pathologist determines that the attachment is severe enough to cause speech problems.

Of greater periodontal consequence is the labial maxillary frenum, a little strip of flesh you can feel if you stick your finger under your lip above your upper front incisors. When there is a large space between the upper central incisors that needs to be closed orthodontically, this frenum may need to be removed surgically. Whether a labial frenectomy should be performed usually cannot be determined until after the permanent canines have erupted, which typically occurs when a child is 11 or 12 years old.

Baby Bottle Tooth Decay (BBTD, Nursing Caries)

A number of professional and nonprofit groups concerned with dental and children's health have adopted this term over others, such as nursing caries or baby bottle caries, in recognition that this type of caries in a child under the age of three years is most often caused by using a bottle filled with formula, milk, or juice as a pacifier. Less commonly, however, it can be caused by demand breast-feeding during the night or sucking on pacifiers dipped in honey. When caries occurs before 20 months, it almost always results from taking the bottle to bed or breast-feeding on demand at night. During sleep, both the flow of saliva and swallowing are reduced. This allows the sugars in milk and juice to pool around the teeth, giving the bacteria in plaque more time to produce the acids that destroy tooth enamel. Most frequently, the upper incisors and canines are affected, although in severe cases the molars can be affected, too.

BBTD can progress and result in rampant caries, which will require extensive restorative treatment for children at an age when usually they are not able to cooperate. As a consequence, the dentist may need to use sedation, physical restraint, or general anesthesia to restore the teeth with fillings or crowns or to extract them. The best way to avoid BBTD is by following the suggestions in Box 8.1.

Nonnutritive Sucking Habits (Pacifiers, Fingers, and Thumbs)

For some babies the innate urge to suck is satisfied through the normal suckling they do while breast- or bottle-feeding. Most infants, how-

---

BOX 8.1

TIPS ON REDUCING YOUR BABY'S CHANCE OF DEVELOPING DENTAL CARIES

• Do not use a bottle filled with formula, milk, or juice or the breast as a pacifier.

• Limit drinking formula, milk, or juice from a bottle and breast-feeding to regular feeding times.

• If you put your child to bed with a bottle, be sure it contains only plain water.

• Never dip a pacifier in syrup, jelly, sugar, or honey.

• Wean your child from the bottle to the cup as soon as possible, preferably by the age of 1 year and at least by 18 months.

---

ever, supplement this with nonnutritive sucking, most often choosing fingers, thumbs, or a pacifier. In children under the age of four, nonnutritive sucking seldom seriously affects the arrangement of the teeth. The usual result is a minor change in the position of the primary incisors that causes them to tip toward the lips. Most often this will resolve without treatment if the child stops the habit before the permanent teeth erupt.

There is no need to worry if your child sucks on a pacifier (except if it is coated in honey or another substance containing sugar) or a thumb or fingers, unless the habit continues after the permanent teeth begin to emerge, usually after five years of age. If it does, the force exerted from the habit and the placement of the finger or pacifier may cause the teeth to move to such an extent that orthodontic treatment may be needed. The longer and more often a child engages in the sucking habit during the day (whether with a pacifier or fingers) and the more intense the force applied to the teeth is, the more severe the problems that can result are. Studies indicate that four to six hours of force per day are required to cause the teeth to move. Intermittent forces for less than this time probably will not produce a malocclusion.

If pacifier, thumb, or finger sucking persists beyond the age of four, the parent and dentist may want to intervene to discourage it for dental reasons or because it is not socially acceptable and can hinder a child's social interactions. For intervention therapy to be successful, though, the child must be willing to give up the habit and must be a part of the decision to treat.

Three treatment approaches are commonly used. Reminder therapy involves placing something, such as a bandage or unpleasant tasting coating on the finger or thumb to remind or discourage the child not to suck on it. With the reward system, the child is rewarded with something special (e.g., a toy, trip, or event) if the habit is stopped after a time agreed on mutually between the child and parent, or the child and dentist. During the time of the contract, the child can be rewarded with stickers or stars placed on a calendar or chart for making it through that day without thumb or finger sucking. For recalcitrant children, it may be necessary for a dentist to place an appliance in the child's mouth to serve as an interfering device or reminder not to place the finger or thumb there.

Nipples. Studies have shown artificial nipples designed to resemble the contours of a breast nipple and touted frequently as orthodontic by the manufacturers to be no better for a child's teeth than regular ones. The hole in a nipple for a nursing bottle should be designed so that it is small enough that the liquid inside does not pour out too freely and the child is required to exercise the tongue and chewing muscles to extract it. A pacifier can serve the same function. If you give a pacifier to your child, follow the safety precautions outlined in Box 8.2.

Tongue Thrusting

When suckling (to obtain nourishment), infants place their tongue underneath the nipple, touch the lower lip, raise it against the palate, and swallow with the lips held together and the jaws apart. This action develops the muscles of the tongue and cheeks and strengthens the swallowing reflex. Between the ages of three and ten years, a child usually makes the transition from this infantile swallowing pattern to the adult swallowing pattern (in which the tip of the tongue is held against the palate, the teeth are together, and the lips are relaxed).

If the infantile swallowing pattern continues after the teeth emerge,

---

BOX 8.2

CARE AND SAFETY
FOR PACIFIERS

To minimize the risk of a child's choking or strangling while using a pacifier, take the following precautions:

• Never attach a string or ribbon to a pacifier and place it around a child's neck.

• Never coat the pacifier with honey, sugar, or syrup with sugar, which encourage the risk of caries. In addition, honey poses a small but fatal risk of botulism for some infants when it is contaminated with *clostridium botulinum* spores.

• Test the nipple frequently by pulling on it to be sure it does not pull away or tear off. Discard it if it does.

• Throw away a pacifier the moment a crack or split develops or when it becomes worn.

• Keep the pacifier clean by washing it frequently in warm water and mild soap and rinsing it thoroughly.

---

the thrusting of the tongue between the upper and lower front teeth can push them out of position and create orthodontic problems. This is a difficult habit to stop because it is unconscious (as opposed to thumb sucking, which is usually conscious). Closing teeth spaces with braces and sometimes speech or swallowing therapy may be recommended if the habit continues after the permanent incisors have erupted.

Bruxism

About 15 percent of children in the United States grind their primary teeth, some almost down to the gum line. Although this tension-releasing habit is annoying and extremely difficult to treat, usually it does not affect the development or eruption of the permanent teeth and seldom continues after the permanent teeth have emerged. Appliances that are used to prevent it often prove more detrimental than the habit.

Mouth Breathing

There has been considerable debate among dentists over whether malocclusions develop as a consequence of children breathing through the mouth or whether they result from a physical condition that causes the mouth breathing. The consensus is that there is a weak relationship between mouth breathing and the malocclusion that is most often characterized by a long lower face, a constricted upper jaw, and a smaller-than-usual upper dental arch. Because mouth breathing can be caused by a restricted airway and/or enlarged tonsils and/or adenoids, a consultation with an otolaryngologist may be advised.

Cleaning and Brushing

In the first few weeks after a baby's birth and before the teeth appear, the gums should be wiped daily with a clean damp cloth or gauze pad. When a baby's teeth erupt, they should be cleaned at least once a day with sterile gauze or a washcloth or a brush with soft bristles, with or without toothpaste, to remove plaque. Be sure not to use more than a pea-sized amount of fluoride-containing toothpaste on the brush or gauze. A one-inch strip of fluoride toothpaste contains the daily dosage of fluoride recommended for a child over six years whose drinking water does not contain any fluorides, and children usually swallow 35 to 65 percent of the toothpaste used.

Visiting the Dentist

The American Academy of Pediatric Dentistry recommends that a child's first dental visit be within 6 months after the first tooth erupts and no later than 12 months of age. Children who visit at this early age will be best served by a pediatric dentist who is trained to evaluate and treat infants. Subsequent visits should be scheduled for examination and tooth cleaning, as determined by the examining dentist, depending on the presence or absence of dental disease. Children who have no evidence of caries may visit less frequently; those who have severe caries should be examined more frequently. Topical fluoride treatments may be applied every six months after a child has reached two years.

The point of the first visit at this early age is not so much for the dentist to look for caries, although early signs of BBTD can be identified, but to counsel parents in the prevention of dental diseases. It is also a good time to assess whether the amount of fluoride the child is receiving is appropriate for optimum enamel development.

Who Should Treat Your Child?

Because of the additional years of training they spend studying child development and learning behavior modification techniques to introduce dental procedures to children in comfortable and nonthreatening ways, pediatric dentists are best able to deal with young children, as well as older children and adolescents who have emotional, mental, or physical disabilities. The training pediatric dentists receive also emphasizes the importance of preventive measures. As an example, studies show that pediatric dentists apply sealants more frequently than general dentists do. Nevertheless, most children over the age of three years visit general dentists. One reason may be that pediatric dentists are not available in many communities: there are only about 3,500 in the country, and most of them are concentrated in urban areas. Another reason may be that many parents want their entire family to be treated by the same dentist and choose a general dentist. If your child has special medical or dental needs, however, a pediatric dentist may be necessary.

Parents in the Operatory. The decision about whether to permit parents in the dental operatory (treatment room) is best made by the professional. (Many dental offices do not allow it.) If you remain in the operatory during your child's treatment, you should resist the urge to help by interfering with the questions the dentist asks your child and trying to explain the procedure to your child. The explanation of what the dentist is doing should be left to the dentist. By communicating directly to your child, a dentist establishes a trusting professional relationship, which can help make treatment proceed more smoothly.

Although as a parent you are within your legal rights to decide how your child is to be treated, dentists, in turn, have a professional right to refuse treatment if you insist on accompanying your child in the operatory when the dentist believes it is not in the best interest of the child's care. If you feel strongly about this controversial issue, you should discuss it with prospective dentists when selecting one for your child before treatment is begun.

What to Tell the Dentist

To prevent dental and medical complications that can result from some dental procedures, be sure to tell the dentist whether your child has any allergies or medical conditions, such as heart murmurs or diseases, immune-system problems, respiratory diseases (e.g., asthma or cystic fibrosis), neurological disturbances, seizure disorders, cancers, mental retardation, or infectious diseases. Children with certain heart conditions and some other medical conditions need antibiotics before and after dental treatment to prevent systemic bacterial infections. Children with some other conditions, such as Down syndrome, can have increased susceptibility to specific dental problems and may need more frequent exams and special treatment. You should also forewarn the dentist if your child is fearful about the visit.

Treating the Anxious Child

Dentists understand that anxiety and fear are learned behaviors, and for anxious children with special medical problems the pediatric dentist may be the dentist of choice. The majority of children can be treated well by general practitioners; however, if your general dentist determines the child to be a behavior or management problem, the dentist will refer the patient to a pediatric dentist. Before invasive or painful treatments, such as restorations or extractions, the child should be seen for a preventive appointment.

The Exam

When examining a child, a dentist inspects the teeth and soft tissues of the mouth and other areas of the head and neck, noting the alignment of the teeth, jaws, and dental arches. Although dentists use many of the same instruments (e.g., hand mirrors, explorers, periodontal probes, and

BOX 8.3

WHAT TO TELL YOUR CHILD
BEFORE VISITING THE DENTIST

• Be matter of fact about the visit. Do not offer more explanations than are necessary to answer the questions your child asks.

• Do not bring up the concept of pain or hurting.

• Explain that a dentist is a "doctor for the mouth" whom we need to visit regularly "to keep our teeth and gums healthy."

• Do not bribe your child to get him or her to go to the dentist.

• If you are unsure about a question your child has concerning the procedures and tools used or whether "it will hurt," ask the dentist to explain to the child.

• Let your child form his or her own impressions. Do not tell about your own experiences with the dentist, especially if they have been unpleasant.

sometimes radiographs) on children as they do on adults, they frequently employ different techniques to elicit cooperation and compliance since children do not, in general, respond as well to logical, spoken commands. At this appointment, the general dentist can best determine whether your child is best treated by him/her or a pediatric dentist.

A popular method pediatric dentists use to allay children's fears and to get the response they want is "tell-show-do," in which the dentist explains about a dental instrument and demonstrates it before using it for treatment, such as by running the drill on a child's fingernail. When children are not able to understand an explanation because of age, disability, medication, or emotional immaturity or are being uncooperative or inattentive, the dentist can modulate voice volume, pace, and tone to establish authority, gain attention, and head off undesired behaviors. Praise or a small reward (e.g., a toy, sticker, or toothbrush) is also used to reinforce desired behavior. Body language and facial expressions are effective nonverbal methods of communication. For children who are so defiant or noncompliant that their actions jeopardize their safety or that of the dentist, the dentist may put a hand over the child's mouth to gain his or her attention while explaining the behavior that is expected. For invasive procedures or extremely anxious children, restraining devices, conscious sedation, or general anesthesia may be necessary to complete treatment. If restraints, sedation, or general anesthesia are recommended to treat a child, the parents should be provided with the necessary information regarding the risks and benefits of such procedures so they can give informed consent prior to treatment.

Radiographs (X-rays)

As with adults, radiographs for children are used to detect more than dental caries. They are aids for assessing the presence and eruption of teeth, detecting and evaluating bone diseases and injuries, assessing growth, and conceptualizing orthodontic treatment.

A child's first dental radiograph should be made if the spaces between the primary teeth are so tight that the surfaces between them cannot be examined visually. In addition to bitewing films of the molars, a radiograph of the upper front teeth should be made when a child is between the ages of three and five years to determine whether any extra teeth are developing. Some persons, such as those with high dental disease rates, regardless of age, need dental radiographs more frequently than others. Children often require radiographs more frequently than adults because their mouths are growing and changing rapidly. For children who have a history of no caries or no recurring caries, one set of bitewing films every two years may be sufficient, unless there are other dental problems that require more films. While they are being made, a child always should be protected from radiation by a lead body apron and/or shield, and a thyroid collar.

Fluoride

Systemic Supplements. The effect of ingesting fluoride is cumulative. In recent years there has been an increase of mild fluorosis, a condition in which concentrations have exceeded established optimum levels. This can result in white or brown defects in the enamel of the teeth. Because some children may be ingesting too much fluoride from the many

BOX 8.4

SCHEDULE FOR
FLUORIDE SUPPLEMENTATION

This table lists the current dosage schedule, approved April 1994 by the American Dental Association, the American Academy of Pediatric Dentistry, and the American Academy of Pediatrics for supplementing children between the ages of 6 months and 16 years who are living in areas where the water they consume is deficient in fluoride.

| | *Fluoride Ion Level in Drinking Water (ppm*)* | | |
Age	*Less than 0.3 ppm*	*0.3–0.6 ppm*	*More than 0.6 ppm*
Birth to 6 months	None	None	None
6 months to 3 years	0.25 mg/day†	None	None
3 to 6 years	0.5 mg/day	0.25 mg/day	None
6 to 16 years	1.0 mg/day	0.50 mg/day	None

*1.0 ppm (parts per million) = 1 mg(milligram)/liter.
†2.2 mg sodium fluoride contains 1 mg fluoride ion.

sources from which it is available, among them foods high in fluoride, toothpastes, drinking water, and other beverages, the dosage schedule for fluoride supplementation recommended by the American Academy of Pediatric Dentistry, the American Dental Association, and the American Academy of Pediatrics has been revised recently (see Box 8.4).

Using drops or tablets as the vehicle to deliver fluoride can be as effective, although not as convenient, in preventing caries as supplementation through the drinking water supply. Before prescribing fluoride supplements, your pediatrician and/or dentist must evaluate your child's total fluoride intake to determine whether sufficient quantities already exist. Included in this evaluation should be a chemical analysis of your child's drinking water (whether from a private well or a municipal source), by a local or state health department or a local water authority to determine its fluoride content. A diet high in fish and certain vegetables and drinks made from fluoridated water usually will be high in fluoride. If and only *if* the *total* intake of fluoride is deficient should supplementation take place.

To maximize topical effect, fluoride supplements should touch the teeth before they are swallowed. Place the drops on your children's teeth or put them in their food or drink. Do not add them to milk because the calcium in the milk binds with the fluoride and reduces the amount of fluoride available to protect the teeth. Older children should be encouraged to chew and swish the tablets around in their mouths to prolong contact with the teeth before swallowing. Daily fluoride mouthrinses for home use are *not* for children who are under six or unable to spit out all the rinse.

Dentist-Applied Fluoride. The topical fluoride dentists and hygienists apply in the office is an 8 percent solution of stannous fluoride or, more often, 1.23 percent of acidulated fluoride in a gel or foam. To prevent swallowing and the potentially harmful effects of fluoride, a saliva ejector should be used.

Bottled Water. Many parents concerned about the quality of their tap water purchase bottled water. The present labeling regulations make it difficult to determine whether a specific brand of bottled water contains fluoride and, if it does, how much. According to the Food and Drug Administration (FDA), producers of bottled water are not required to indicate the fluoride content of water if it is from natural sources. If, however, the producers *add* fluoride, they must state so and the amount must be in accordance with levels set by the FDA. The FDA also requires the producers to test their bottled water annually for a number of chemicals, including fluoride, to be certain it remains within the standard. In general, analyses of bottled water have found most to contain less than the maximum permissible concentration of fluoride. To find out whether a particular brand contains fluoride and, if so, how much, you need to contact the producers.

Dental Caries

To avoid transmitting this infectious disease, parents and other young children's caregivers who have high rates of caries should not share utensils, suck a pacifier and then give it to a child, or engage in other actions with a child that transfer saliva. In addition, parents who have high rates of caries may want to have the dentist monitor the levels of bacteria associated with it, with one of the caries activity tests described in Chapter 5. To prevent creating an environment conducive to the growth of caries-promoting bacteria, you should restrict the frequency of your child's consumption of highly cariogenic foods, such as cookies, candies, chips, sweet baked goods, raisins, and other dried fruits. You should be sure your child eats a variety of food from the major food groups: fruits; vegetables; milk, cheese, and yogurt; meat, poultry, fish, dried beans, peas, eggs, and nuts; and breads, cereals, and other grains.

Treatment. Of the many new filling materials available, some have properties that lend themselves especially for the treatment of primary teeth. If appearance is the chief concern for restoring (filling) your child's teeth and payment is not covered by your insurance carrier, ask your dentist to inform you of all possible choices in materials and not just the ones your insurance will cover. Composite resins (plastic) may be more acceptable esthetically for filling and capping some primary teeth than silver amalgam materials or stainless steel crowns. Glass ionomer resin materials also offer advantages as pediatric dental filling materials. They contain fluoride that will be released to offer protection against caries that may develop around the edge of the fillings.

Primary Tooth Loss

Young children can lose their primary teeth prematurely for a number of reasons, among them uncontrolled caries, injury, or extraction. Although primary incisors that are missing or lost prematurely are sometimes replaced prosthetically for better function and speech, appearance is the most compelling reason to replace them, usually with either a fixed or a removable partial denture. But when primary molars are lost, the space does need to be maintained by any of a variety of dental appliances (four of which are explained here) to prevent future problems in alignment and crowding. Before placing any appliance, all teeth with caries need to be restored. If there has been damage to the pulp, endodontic therapy should be performed, whenever possible, in an attempt to save the natural teeth.

Band and Loop. This appliance is used most frequently for the loss of a single primary molar. It is relatively inexpensive and easy to make but does not restore the biting surface of the tooth. A band is cemented to one of the teeth next to the space. The space is encircled by a wire soldered to the band. When the permanent tooth begins to erupt, the appliance is removed.

Passive Lingual Arch. This valuable appliance consists of a round wire that lies along the tongue, or back (lingual), side of the lower front teeth. It is attached to bands on either the permanent first molars or the primary second molars. Although this appliance is usually used to prevent the permanent first molars from drifting into the space for the second premolars in the lower arch, it also can be bent and used to reposition teeth orthodontically.

Transpalatal Arch. This fixed appliance is placed when two or more teeth, for example, left and right primary molars, have been lost in the upper arch. It consists of a large wire that crosses the palate and connects to bands on two back permanent molars on either side of the dental arch.

Distal Shoe. The construction of this appliance is similar to the band and loop. It is used to maintain the space of a single primary second molar before the permanent first molar erupts. An extension of stainless steel is soldered to the back end of a loop of wire or steel bar and is placed into the missing space to guide the eruption of the permanent first molar. To be sure that the extension is placed properly, a periapical radiograph should be made.

Removable. These devices are similar to partial dentures and are sometimes the choice when two or more teeth within an arch are lost. When young children will not tolerate a partial denture, the dentist will sometimes wait until the permanent molars erupt and a fixed space maintainer can be placed to save the space for the lower permanent teeth. This consists of a heavy wire soldered to bands cemented on the permanent molars.

AGES 6 THROUGH 12

During these middle childhood years, most of the permanent teeth erupt and children exhibit a greater interest in and ability to care independently for their teeth and a greater awareness of how they look. The risk of injury to teeth, especially the upper central incisors, from athletic activities in which children of these ages often engage, increases. Since children still spend much of their time at home, these years provide opportunities for parents to instill in them the importance of eating a balanced diet, not consuming too many sugary foods or processed beverages, and practicing good oral hygiene.

Appearance of Incisors

In comparison to the white color and small size of the primary teeth, newly erupted upper permanent incisors often appear yellow and large, even when they are of normal size and color. The space that frequently exists between them usually closes when the permanent canines emerge and push them together.

Personal Cleaning

By the time children are eight years old, most have the manual dexterity and the perseverance to brush their teeth adequately on their own. Even so, adults should continue to supervise. Children over the age of six years who can rinse and spit without swallowing can start using fluoride mouthrinses, which provide a good source of topical fluoride to protect the erupted teeth.

Professional Cleaning

The fluoride content in teeth increases with age until it reaches a saturation level during a person's twenties. Because the content in children's teeth is not yet at an optimal level, a dentist should apply topical fluoride after a professional cleaning in which the teeth are polished with pumice and a rubber cup or rotary bristle brush to replenish any that might have been removed from the outer layer of enamel. To prevent removing fluoride on the surface of the teeth, many dentists instead use a toothbrush and dental floss to dislodge plaque before applying topical fluoride for children whose teeth have no calculus or stain.

Fluoride

Regardless of whether or not fluoride is added to the drinking water, professional topical applications twice a year should be part of every child's dental regimen.

Sealants

Sealants are highly effective at preventing caries on the biting surfaces of permanent first molars. Dentists also recommend them for permanent second molars and premolars or primary molars with deep grooves in children who are prone to caries. They should be applied as soon as these teeth are erupted fully. (See Chapter 5 for a detailed discussion.)

How long sealants remain on the teeth depends, in large part, on the skill of the practitioner and the cooperation of the patient. Having them applied by someone who does the procedure regularly, such as a pediatric dentist or a trained dental hygienist, increases their rate of retention. In a recent study, the retention rates of sealants (on permanent first molars) varied, from 92 percent after 1 year to 28 percent after 15 years; their effectiveness in preventing caries was 83 percent after 1 year and 53 percent after 15 years.

Lip Habits (Licking, Pulling, Sucking, and Biting)

As disconcerting as these habits may be, many children lick or pull their lips with few, if any, dental effects. The chapped, inflamed, and red lips that result frequently occur during cold weather and are remedied easily by using moisturizing ointment on the lips.

Whether sucking or biting the lips can create a malocclusion is not clearly understood. What is known is that these habits can exacerbate an existing malocclusion if they are done with enough intensity, frequency, and duration. Most commonly, the lower lip is inserted under and behind the upper incisors. This places pressure on the lower and upper incisors and can result in an overjet or vertical space between the upper and lower teeth, with the upper incisors tipped forward and the lower ones tipped backward. Depending on the extent of the problem and related factors, treatment will involve either fixed or removable orthodontic appliances and may include more complex orthodontic treatment.

Iron Stain

Some children ingest iron from vitamin supplements they are given by their parents or from supplements their physicians prescribe. When more iron than the body can use is present in the system, much of the excess is secreted through the saliva and deposited on the teeth, where it can stain the surfaces gray or black. These stains can be removed, but only by professional cleaning.

Malocclusions

Between 6 and 18 years of age, approximately 75 to 90 percent of children have some kind of malocclusion. About 10 to 12 percent of them require treatment by an orthodontist for either oral health or aesthetic reasons. (See Chapter 15 for more information.)

Because the wires and brackets of orthodontic appliances can trap food particles and bacteria that set the stage for the development of caries, children who wear braces must be thorough about brushing and flossing and conscientious in keeping all dental checkups and orthodontic appointments. If an appliance breaks or bends, the child should be brought promptly to the orthodontist or treating dentist.

Most children need parental or other adult guidance to help them avoid eating the sticky foods (caramels, sticky candies, gum) and large, hard foods (nuts, ice, popcorn) that can damage orthodontic appliances. Athletic or recreational activities usually do not need to be restricted, although a mouthguard might be recommended for some activities.

THE TEEN YEARS

Adolescence is a sensitive time for oral health. With all the permanent teeth erupted, except the four third molars, and with most children now responsible for their own oral hygiene, preventing caries becomes of paramount importance. With more independence in their lives and eating habits, taking optimal care of their teeth seldom tops the list of teenage priorities. Fatigue from school and home activities can bring on stress-related oral problems, such as cold sores (herpes simplex) or necrotizing ulcerative gingivitis. Because of the dental anatomy during adolescence (the gums cover more of the crown of the tooth and the pulp chambers are relatively large), some restorative treatments, such as crown and bridge procedures, are more problematical than during adulthood and place the teeth at increased risk, sometimes necessitating the placement of less invasive interim restorations.

Dental Caries

At the age of 12, 58 percent of children in the United States have some caries in their permanent teeth. By age 17, the figure jumps to over 84 percent.

The Teen Diet. Studies show that teenagers eat on average nine times a day, much of it sweet and sticky foods that adhere to the teeth. Caries can also be caused when the enamel is damaged by the acids in foods like lemons, which cheerleaders sometimes suck to clear their throats during athletic games.

As a society we send children mixed messages about nutrition. Although school health curriculums teach the importance of eating well, sugar-laden soft drinks and other sweets are readily accessible to students in school. Parents and educators should encourage teens to snack on nutritious and noncariogenic foods (listed in Chapter 5), to brush with fluoride-containing toothpaste, to floss every day, and to use fluoride rinses, especially if they are wearing braces or other orthodontic appliances. Teens who turn a deaf ear to a discussion about dental health often will listen when the aesthetic consequences of dental diseases are stressed.

Eating Disorders. The serious and sometimes life-threatening eating disorders anorexia nervosa and bulimia nervosa frequently surface during adolescence. They can have significant oral repercussions, which are detailed in Chapter 11.

Periodontal Problems

According to the latest data, 60 percent of 15-year-olds have gums that are inflamed. These figures predominantly reflect gingivitis, the least serious of the periodontal diseases. For girls, this is often a result of hormonal fluctuations (see Chapter 11).

Despite these statistics, the overall periodontal health of teenagers is basically good. These years remain critical, however, because if poor oral hygiene habits are developed and continued, they can set the stage for serious oral health problems and periodontal destruction later.

Sports Injuries

If every child who engaged in sports or activities that pose a potential for harm to the face and head were to wear a mouthguard, tens of thousands of dental injuries would be prevented. These devices already prevent an estimated 200,000+ injuries each year in high school and college football. Although a number of amateur, high school, and collegiate sports associations require mouthguards for ice hockey, lacrosse, football, and boxing, they should also be used for basketball, soccer, baseball, skateboarding, surfing, gymnastics, and other activities in which there is a risk of injuring the teeth.

Mouthguards help prevent teeth from becoming chipped, dislodged, fractured, or nerve damaged and help shield lips, tongue, and cheeks from injury. In addition, they can soften the impact of falls and blows that could cause concussions and fractures of the jaws.

Stock mouth protectors can be purchased inexpensively at sporting goods stores. They must be held in place by clenching the teeth and, as such, can interfere with breathing. Mouth-formed guards may be the best choice for younger children who have both primary and permanent teeth. They are made with a moldable plastic that can be reformed repeatedly by softening it in warm water. When inserting them, children must be careful not to burn their mouths. To provide optimal fit and comfort, mouthguards should be custom-made by a dentist. Although most only cover the upper teeth, they can be made to cover the lower teeth for individuals who have protruding jaws, wear braces, or have special needs.

BOX 8.5

SOME COMMON ORAL PROBLEMS CAUSED BY SOME SEXUALLY TRANSMITTED DISEASES

Sexually Transmitted Disease	Oral Problems	Locations
Acquired immune deficiency syndrome (AIDS)*	Candida infection, necrotizing ulcerative gingivitis, hairy leukoplakia	Gingiva (gums), palate, tongue
Condyloma acuminatum (venereal) wart)	Pink lesion	Lips, gingiva, palate, tongue
Gonorrhea	Tonsillitis, inflammation, ulceration	Mucous membranes
Herpes simplex virus I	Blisterlike sores	Lips, gingiva, palate, tongue
Syphilis	Red and sometimes ulcerated gingiva	Gingiva, oral mucosa

*HIV infection and AIDS cause a number of oral problems. Their appearance is often the first indication of the development of AIDS, and they are related to the degree of immunosuppression. If the reader is especially interested in this area, several good books are available, including *Oral Manifestations of HIV Infection,* John S. and Deborah Greenspan (Carról Stream, Ill.: Quintessence, 1995).

Removal of the Third Molars (Wisdom Teeth)

Between the ages of 12 and 18 years and before orthodontic treatment, the third molars, which usually emerge during the late teen years, should be evaluated by radiographs. If removal is recommended, patients should seek a second and possibly a third opinion, preferably from an oral surgeon. Although it is easier and less painful to remove them before the alveolar bone in the jaws hardens significantly (prior to age 25 years), they should never be extracted routinely or removed simply to prevent the possibility that they might have to be taken out later when it would be more difficult.

Sexually Transmitted Diseases

An increase in the number of teenagers who lead early and active sex lives leaves these teens more vulnerable to sexually transmitted diseases. (See Box 8.5 for their effects on oral health.)

Chewing Tobacco and Snuff

In 1991 20 percent of high-school-aged boys either chewed tobacco or placed it in their cheeks. This represents an eightfold increase from 15 years earlier. Smokeless tobacco contains a higher nicotine concentration than that found in cigarettes and, as a result, has serious medical and dental consequences. Chronic users have 50 times the risk of developing cancers of the gums and lower lip, 4 times the chance of developing oral cancer, and an increased risk of developing high blood pressure, heart attacks, kidney disease, and strokes. Smokeless tobacco can erode the enamel of teeth and irritate the gums, and so cause them to whiten and recede; this exposes the roots of the teeth and sets the stage for root caries. A study of major league baseball players showed the use of smokeless tobacco does not enhance a player's performance. This is contrary to what some athletes believe. Parents, educators, dentists and physicians, athletic coaches, and all other adults should do what they can to discourage this very harmful and addictive practice, especially among teenagers.

CHAPTER 9

——

The Adult Years

DENTAL CHANGES

Many people notice changes in the appearance of their smiles or in their dental health or comfort as they grow older. Although many of these can be attributed to diseases or medications, some are due to age-related changes in the oral tissues.

Changes Related to Age

There are physiological reasons why teeth during the adult years are not as "white" as they were in youth. With age, the enamel becomes more brittle and reflects light differently. Caries and wear cause the tooth to produce additional dentin, which is yellower in color. With the enamel less luminous, this secondary dentin shows through and the teeth take on a yellowish tinge. With age, the cells in the gingiva do not replenish themselves as rapidly, nor do they keratinize as well to form a tougher and protective surface. As a result, the gingiva's ability to resist bacteria and mechanical irritants and to repair itself is reduced and the gums may recede. As they do, the cementum of the tooth beneath the gumline shows and the tooth appears longer. Gum recession caused by aging alone is modest. Most of the gum recession adults experience as they grow older is a result of periodontal disease and overzealous brushing. Without these, some researchers believe most adults would not look "long in the tooth" until they were at least 65.

The tooth inside also changes. The secondary dentin invades the pulp chambers and root canals and compresses them so they become smaller. The blood supply to the pulp is diminished; this makes it less sensitive.

Changes Related to Disease

Although the probability of experiencing some specific dental problems increases with age, the act of growing older itself is seldom wholly responsible for them. As an example, it is now known that dry mouth (xerostomia) is a consequence of diseases or the medications taken for them and not aging, as had long been assumed. We also now know that periodontal disease is an infectious disease, as preventable and treatable in adults as it is in younger persons.

Wear and Tear

Throughout life, our teeth are subjected to repeated chewing, brushing, and flossing. Although a certain amount of attrition from chewing is inevitable, brushing and flossing the teeth properly will not wear away the tooth surface. Yet if done improperly or with too much force, they can cause wear, as well as recession of the gums. If the abrasion or attrition (explained below) is significant and the tooth does not respond by depositing secondary dentin rapidly enough, the pulp may become exposed; this will threaten the vitality of the tooth.

Damage to the teeth by attrition, abrasion, and erosion can be prevented or minimized by modifying the diet, maintaining good oral hygiene, and avoiding certain habits and offending substances. (Box 9.1 lists some causes of tooth wear.)

Attrition. From years of chewing, teeth wear down where they are in contact with other teeth, especially on the biting surfaces. Depending on the consistency and texture of an individual's diet, some teeth wear more than others. The teeth of primitive humans, who ate coarse-ground materials and used their teeth as tools, wore down at a rate greater than most of ours will.

With attrition, the cusps of the teeth flatten. This leveling usually occurs faster in men than women, it is believed, because men exert more force when chewing. For some people, enamel and dentin wear away from the force exerted with normal chewing of food or tobacco. For others, the attrition is hastened by bruxism (grinding) or other oral habits, such as using their teeth as bottle openers or scissors.

BOX 9.1

SOME CAUSES OF TOOTH WEAR

The following substances can cause overall corrosion of the enamel:

• Fruits and fruit juices containing citric acid (lemons, oranges, bananas, etc.)
• Carbonated drinks (both diet and regular)
• Chewable vitamin C, aspirin, or iron tablets
• Vinegar
• Sucking on lemons
• Abrasive toothpastes, some of which are marketed for whitening teeth and/or removing stains on teeth
• Repeated vomiting from bulimia or chronic alcoholism
• Refluxed gastric acids from hiatus hernia
• Exposure to industrial acids
• Hydrochloric acid used to treat achlorhydria, a condition in which there is either no or a reduced secretion of gastric acids

Tips:

• Instead of drinking from a glass, use a straw to suck up acidic drinks or medicines to reduce their contact with the teeth.
• Use regular tablets that can be swallowed instead of chewable tablets when taking vitamins or aspirin.

The following can cause notches or grooves in the teeth:

• Habitual biting on pipe stems, pins, tacks, toothpicks, etc.
• Improper use of floss, interproximal brushes, toothbrushes

Abrasion. Nonchewing mechanical force, most commonly caused by brushing too hard or improperly (horizontally) with a hard-bristled brush or gritty toothpaste, especially some very abrasive toothpastes marketed for whitening teeth or removing tobacco and other stains, can cause the structures of the teeth to wear away. Abrasion can also result from malocclusions, dental appliances, or chronic use of toothpicks.

When the teeth show wear at a specific site, it probably is caused by a habit or by improper oral hygiene. Grooves or notches can form in the teeth from holding pins, tacks, or pipes repeatedly in one place in the mouth. Quadraplegics frequently sustain abrasive damage to their teeth because they use them as tools or to hold pencils or brushes to draw or paint. Brushing too strenuously and too frequently with a hard-bristled brush, sometimes in conjunction with an abrasive toothpaste, can cause V- or U-shaped indentations. This occurs most often on the premolar and canine teeth. At the gumline, the enamel may be worn away and the dentin exposed. With abrasion on the front incisors, the gums may recede and expose the cementum. In severe cases, the alveolar bone may be affected.

The tooth surfaces of people who work in the presence of abrasive dust particles (e.g., in coal mines, brick factories, or some types of construction) can become abraded when they are exposed during speech or at other times when the mouth is opened. Wearing a protective mask can help prevent this. The first step in treating abrasion is to stop the habit. (See Chapter 5 for tips on cleaning teeth without damaging them.) There are devices the disabled can use to reduce reliance on their teeth. To prevent caries from developing, your dentist may apply topical fluorides. If the pulp is threatened, the tooth may need to be restored.

Erosion. If teeth are bathed in too much acid (from lemons, carbonated beverages, or repetitive vomiting, as with alcoholism or bulimia), the enamel and dentin can wear away. Treatment consists of stopping the habit, applying topical fluorides and sealants with fluorides, and using alkaline mouthwashes. Because erosion happens rarely when there is no chemical reaction, a dentist needs to evaluate the cause to rule out any hereditary or congenital factors.

When vomiting occurs as a result of a medication, medical condition (such as the reflux of gastric acids resulting from an incompetent sphincter at the base of the esophagus), or medical treatment, the dentist should contact the patient's physician to see whether alternative medications or treatments can be substituted. If the vomiting or reflux occurs at a specific time, a soft splint (sometimes with a fluoride gel or antacid on the inside of it) can be effective in shielding the teeth. A mask worn to protect the mouth can be helpful for individuals who work with industrial acid vapors.

Crowns should not be put on the teeth until the cause of the erosion is identified and treatment is undertaken. If crowns are placed and the erosion continues, the acid might attack the margins and cause extensive caries.

DENTAL PROBLEMS

Dental Caries

Root Caries. Before the age of around 50, most caries affects the biting surfaces of the back teeth, between the teeth where they touch, and along the gumline. After this age, caries occurs most frequently where the roots are exposed from recession of the gums. Dentists usually fill carious lesions on the root surfaces with glass ionomer cement because its fluoride content leaches out effectively to protect the cementum from further attack of caries.

Re-restorations. Restorations (as do teeth) must endure multitudes of bacteria, extreme fluctuations in temperature, pressures from chewing foods with different textures, and sometimes their use as tools. Even though some dental materials, such as gold and amalgams, are very durable and provide long-lasting restorations for many individuals, none should be considered permanent. Most adults who have amalgam fillings may have to have them repaired or replaced after a number of years. When this is recommended, there are a number of factors to consider.

Each time a filling or other restoration needs to be replaced, more of the tooth needs to be removed. Therefore, when having a filling placed initially, it is important to consider the longevity of the material. The longer the material lasts, the greater chance you have of retaining more of your tooth longer and the longer you put off the likelihood of having a more extensive and expensive restoration, like a crown.

Repair of an existing amalgam filling may, at times, be preferable to replacing it. If the defect is minimal, ask your dentist whether a filling you have already can be repaired, saving you, at least temporarily, from losing additional tooth structure. A problem inherent in repairing a filling is that when new material is added on top of old, it is not as strong as the bulk of the original. The use of a bonding agent can improve the strength of the repair, but it still will not make it as strong as a new filling would be.

For many, aesthetics may be a factor in the decision. Some choose to replace a defective amalgam filling with composite resin because it will look better and not be as noticeable. Another factor is cost. As a general rule, each time a restoration is replaced and more of the tooth is lost, the cost of the replacement is higher.

Periodontal Disease

According to findings from a recent survey conducted by the National Institute of Dental Research, serious periodontal infections in adults are not as widespread as they were believed to be. Almost 44 percent of adults have bleeding gums, an indication of gingivitis; about 15 percent have gum pockets greater than 4 millimeters; and fewer than 2 percent have a pocket depth greater than 7 millimeters.

One's predilection for periodontal disease does increase with age, as many of the habits, diseases, and medications that raise the risk of developing it and increase its severity are present during adulthood. Ill-fitting bridges, defective restorations (fillings, crowns, bridges), and sometimes teeth that are poorly aligned, are prone to accumulating plaque, which contributes to periodontal disease. To prevent the progression of periodontal disease, these dental problems need to be corrected. In addition, at different ages different strains of pathogens are more dominant. In children, the bacteria that causes caries, *Streptococcus mutans,* predominates in plaque, whereas the strains of bacteria in the mouths of adults are associated more often with periodontal disease.

Chronic adult periodontal disease, which often takes years to progress, usually begins in adults over the age of 35. It is a direct response to the accumulation of plaque and tartar. Individuals who seem most afflicted are those whose habits or the condition of whose teeth encourage the accumulation of plaque. These are adults with missing teeth, many restorations, and medical conditions or medications taken for them that depress the production of saliva.

Some research has also shown that the gingiva of older persons become inflamed more quickly and more severely in the presence of plaque than they do in younger persons. The good news, however, is that when good oral hygiene measures are taken, any inflammation or other symptoms of gingivitis reverse as quickly as they do in younger persons.

Oral Cancer

In the United States men between the ages of 40 and 65 have the highest rate of oral cancers. The most common sites are the lip, the floor of the mouth, and the lateral tongue. Although the cause of oral cancer is not completely understood, it is often associated with the use of tobacco or alcohol or, for the lower lip, with sun exposure. Exposure to industrial chemicals or viruses also may play a role.

Oral cancer is not a rare cancer (it makes up between 2 and 5 percent of all cancers). It is more common than leukemia, melanoma, and cancers of the brain, thyroid, stomach, kidney, ovary, or cervix. All dentists are

---

B O X 9.2

SIGNS OF ORAL CANCER

See your dentist promptly if you experience any of the following:

• A sore in your mouth that bleeds easily and does not heal
• A lump or thickening in your cheek that you can feel with your tongue
• A white or red patch on your tongue, gums, or oral mucosa
• Soreness of the throat or the sensation that something is caught in your throat
• Difficulty chewing or swallowing
• Numbness in your tongue or elsewhere in your mouth

trained to identify oral cancer. For this reason, they frequently are the first healthcare professionals to detect it. Even so, the condition is sometimes overlooked by dentists. Having routine dental exams, as well as heeding the signs of oral cancer (listed in Box 9.2) can aid in early detection, which, along with early treatment, can improve its generally poor five-year survival rate of approximately 50 percent.

Oral cancer usually first appears as a red, white, or red-and-white sore with a raised, rolled margin. In general, if you have any sore in or around your mouth that does not heal within 10 to 14 days, you should have it checked by your dentist. Pain and numbness are symptoms that develop much later and can indicate that the tumor has spread to the bone or other deeper structures. When the cancer spreads to the lymph nodes in the neck, the nodes frequently become enlarged and are painless and firm. A loose tooth or a tooth socket that does not heal after an extraction can occasionally be a sign of a tumor within the jaws.

If not treated, the cancer spreads, first to the surrounding soft tissues, then into the bones of the jaws and to the lymph nodes. Survival time usually is reduced if the lymph nodes become involved. Approximately 10 to 20 percent of patients with oral cancers develop cancer in the pharynx.

Between 70 and 90 percent of oral cancers are squamous cell carcinomas. This type of oral cancer is treated most often surgically by a head and neck cancer specialist. In many instances surgery is followed with radiation therapy and chemotherapy. (For more information on surgery, see Chapter 18.)

Halitosis (Bad Breath)

Although the causes of bad breath are many, the reaction to it is singular. Bad breath is unacceptable socially and can subject the person who has it to social and professional ostracism.

Most foul breath odors are caused by the breakdown of sulfur-containing proteins by gram-negative bacteria in an alkaline environment. Bad breath often becomes a problem during the adult years when the oral conditions that contribute to it usually develop. These include reduced salivary flow resulting in xerostomia and periodontal disease, which encourage the growth of gram-negative bacteria and a rise in the pH in the mouth. Among the causes of xerostomia are the use of medications, aging, stress, head and neck irradiation, diabetes, anemia, multiple sclerosis, and AIDS.

Other dental causes of halitosis include caries, poorly fitting dental appliances and prostheses, defective restorations, diseases of the dental pulp, candidiasis, and a tongue with fissures, which trap food debris and bacteria. Infected sinuses, nasal cancers, and lesions of the nose, sinuses, and nasopharynx are additional causes, as are hiatus hernias, esophageal strictures, liver failure, and chronic respiratory problems, such as bronchitis and pneumonia.

Breath also becomes unpleasant smelling during sleep and mouth breathing when the production of saliva is reduced and the alkalinity in the mouth increased. Dieting, which increases the metabolic breakdown of fats and proteins, contributes to bad breath, whereas eating reduces it. The act of chewing stimulates salivary flow and helps clean the mouth. If you experience persistent bad breath, see your dentist.

Examination. Your dentist will review your dental, medical, and medication histories and examine you to determine whether the odor is emanating from your mouth or from your upper digestive tract. Radiographs to diagnose diseases of the teeth, jaws, or related structures and biopsies may be made. If an infection of the mouth is believed to be the cause, culture and sensitivity tests may be performed. If your dentist suspects that your halitosis results from a medical condition, you will be referred to a generalist or specialist physician. Patients for whom no physical cause for their bad breath can be found may be referred to a physician to rule out psychological or mental causes, among them depression, schizophrenia, organic brain syndrome, neurosis, and difficulties in interpersonal relationships.

Treatment. Oral hygiene should be improved by removing plaque and using mouthrinses and other agents to reduce oral bacteria. Dental problems, such as candidiasis, xerostomia, or carious lesions, should be treated with appropriate measures. Faulty restorations and defective crowns, appliances, and prostheses should be replaced or repaired. Teeth with diseased pulp require endodontic treatment or, if necessary, extraction. Antibiotic therapy may be given for infections, and antifungal medications for candidiasis.

Bruxism (Tooth Grinding and Clenching)

It is estimated that as many as 96 percent of adults grind their teeth. While most bruxers engage in the habit while sleeping, only 5 to 20 percent are aware of it.

Although the causes of bruxism are not understood entirely, the condition is related to many factors, among them stress, sleep disorders, and possibly problems with occlusion. Because bruxism occurs more often in members of the same family, it may be genetically related.

Bruxism can cause a number of dental problems, including tooth attrition, inflammation of the gingiva, sensitivity of the teeth to extreme temperatures, broken restorations, limited jaw opening, and tenderness of facial muscles. The damage to permanent teeth happens slowly but is irreversible. The upper canines, followed by the back teeth, are the teeth worn down most commonly. If bruxism continues, the periodontal ligament can be damaged. This makes the teeth looser and can interrupt the blood supply to them and result in loss of the alveolar bone. Bruxism can also be responsible for headaches and myofascial pain syndrome.

To detect the disorder, dentists ask their patients a series of questions, measure the maximum jaw opening, palpate the temporomandibular joints and facial muscles, and look at the teeth for abnormal signs of wear.

With appropriate therapy, the symptoms of bruxism can be treated, but the disorder usually cannot be cured. Treatment may involve a combined effort between the patient's physician and dentist. Treatments include biofeedback, changing sleep positions, medications to suppress the REM (rapid eye movement) stage of sleep (the sleep stage during which the most damage to the teeth from grinding occurs), visual imagery, and autosuggestion. Using an intraoral appliance to protect the teeth from further abrasion has been shown not to be effective, although using one to relieve temporomandibular joint and myofascial pain may be. Correcting the dental problems that result, such as repairing fractured tooth cusps and reducing tooth mobility and sensitivity, are most effective after the teeth grinding is controlled.

Dental Aesthetics

Whatever the individual reasons for adults to seek out cosmetic dental procedures, age frequently is an underlying factor. Some adults seek cosmetic dental treatment to camouflage changes in tooth color and repair the other minor aesthetic imperfections in their teeth caused by the wear and tear of aging. Others undergo it for economic reasons. Adults today face stiff competition professionally, especially in a market geared to younger consumers. To stay competitive, many want to maximize their possibility of securing and keeping a job by appearing as attractive and young as they can. For others, the motivation to enhance the aesthetics of their smile is their reentry into the social or romantic market, following divorce or the death of a spouse or loved one.

Practicing good oral hygiene and having carious lesions restored before they spread is a good start in enhancing your smile by helping preserve your teeth and gums. For adults who find growing older difficult in a culture that extols youth, cosmetic dental procedures, such as having their teeth bleached, veneered, bonded, or reshaped, can impart a needed psychological lift. (See Chapter 14 for a detailed discussion of cosmetic dental treatments.) The appearance of your smile can also be improved with orthodontics and prosthetic appliances or implants.

CHAPTER 10

The Elder Years

Many people over 65 lead healthy and active lives. Even so, on average, seniors suffer from higher rates of dental caries, periodontal disease, and tooth loss than those who are younger do. Many of these problems can be attributed to a longer life span, which provides more opportunities for them to develop. The advances in medical care enabling more older persons to lead productive lives also allow more to live longer with acute and chronic conditions requiring medications that can complicate dental treatment. This chapter discusses some of the specific dental challenges seniors face, many of which can be forestalled or prevented with quick intervention and by following many of the same preventive measures recommended for younger persons. For more detail on many of them, you need to consult other chapters.

AGE-RELATED DENTAL CHANGES

As we grow older, the condition of the teeth and gingiva change. Because most of these alterations begin early in our adult lives, they are described in Chapter 9.

In more advanced years, the tongue also changes. The natural fissures become deeper and more pronounced. Although this does not affect health, it may look unattractive and trap bacteria. Due to either the loss of elasticity in a vein wall or a blockage in a vein, varicosities (varicose veins) can develop underneath the tongue along the course of a vein. They produce a dark bluish to black enlargement. These are benign changes and require no treatment.

The physiological effects of aging in other parts of the body can affect dental health. As we age, the immune system weakens; this makes us less resistant to infections and more susceptible to diseases, including those in and affecting the mouth. As a consequence, recovery from surgery or illness may take longer and wounds and bruises may heal more slowly. Even so, many older people do recover completely and quickly from surgeries and illnesses.

Osteoporosis, loss of bone density, is common in the elderly. When it effects the alveolar, or jaw, bone, wearing dentures and securing implants is more difficult. Compounding this, the temporomandibular joint is more prone to degenerative changes.

DENTAL CONCERNS

Dental Caries

Over 60 percent of those over age 65 have root caries, three times the rate of younger adults. One-half of these lesions have not been filled; this leaves teeth vulnerable to further caries and pulp death. Older adults also experience caries on the crowns of the teeth, especially around the margins of fillings.

Dental caries in the elderly is exacerbated by dry mouth caused by disease, such as Sjögren's syndrome, irradiation of the head and neck from cancers, and medication use. Difficulty in brushing and flossing because of loss of manual dexterity, mental disorders, and depression also can contribute to the problem.

Periodontal Disease

Most adults have some of the signs of periodontal disease. Almost all seniors (95 percent) have at least one area where the gum has lost its attachment to the tooth. Nearly 70 percent have more severe periodontal pockets (over 4 millimeters). The severity of periodontal disease in older adults is increased by (and can be curtailed by remedying) ill-fitting dentures and bridges, poor diets, some medical diseases and medications, and inadequate oral hygiene.

Tooth Wear

Although the mechanical and chemical forces (described in Chapter 9) that can wear away tooth structure can occur at any age, older persons are more prone to them for a number of reasons. First, the longer teeth remain in the mouth, the more opportunities there are for wear. Second, gum recession, more prevalent with age, exposes the softer tissues of the cementum and dentin. These are eroded more easily by the acids in fruits, fruit juices, and candies containing phosphoric or citric acids. Finally, reduced flow of saliva resulting from medications and diseases results in less lubrication and less pellicle, the protective coat of nonbacterial film deposited by saliva on the teeth. This makes the teeth of older persons more vulnerable to erosion from the use of sugar-containing candies to help relieve oral dryness.

Dentin Hypersensitivity

As a result of abrasion and erosion, the necks or the areas around the tooth where the cementum has been exposed become overly sensitive. If the sensitivity is pronounced, many people avoid removing plaque, which increases their risk for caries and periodontal disease. They also may not go to the dentist for fear of having their teeth touched. A toothpaste or gel made for sensitive teeth, containing potassium nitrate or strontium chloride, can help alleviate the discomfort. Topical fluorides, in rinse or gel form, also can be helpful.

Tooth Loss

Despite the encouraging news that more older people are retaining their teeth, a significant number are toothless. Only 2 percent of seniors have the full set of 28 permanent teeth still intact. And although too many still lose their teeth (32 percent of the 65- to 69-year-olds and 49 percent of those over 80), those who do have more and better options, including bone-integrated implants, to replace them. To prevent the problems caused by tooth loss, it is recommended that all missing teeth be replaced quickly by bridges, dentures, or implants. There may be times, however, depending on an individual's age, medical condition, and the costs of treatment, when an older person may not need to replace a certain tooth, for example, a back molar. Patients need to discuss this with their dentists. For detailed information about the problems associated with tooth loss and options for replacing lost teeth, see Chapter 16.

Denture Problems

Older persons with dentures need to have them checked regularly. Loss of sensitivity in the mouth due to aging and a reluctance to complain can cause seniors to tolerate irritating and ill-fitting dentures. This tolerance, along with having a foreign appliance in the moist environment of the mouth, can result in problems, among them:

Candidiasis. This is a fungal infection of the mouth (as well as the gastrointestinal tract and vagina). Its incidence has increased significantly with the widespread use of antibiotics, which interfere with the oral environment and destroy bacteria that inhibit the growth of *Candida albicans,* the fungal species most responsible for it. Although it can occur at any age, *acute pseudomembranous candidiasis,* the most common form of the disease, especially afflicts people who are older and frail or who use immunosuppressive drugs for the treatment of leukemia and other malignant diseases, have had organ transplants, or have AIDS. The soft, white, slightly raised lesions that result may appear on the insides of the cheeks, palate, gums, tongue, and floor of the mouth. Because candidiasis sometimes can be life threatening, it is essential to treat it with antifungal agents.

Denture Stomatitis (denture sore mouth). This is an inflammation of the areas in the mouth dentures rest on. Possible causes include candida infections, allergy to dental materials, reaction of the tissues to poorly fitting or unclean dentures, systemic disease, or residue of denture cleanser.

Cleaning the dentures with an ultrasonic device or soaking them in an antifungal solution and applying antifungal ointment to them and to the mouth, along with a tissue conditioner, may reduce the inflammation. If it does not and the dentures still do not fit well, a new set should be made and kept clean.

Papillary hyperplasia. This is a red inflammation under dentures (usually full ones). It can usually be lessened by relining the dentures with a soft liner. In some cases, the lesions must be removed surgically, chemically, or with electrocautery, after which new dentures are fabricated and must be kept scrupulously clean.

Epulis fissuratum. This is small folds of tissue in the gums that accumulate and grow in response to an irritation from ill-fitting dentures. Adjusting the dentures may cause early lesions to disappear. If the lesions persist, they should be removed surgically and new dentures made. The lesions are benign, but all abnormal structures in the mouth should be biopsied to verify the diagnosis.

There are other problems older persons with dentures encounter. Inadequate or painful muscle control from a stroke, Parkinson's disease, arthritis, or other medical condition can make controlling complete dentures difficult. A significant loss of weight or a nutritional imbalance can cause the jaw ridges to shrink and the dentures to loosen. While the reason for the shrinkage is investigated, the dentures should be relined.

Whether people who have been without teeth and replacements for a while will be successful wearing dentures depends on how motivated they are to making the muscular and hygienic adjustments necessary. Much of this depends on their psychological attitude (discussed later in "From Attitude").

Glossitis or Burning Tongue

A common complaint among older persons, especially women, is a burning or painful sensation in the mouth or on the tongue, which may be accompanied by redness, swelling, sores, or systemic disease (see Chapter 11).

Oral Cancer

For a number of reasons, including the loss of teeth, dependence on caregivers, and difficulty getting to appointments, many older persons do not routinely visit the dentist. As a result, they miss regular screenings for oral cancer in which early lesions can be readily detected.

To help prevent cancers of the lip, tongue, mouth, and throat, older persons should eat a balanced diet with an adequate intake of nutrients, avoid or restrict the use of tobacco and alcohol, reduce irritation from removable dentures, and apply sunblock to their face and lips.

Angular Cheilosis

Sometimes a painful crack or split develops in the skin at the corners of the mouth. Because the moistness from the mouth provides a conducive environment for the growth of fungus, candida infections frequently develop here.

Although this condition can develop regardless of age, it is found more frequently in older persons who have the factors associated with it, among them prolonged antibiotic therapy, anemia, and B-vitamin and iron deficiency. Other causes are herpes simplex virus type I and syphilis. Depending on what is causing the condition, treatments can include vitamins or antifungal drugs.

Xerostomia (Dry Mouth)

Seniors experience increased rates of all three of these most common causes of salivary gland dysfunction: certain systemic diseases, usually Sjögren's syndrome; medications; and irradiation to the head and neck for cancer therapy. The most common cause of diminished salivary flow and dry mouth is the use of medications, which is greatest in persons over 65. About 400 medications have been associated with dry mouth (see Box 10.1 for a list). (See also Chapters 6 and 11.)

BOX 10.1

SOME KINDS OF DRUGS
THAT CAN DRY THE MOUTH

Amphetamines	Anticonvulsants	Decongestants
Antianxiety drugs	Antihistamines	Diuretics
Antidepressants	Antipsychotics	Hypnotics
(tricyclics)	Antispasmodics	Muscle relaxants
Anticholinergics	Appetite suppressants	Opioid (narcotic)
(atropine)	Barbiturates	analgesics
Antiparkinsonians	Bronchodilators	

DENTAL COMPLICATIONS

From Medications

Older persons have twice the number of adverse reactions to drugs as younger persons. This is not surprising, given both their high medication use (representing only 12 percent of the population, people over the age of 65 take 25 percent of prescription medications) and their difficulty tolerating fat-soluble drugs. As described in Chapter 12, many medications can produce oral side effects, complicate dental treatment, and interfere with oral health. For example, the antibiotic erythromycin, recommended before some dental procedures, can interact with the heart medication digoxin to create a toxicity of digoxin.

The physiological alterations that occur with age, among them a decrease in the percentage of body water, the ratio of lean body weight to fat, lung capacity, kidney function, and blood flow to vital organs, make it more difficult for seniors to tolerate and excrete drugs. With a higher proportion of body fat, fat-soluble drugs, such as the antianxiety drug diazepam (Valium), have a longer half-life. As a consequence, their effects linger longer in older persons (especially in women who naturally have a higher content of body fat than men) than they do in younger individuals. This intensifies both the effects of the drug given for the dental treatment and the potential for interactions with other medications being taken.

From Disease

Seniors suffer from chronic diseases (those lasting more than three months) in disproportionate numbers. Chronic diseases have numerous implications for dental care: More medications are given to treat them; this increases the potential both for interactions with drugs in dental treatment and for oral side effects. The physiological effects of the disease can interfere with or be a contraindication for dental treatment.

Older persons also are more prone to developing medical conditions that have an impact on their oral health. Others, in addition to the ones covered in Chapter 12, include:

Facial neuralgias. These are disorders affecting the nervous system causing facial pain. Trigeminal nerve neuralgia is characterized by sharp shooting pains along branches of the trigeminal nerve in the face. The two trigeminal nerves are the largest pair of cranial nerves. They are responsible for controlling facial movements and necessary for chewing. Symptoms usually begin with an occasional sharp pain in the face, increasing over the next few years in frequency and severity. The painful episodes typically last no more than five minutes, with a complete abatement of the pain between attacks. Touching the trigger zones of the face can induce an attack. Some persons respond to the drug carbamazepine; for others surgery on the nerve is required.

Carbamazepine is also used to treat glossopharyngeal neuralgia, a less common facial neuralgia. This condition also causes severe pain, most often at the back of the tongue, in the pharynx and tonsils, and, less frequently, within the ear.

Glossitis (painful or burning tongue). This may be a symptom of nutritional problems.

Pemphigus and bullous pemphigoid. These are serious skin disorders, which can cause sores in the mouth and on the gums.

The symptoms of other diseases that afflict the elderly disproportionately, such as arthritis, vision disorders, Parkinson's disease, Alzheimer's disease, and other dementias, interfere with the ability to perform routine oral hygiene by reducing range of motion, manual dexterity, sight, or memory. Box 10.2 offers helpful tips.

From Attitude

Although age alone should not prevent a senior from undergoing any dental procedure, it increases the likelihood of a medical condition or dental problem interfering with treatment. For example, an older person might want dental implants but not be a candidate for them because of bone loss in his or her jaw resulting from osteoporosis or from resorption hastened by tooth loss.

Age also may affect a person's desire, irrespective of a physical problem, to undergo elective dental treatment. Some older persons feel erroneously that they no longer need to take care of their teeth because they "won't be around much longer," whereas others are reluctant to undertake treatment for cost-benefit reasons, not knowing whether they will "get their money's worth out."

BOX 10.2

HELP FOR WEAK GRIPS

The following tips may make caring for your teeth and gums easier if you have limited range of motion in the hands, shoulders, and arms.

To thicken the handle of a manual toothbrush, use:

A washcloth	A handle from a bicycle
Aluminum foil	Elastic bandage
A sponge	Tape
A rubber ball	

To lengthen the handle of a toothbrush, use a piece of wood or plastic, such as a ruler, popsicle stick, broom, or tongue depressor. Select brushes with long handles; there are an increasing number on the market.

If your hand is incapable of gripping, you can attach your toothbrush to it by means of an elastic or Velcro band or cloth.

To make flossing easier, use:

• A floss holder

• A loop of floss (Take approximately 18 inches of floss and tie three knots in it to make a circle. Place your fingers [except thumbs] within the loop, spreading them about 1 inch apart. Use your index finger and thumbs to guide the floss through your teeth. Rotate the loop as you floss, so that you use a new section between different teeth.)

Other tips:

• Use a toothbrush with an angled handle to reach back teeth. To bend your toothbrush, run the handle under hot water.

• Use an electric or sonic toothbrush.

From Depression

Older persons encounter many losses, of spouses, friends, children, employment, independence, driving. A decline in physical condition brings declines in other areas: motor function, cognitive abilities (memory, problem solving skills, attention, intelligence), vision, taste, hearing. These losses can contribute to depression.

By being alert to the oral symptoms of depression, dentists, family members, and caregivers can intervene to get the older person appropriate medical and dental treatment. The symptoms are:

- Less attention to oral hygiene
- Ignoring caries and poorly fitting dentures
- Reduced saliva flow
- Painful or burning sensation in the mouth
- Increased periodontal disease
- Vague facial pains

PREVENTIVE CARE

The prevalence of disease, depression, medication use, and difficulty using toothbrushes makes preventive oral care especially critical for seniors. The basics (see Chapter 5) do not change, but the emphasis and mode of delivery may.

Even in the senior years, fluoride applied topically at home and professionally, and systemically from water and other beverages remains a significant caries preventive. Artificial salivas with fluoride help those who suffer from dry mouth. Counseling to reduce high intake of sugary foods may aid older persons, who, because of loss of taste, denture problems, or missing teeth, too frequently consume soft, sugary foods.

An electric toothbrush can benefit seniors with limited dexterity. Their large handles are grasped easily, and the power from the motor reduces the number of arm and wrist movements required. Electric toothbrushes with override mechanisms that shut off when excess pressure is applied prevent damage to gums and teeth. The lighter, rotary-driven brushes are preferable for individuals who have rheumatoid arthritis or back problems and find lifting a strain.

BOX 10.3

WHAT TO LOOK FOR
IN A DENTIST

If you are a senior, you may want a dentist who:

- Treats you with respect.
- Does not finish your sentences.
- Listens to you.
- Does not treat your age as a reason not to have dental treatments.
- Takes a complete medical, as well as dental, history.
- Keeps current on the medications you are using.
- Will work in conjunction with your physician and other healthcare professionals.
- If you need it, has handicapped access to office and special equipment to treat wheelchair-bound patients (head rests to clamp on the back of the wheel chair or a base to turn the wheelchair into a dental chair).

THE DENTIST

Although the attributes of a good dentist—competence, communicativeness, and courtesy—remain the same for patients of all ages, dentists treating older persons need more patience. Taking a medical and drug history for an older dental patient takes longer than it does for a younger patient because of the greater incidence of chronic conditions and prescription medication usage. The dentist may also need to spend time discussing proposed dental treatments with an adult child, spouse, or other family member who has the responsibility for making medical and dental decisions (and sometimes for paying for them) for older patients who are unable to do so themselves. Paying for dental care can be a hurdle for some older patients, especially those who have retired and are less likely to have dental insurance. Medicare, in general, as explained in Chapter 4, pays for very few dental treatments. As a consequence, older patients and/ or those responsible for them may prefer consulting a dentist who accepts a monthly schedule of payment.

Dentists for older patients may, depending on the setting (sometimes hospitals and long-term care institutions), act more in concert with other healthcare professionals, among them physicians, geriatric nurse practitioners, social workers, and physical and occupational therapists. Box 10.3 lists the traits older patients may desire in their dentists.

CHAPTER 11

———

For Women Only

D uring different stages of their lives women are predisposed to certain health conditions, some of which may affect dental health.

HORMONAL INFLUENCES

The dental changes women are especially vulnerable to during puberty, menstruation, pregnancy, menopause, postmenopause, and oral contraceptive use most often involve the gums (gingiva). Although researchers are not sure why this happens, most believe it is related to hormones.

Puberty

Gingivitis. At puberty, the hormone gonadotropin stimulates the ovaries to produce other hormones, estrogen and progesterone, that result in a girl's menstrual periods, as well as her secondary sex characteristics. The gingivitis that may occur at this time is not related to an increase in plaque. Studies have revealed that even when the amount of plaque on a girl's teeth and restorations remains low and constant, the frequency and severity with which the gums become inflamed can increase from puberty on. These observations have led researchers to speculate that the higher levels of estrogen and progesterone make the gingival tissues more sensitive to bacteria in plaque, food, and tartar that cause gingivitis. Some studies have also found a greater number of a type of bacteria associated with periodontal disease in the plaque beneath the gumline of girls who were undergoing and just past puberty than were found in girls who had not yet reached puberty.

To reduce the swelling and prevent gingivitis from progressing, the teeth need to be brushed and flossed regularly and thoroughly and cleaned professionally at regular intervals.

Periodontal Diseases. Around puberty and soon afterward, two serious but uncommon forms of periodontal disease develop. Juvenile periodontitis most often begins during puberty. It afflicts three times as many women as men and may be genetically transmitted. Women also are afflicted more often than men, at a ratio of 2.5 to 1, by rapidly progressive periodontitis, called type A. This disease occurs later, usually between the ages of 14 and 26 years. Genetics, hormonal influences, or both may be responsible. Both types of periodontal disease need to be treated by a periodontist and are discussed in more detail in Chapter 7.

Menstruation

In general, the hormonal changes during pregnancy, oral contraceptive use, menopause, and postmenopause may cause more significant periodontal problems than those encountered during menstruation.

Gingivitis. Due to the accumulation of plaque and the same hormonal mechanisms present during puberty (and explained in the following section, "Pregnancy"), sore, red, tender, and swollen gums that bleed easily and teeth that may become slightly looser are more common during a woman's menses than at other times during the month. The symptoms either begin before or during the menstrual period and disappear after it is over. If they do not disappear, a woman should see her dentist.

Women who have gingivitis during their menstrual periods show an increase in the fluid that exudes from the gum tissues into the gum crevice. This is called *gingival crevicular fluid* and is released as a response to gingival inflammation: the more fluid, the more inflammation, and vice versa. Before the menstrual period, the amount of gingival fluid increases until it reaches a maximum at ovulation; then it decreases. The rise coincides with an increase in the production of estrogen and, to a lesser extent, progesterone. Women who do not develop gingivitis during their periods have no increase in the production of crevicular fluid. The additional fluid that is released may be related to the small increase in tooth looseness at this time. As with the gingivitis that develops during puberty, good oral hygiene at home and professional care consisting of scaling and root planing help minimize the problem.

Women who experience inflammation in their gums during their menstrual cycle are more likely to develop rapidly progressive periodontitis than those who do not. Although gingivitis does not damage the alveolar bone, rapidly progressive periodontitis does and therefore needs to be treated more aggressively, usually by a periodontist working in conjunction with a general dentist.

Canker and Fever Sores. Although many women believe that they have a greater tendency to develop canker sores (ulcers inside the mouth) and fever or cold sores (blisters on the inside and outside of the lips caused by the herpes simplex virus) during pregnancy or menstrual periods, a recent study concluded that there is little scientific evidence to support this association.

Pregnancy

Gingivitis. Between 30 and 100 percent of the nearly 5 million women in the United States who become pregnant each year experience changes in their gums. They swell, can become deep red in color, and bleed easily. For most women, the changes do not cause discomfort.

The normal pattern is for the gingivitis to begin during the second month of pregnancy, escalate until the eighth month, and decrease in intensity during the ninth month. After birth, the condition of the gums reverts to what it was during the second month of pregnancy, remains that way for between three and six months, and then subsides.

The gingivitis of pregnancy can increase and become more severe irrespective of changes in the amount of plaque or in oral hygiene habits. As with the gingivitis that develops during menstruation, it will not occur when there is no plaque. Because hormone levels are much higher during pregnancy than at other times, the response of the gum tissues to plaque and food particles and bacteria is exaggerated.

Four main hormones are essential to sustain pregnancy: human chorionic gonadotropin, progesterone, estrogen, and human chorionic somatomammotropin. By the end of pregnancy, the concentration of estrogen in a woman's blood is 30 times higher than it is during menstruation and the amount of progesterone is 10 times higher. A number of theories have been suggested to explain how the elevated levels of the hormones during pregnancy promote gingivitis.

One hypothesis is that the hormones encourage the proliferation of anaerobic organisms (those that thrive without oxygen). Some researchers have found a dramatic increase (up to 55 times greater) in the numbers of *Bacteroides intermedius* in the mouths of pregnant women. (Their numbers also rise with oral contraceptive use and during puberty.) These bacteria are seldom found in healthy gums and are associated with adult periodontitis, acute necrotizing ulcerative gingivitis, and localized juvenile periodontitis.

The gingiva contain receptors for estrogen and progesterone. When the levels of these hormones increase in the blood, they also increase in the gingiva and saliva. Elevated levels of estrogen and progesterone stimulate the production of prostaglandins, hormonelike fatty acids produced by some organs for specific functions. A function of some prostaglandins is to promote inflammation in the gums. Progesterone also causes the capillaries in the gingiva to dilate; this results in increased blood circulation to the gums, which causes them to swell. The inflammation, in turn, stimulates the production of crevicular fluid. Both crevicular fluid and blood transport estrogen and progesterone to the gingiva.

Estrogen and progesterone are also believed to alter the structure of the gingiva in ways that make them vulnerable to bacterial invasion and trauma. Normally, gingiva are keratinized, meaning the cells lose their nuclei and cell boundaries and the outer surfaces of the tissues toughen. The estrogen during pregnancy reduces the keratinization in the attached gingiva. When this happens, the gums lose the protective barrier for the soft tissues underneath and are injured or invaded more easily by bacteria.

Finally, high levels of both estrogen and progesterone affect the immune system, suppressing antibody and T-cell responses, as well as interfering with the function of neutrophils, white blood cells instrumental in destroying harmful bacteria. As a result, the normal protective defenses of the gums are compromised and an environment that is conducive to the growth of harmful pathogens is created.

Although a woman clearly cannot avoid being exposed to extremely high levels of hormones during pregnancy, she can minimize gingivitis or avoid it altogether. Studies show that women who are plaque-free before becoming pregnant and who keep their teeth brushed and flossed and professionally cleaned while pregnant have very low incidences of gingivitis during pregnancy. The studies also indicate that women whose gums bleed and swell before they conceive are more likely to develop gingivitis while pregnant.

Pregnancy Granuloma. A small number (up to 5 percent) of pregnant women develop a deep-or bluish-red swelling of gingival tissue that resembles a tumor. The swelling usually begins quickly during the second month of pregnancy and can reach 2 centimeters in size. The lesion is thought to begin when a minor trauma to the gums provides an opening for bacteria to invade the tissues. The increased hormone levels trigger a reaction of the tissues to the bacteria, and a growth of connective tissue results. The growth usually is not painful (nor is it cancerous), but it may be uncomfortable if it interferes with chewing or speaking or if food collects underneath it.

Women who have had a granuloma in one pregnancy can prevent recurrences in subsequent pregnancies by having their teeth scaled and the roots planed before and between pregnancies. If the tumor is removed surgically during pregnancy, it often will regrow. After birth, the granulomas usually diminish in size and sometimes disappear altogether.

Tooth Mobility. Whether or not you have gingivitis and even when there are no signs of periodontal disease, teeth often become looser during pregnancy. The problem disappears after birth.

Tooth Loss. The belief that a woman loses a tooth for every baby she bears has a firm foothold in folklore but not in science. This old wives' tale is based on the fallacy that calcium is taken from a woman's teeth and given to the fetus. This cannot happen as the calcium within the teeth is in a stable, crystalline form that is not accessible to the rest of the body.

Dental Treatment. In the past, women were advised to postpone elective dental visits during the first and last trimesters of pregnancy. During the first trimester, when nearly 80 percent of spontaneous miscarriages take place, the fear was that the stress of dental care might precipitate one. During the third trimester, the concern was that sitting in the dental chair not only would be uncomfortable for a woman but it might prompt premature labor. The second trimester traditionally has been viewed as the best time for a woman to schedule her dental appointments.

In recent years, these caveats have been relaxed. Many obstetricians find no threat to the fetus or the mother from routine dental treatments during any stage of pregnancy provided the woman is not anxious about dental care and she and the fetus are in good health. Because the potential deleterious effects of an infection or severe pain from an infected tooth or gums are greater for mother and fetus than the risks of any treatments for them, emergency dental care should be performed whenever it is required, preferably after consultation with the woman's obstetrician or physician. Women who have a history of miscarriage, who are threatening to miscarry, or who have another medical condition may be advised by both their dentists and obstetricians to avoid elective dental care during the first trimester. Similarly, women who have histories of premature delivery may want to consult their physicians before elective dental care during the last trimester of pregnancy.

Local anesthetics in dental care should not cause problems for mother and fetus. The antibiotics used most frequently in dentistry—penicillin, erythromycin, and the cephalosporins—are generally considered acceptable but should only be administered when they are absolutely necessary, as with all medications during pregnancy. Tetracycline should *not* be given because of its effects on the enamel of the fetus's teeth. Most physicians know not to prescribe it to a woman while she is pregnant or to a child during the first eight years of life. But if you are in the early months of pregnancy when your condition is not apparent, be sure to alert all healthcare professionals treating you, so you can avoid this hazard.

Concerns have been raised about the use of certain analgesics prescribed for dental treatment during pregnancy and while breast-feeding. Codeine, prescribed for pain, is associated with several congenital anomalies. Nonsteroidal anti-inflammatory drugs, such as ibuprofen, used to treat pain and inflammation, are not recommended because they interfere with prostaglandins, which, among other things, stimulate uterine contractions. Many obstetricians recommend that women avoid aspirin during pregnancy and breast-feeding. Some other medications, sometimes prescribed by dentists, that should not be taken as they are known to cause complications in pregnancy are diazepam (Valium), flurazepam (Dalmane), chlordiazepoxide (Librium), tetracyline, and streptomycin. In fact, current practice is to avoid all drugs (including alcohol) if possible.

The use of dental radiographs for persons of all ages has decreased in the last 20 years. The amount of radiation that the uterine region receives (when protected by a lead apron) during a full-mouth series of radiographs is nearly zero. Yet even though the risk from radiation is small and concentrated on the mouth, far from the fetus, many pregnant women and their obstetricians feel more comfortable postponing radiographs for nonemergency care until after birth. When they are taken, all patients should wear a lead apron.

Early in pregnancy you should ask your obstetrician or physician what dental treatments you should consult them about before having. Many physicians ask their pregnant patients to consult them before:

- Undergoing dental treatment, especially those with a risk of bacteremia (bacteria entering the blood)
- Having a dental radiograph
- Taking any medication

By taking preventive measures and being in good dental health before becoming pregnant, you can reduce your need for dental treatment during pregnancy. If you plan on getting pregnant, have your teeth cleaned professionally, all caries restored, and any other elective procedures performed. Practicing a good oral hygiene regimen at home and having your teeth cleaned by your dentist during pregnancy minimize the gingivitis associated with elevated hormone levels.

Nutrition. Nutritional deficiencies that affect the development of the teeth are uncommon in the United States. Nevertheless, you should eat a well-balanced diet during pregnancy to prevent any potential problems to your fetus's teeth and general health.

Oral Contraceptives

Gingivitis. Birth control pills cause the body to mimic pregnancy by providing synthetic doses of the female hormones estrogen and/or progesterone. As a consequence, women who take them are prone, as when pregnant, to developing gingivitis. This occurs most often around the front teeth and in the gingival tissues between the teeth. The gingivitis results from the same exaggerated response of the gingival tissues to irritants that occurs during pregnancy and menstruation and is not necessarily related to the amount of plaque.

Different formulations of birth control pills contain different drugs at different doses, with the result that some may cause more oral problems than others. If you are experiencing red and swollen gums, you should ask your physician to consider another type of oral contraceptive.

Most often, the alterations in the gingival tissues manifest during the first three months after starting the oral contraceptives. Some women who have taken oral contraceptives for years develop chronic gingivitis. For others, prolonged use increases the severity of their existing gingivitis. The same home-care regimen that is recommended during pregnancy, along with scaling and root planing by a dentist, if necessary, helps control the gingivitis induced by birth control pills.

The Effects of Antibiotics. Dentists sometimes prescribe antibiotics to combat refractory periodontitis and to reduce the harmful bacteria in the plaque that could be irritating the gums and contributing to the swelling. In other instances, antibiotics are given before dental treatments to individuals with specific medical conditions (described in Chapter 12) to reduce the likelihood of developing bacterial endocarditis, a potentially fatal inflammation of the heart valves and tissues.

Some antibiotics can inhibit the effectiveness of oral contraceptives, especially the low-dose varieties. To prevent this possibility, be sure to tell your dentist if you are taking birth control pills. While taking antibiotics, you should use another method of birth control to prevent an unwanted pregnancy or breakthrough menstrual bleeding.

Other Dental Consequences. Very rarely, the estrogen in oral contraceptives can prevent the blood from clotting properly and increase the risk of osteitis, a painful bone inflammation. This can pose a potential hazard for oral surgery. To reduce this possibility, extractions or other dental surgery should be scheduled during the nonestrogen days 23 through 28 of the menstrual cycle.

Menopause and After

Menopause, or the cessation of menstruation, usually occurs around the age of 50. (Illnesses or surgical removal of the uterus and ovaries can cause menstrual periods to end earlier.) Menopause is characterized by a precipitous drop in estrogen levels. Many women during and after menopause undergo a host of physical changes, including some that occur in and around their mouths.

Oral Discomfort. Between 20 and 90 percent of women during and after menopause experience unpleasant sensations in their mouths: pain, dryness, or a burning feeling; or a change in the sense of taste, some foods tasting especially spicy or salty. Of the persons who experience burning mouth syndrome, 80 percent are postmenopausal women, whose symptoms started between 3 and 12 years after menopause. The cause of these problems has been attributed to a number of factors, including changes in hormone levels and increased anxiety and depression.

Occasionally, the gums of women who are going through menopause will become dry and shiny and bleed easily. They can range in color from unusually pale to very red. Sometimes fissures may develop on the inside of the cheek. Women with this condition, called *menopausal gingivosto-matitis,* also usually complain of dryness and a burning sensation in the mouth. Practicing good oral hygiene may relieve some of the symptoms and control the inflammation of the gums. Although not substantiated by scientific studies, some women have claimed relief from supplements of vitamins C and B complexes.

Recent studies found that a little over half the postmenopausal women who complained of dryness or a burning sensation in their mouths and had gum tissues that had receded experienced relief of their symptoms with hormone replacement therapy. Whether hormone therapy is effective seems to depend on the presence of estrogen receptors in the gingival tissues. In one study, women who had estrogen receptors in the gingiva were helped by the hormone treatment, while those who did not were not affected by hormone replacement. Some but not all women have estrogen receptors in their gingiva, which enable the hormones to accumulate there. Identifying the postmenopausal women whose gingiva contain receptors for estrogens may make it possible to determine which women will find relief from their oral problems with hormone therapy. If testing is not feasible, you may want to ask your physician about trying hormone replacement therapy for a limited time to find out whether you will respond. Whether to take hormone replacement therapy for dental or other reasons is a complex and individual decision that each woman must make for herself under her physician's guidance.

Some researchers have suggested that there is a relationship between the reduction of hormones and output of saliva. However, a study by the National Institute on Aging found no relationship between postmenopausal women (on or off hormone replacement therapy) and dry mouth (xerostomia). The xerostomia many women experience after menopause may instead be a side effect of an increasing use of various medications (see Chapter 10) and a symptom of some medical disorders, including Sjögren's syndrome. Hormone replacement therapy will not have an effect on a woman's rate of salivary flow. For information on treatments for xerostomia, see Chapter 6 and the section "Sjögren's Syndrome" in this chapter.

MEDICAL CONDITIONS

Anorexia Nervosa and Bulimia Nervosa

These two illnesses are the most common eating disorders. Both affect women disproportionately, and both can have serious consequences on oral health.

A recent study found anorexia nervosa to be a common chronic illness among girls between the ages of 15 and 19. An anorectic has a deep fear of gaining weight. By restricting her intake of food (and sometimes also by binging), she maintains a body weight about 15 percent or more below what is normal for her age and height. The disorder is also characterized by a distorted perception of body image. Anorectics frequently view themselves as heavy when they are emaciated.

The term "bulimia" comes from the Greek for "ox hunger." It is an apt description for the periodic episodes of binge eating, during which large amounts of food are eaten in a short time, and it characterizes bulimia nervosa. To prevent metabolizing the great numbers of calories consumed during a binge, the bulimic induces vomiting or takes laxatives or diuretics. Other preventives to gaining weight include fasting and exercising strenuously.

The overwhelming majority (between 90 and 95 percent) of bulimics are females, white, and from middle- and upper-class homes. The syndrome usually manifests between the ages of 17 and 21.

Enamel and Dentin Erosion. The frequent vomiting that bulimics and some anorectics induce brings up acidic gastric juices that erode the enamel and dentin, especially on the surfaces of the front teeth that face the tongue. This produces a characteristic glassy, smooth surface. If the erosion is severe, the pulp may be visible and the teeth can become very sensitive to temperature. Although it depends on the frequency of vomiting, the erosion usually becomes apparent after a woman has been binging and purging for at least two years. When the back teeth are involved, the biting surfaces become smoothed and rounded. When the erosion is significant, the edges of the restorations will be higher than the teeth and the occlusion can change.

Since anorectics are extremely thin, dentists may be more vigilant about looking for and realizing the cause of their dental problems. Bulimics are frequently of normal weight, and therefore the erosion on the enamel may be the first recognizable sign of the disorder.

Salivary Gland Enlargement. An estimated 10 to 50 percent of persons who frequently engage in the binge-purge style of eating experience enlargement of the parotid (and occasionally the sublingual) salivary glands. The inflammation is most often painless. The glands usually swell between two and six days after an episode of purging by vomiting. If the binging-vomiting cycle continues, the swelling can become persistent, and the jaw takes on a squarish look. The alteration in appearance may further distort the perception a woman has about her appearance and intensify her eating disorder.

Saliva. Purging by vomiting and taking laxatives and diuretics can reduce the flow of unstimulated saliva. The decreased saliva flow can contribute to dry mouth, which also may be a side effect of the psychoactive medications, especially the antidepressants, that are frequently prescribed for eating disorders.

Gingivitis. Depression, apathy, and feelings of hopelessness frequently accompany eating disorders. When these moods are present, oral hygiene may be lax and infrequent and, as a consequence, plaque accumulates and gingivitis develops. Due to the more severe psychopathology of anorexia nervosa, inattention to brushing and flossing is more common with anorectics than it is with bulimics.

Oral Mucosae. In the process of rapidly eating large amounts of food and then eliciting vomiting, the oral mucous membranes and pharynx can become inflamed and injured. A woman also can injure her soft palate when she uses her fingers or other objects to provoke vomiting.

Treatment. Both anorexia nervosa and bulimia nervosa can have serious medical consequences. With the specter of starvation and suicide hanging over them, the mortality rate for anorectics is estimated to be between 7 and 21 percent. Individuals suffering from eating disorders should be under the care of a physician and psychiatrist or other mental healthcare professional. Dentists who are alert to the symptoms may be the first to detect them and refer the patient for medical help.

To stem further destruction of the teeth, a woman who has an eating disorder (and is undergoing appropriate medical treatment for it) needs to establish and follow a thorough and consistent regimen of oral hygiene. A dentist should clean and apply topical fluoride regularly to her teeth to prevent further erosion and to reduce their sensitivity. At home, she can use a toothpaste designed for sensitive teeth and can apply fluoride via trays. Brushing the teeth right after vomiting can spread the regurgitated acids over their surface. Rinsing with water and then a fluoride mouthrinse might be a better tactic to neutralize the stomach acids.

Teeth damaged by erosion may require restorations to reduce their sensitivity, to correct a malocclusion, and to improve their appearance. Porcelain laminates may be the preferred choice for front teeth that have been eroded significantly because little tooth structure needs to be removed to place them and endodontic therapy is less likely to be involved. If enamel has been lost on the back teeth, fixed prosthetic devices may be required to correct the occlusion. When restorations are placed primarily for aesthetic reasons, their effectiveness may have psychological benefits, beyond the merely cosmetic. By improving her appearance and therefore her self-esteem, a woman suffering from an eating disorder may become more cooperative in her recovery.

Women and Aging

American women, on average, live longer than their male counterparts. Of the more than 30 million Americans over the age of 65, over 18 million of them are women.

Living to an older age, women are more likely to develop and live longer with chronic diseases that affect their dental and overall health. A number of these afflict women in disproportionate numbers compared to men. Women experience rheumatoid arthritis three times as often as men do, and they suffer from depression and osteoarthritis twice as often. The medications taken for these and other disorders can have oral consequences. For example, nonsteroidal anti-inflammatory drugs and gold salts, given for arthritis, can cause oral stomatitis, painful lesions that occur on the oral mucosa, tongue, soft palate, and floor of the mouth. Arthritis can also make it more difficult for women to care for their teeth and dentures. (For more information, see Chapters 10 and 12.)

Sjögren's Syndrome

Of the estimated 1 to 4 million Americans (most of them undiagnosed) who have this autoimmune disease, more than 90 percent are women, most of whom are diagnosed during their fifties. The causes may be genetic factors or a virus, such as Epstein-Barr, that is responsible for the immune system's attacking the exocrine glands (which include the salivary glands).

In both the primary and secondary forms of Sjögren's, the mouth and eyes become extremely dry from either the partial or complete lack of function of the salivary and lacrimal (tear) glands. Individuals with the secondary form have, in addition, a major rheumatic disease, such as rheumatic arthritis, lupus, or scleroderma.

Since sarcoidosis (age-associated dryness of the eyes) can cause dry eyes, and other diseases, including HIV infection, diabetes, hypertension, cystic fibrosis, and depression, as well as medications, can reduce the flow of saliva, these other possible causes of dry mouth or eyes need to be ruled out first. Diagnosis is made from a biopsy of the minor salivary glands, an examination of the eyes, and blood tests.

Symptoms of Sjögren's disorder include difficulty in speaking and swallowing dry food like crackers; a gritty sensation in the eyes; a dry, burning, or sticky feeling in the mouth; and enlargement of the salivary glands. Many find dentures difficult to wear. The decrease in saliva, along with an increase in the strains of destructive bacteria in the mouth, can cause discomfort, an increase in periodontal disease and its rate of progression, caries, and candidiasis.

Treatment. There is no cure for Sjögren's syndrome, but the symptoms and dental damage it produces can be reduced with the measures discussed in Chapter 6. Because they lack sufficient saliva to protect their oral mucosa, people with this condition often avoid eating acidic foods, such as citrus fruits, that can burn their mouths. Eating a balanced diet or taking a vitamin supplement is recommended to correct any nutritional imbalance or deficiency that can result. Candidiasis is treated topically with antifungal medications (such as nystatin) and systemically (amphotericin B) if it becomes severe.

Treating the reduction in or lack of saliva is difficult. A mouth that is dry from Sjögren's syndrome is dry both at rest and when stimulated. (A mouth that is dry as a side effect from medications may be dry at rest but can be stimulated to produce saliva.) Individuals who still retain some ability to produce saliva may benefit from chewing sugarless gum, sucking on hard sugarless candies, or drinking beverages with citrus.

For some patients who can tolerate it, the drug pilocarpine, a saliva stimulant in gel form that works systemically, can increase saliva for a short period. Because it is not recommended for people with certain medical conditions, patients need to check with their physician before taking it. Side effects of pilocarpine can include sweating, desire to urinate, and, very occasionally, nausea. Anethole-trithione and bromhexine, two other saliva stimulants, are available in Canada and Europe but are not yet marketed in the United States.

Osteoporosis

One-third of women over the age of 60 have osteoporosis, a condition in which the bones lose tissue and become weaker and more porous. Some researchers have suggested that the loss of alveolar bone (the part of the jaw in which the roots of the teeth are embedded) that some women experience with age may be a consequence of osteoporosis. Studies have shown that postmenopausal women with osteoporosis have less bone mass and density in their lower jaw and more missing teeth than do postmenopausal women without osteoporosis. Women with the condition also experience more problems with their dentures and require new ones more frequently than women without osteoporosis do.

For dental and other health reasons, women should take precautions to prevent osteoporosis and to reduce bone loss. Measures recommended most frequently include eating calcium-rich foods and taking a calcium supplement (in conjunction with vitamin D to enhance absorption) and engaging in weight-bearing exercise. The acceleration of bone loss after menopause can be slowed (but bone cannot be formed) by estrogen therapy, a mainstay of most treatments to prevent osteoporosis.

MEDICATIONS

Due to the physiological differences between men and women, some medications used in dentistry affect women differently than men. One of the significant distinctions between the genders in this regard is the difference in the ratio of body fat to body mass. Women have a larger proportion of body fat in their bodies than men do. As a consequence, drugs that are stored in fat, such as diazepam (Valium), which is given frequently before treatment to reduce anxiety, will linger in women's bodies longer. If a woman has taken diazepam before the dental visit and is then given an additional dose(s) by the dentist, it could result in an overdose, leading to confusion and hallucinations. For this and other reasons, you must tell your dentist which medications (type and brand) you are taking.

Antibiotics, which are sometimes given for dental treatments, suppress the flora in the vagina that keep the fungus *Candida* in check. When the balance is disturbed, candidiasis can result. Knowing that antibiotics may cause vaginitis, an inflammation of the vaginal tissues characterized by itching, premenopausal women may want to avoid taking them frequently. (Postmenopausal women are less likely to develop vaginitis, as their vaginal flora have been altered already by the lack of estrogen.) Vaginitis can be eradicated by using antifungal medications, such as nystatin, miconazole, or clotrimazole. Nystatin can be given prophylactically before antibiotics are given.

CHAPTER 12

Dental Care for
the Medically
Compromised and
Physically Challenged

Medical conditions can affect your dental health in many ways. Some medications taken for medical disorders cause changes in the mouth; others interact with drugs used in dentistry. Certain dental procedures can produce, for example, high levels of stress, bleeding, or infections. For some individuals, maintaining oral hygiene poses physical difficulties. For the disabled, the logistics of visiting the dentist and the ability to pay for services present problems.

Listed below are some of the dental and medical dilemmas posed by some medical conditions. Within the scope of this book it is not possible to enumerate every risk or precaution for all disorders. If you suffer from any medical problem, you should consult your physician and inform your dentist before seeking dental treatment. But you can relax with the knowledge that your dentist undoubtedly has successfully treated patients with similar medical conditions.

BEFORE TREATMENT

Prior to treatment, your dentist will take a detailed medical and dental history. Tell your dentist about your past and present medical problems and include the medications you are taking, allergies you have, and recent surgeries you have undergone. Your dentist will take your blood pressure and may order different tests, such as blood cell counts, glucose levels, and blood clotting times. Depending on their results, the severity of your ailment, whether you are currently under medical treatment, and the dental treatment required, the dentist may consult with your physician for further evaluation before proceeding with your treatment.

AIDS

Infection with the human immunodeficiency virus (HIV) almost always leads to the complications associated with AIDS (acquired immune deficiency syndrome). Patients are considered to have AIDS when they have a life-threatening infection or malignancy associated with the virus. With the viral infection, a wide range of oral problems can develop. These include candidiasis (a fungal infection), periodontal disease, a variety of ulcers including cold sores, hairy leukoplakia (white patches on the tongue), salivary gland swellings, and head and neck lymph node enlargement. Malignancies, which include the purple mouth lesions from Kaposi's sarcoma, and others, may also be seen. An observant dentist is often the first person to see the oral manifestations of HIV infection. This is very important because the patient may be unaware of the infection. The dentist can then refer the patient for medical consultation and valuable medical treatment that may slow the progress of the disease.

Dentists can treat persons who have HIV infection or AIDS normally. It is only when patients become severely ill that it is advisable to treat them in a hospital setting or special clinic. (As healthcare professionals have become more comfortable with HIV infection and since the passage of the Americans with Disabilities Act, an increasing number of dentists treat patients with HIV infection without question.)

When a dentist practices adequate infection control (explained in Chapter 21), it is virtually impossible for dental patients *not* infected with

HIV to contract AIDS from an office in which HIV-infected patients are treated. In an epidemiological study that has been going on since the beginning of the AIDS epidemic, there has been no documented case of HIV transmission from one dental patient to another dental patient.

ALLERGIES

Normally the body responds to foreign substances (e.g., animal dander, pollen, mites in house dust) by ignoring them. If you are allergic, your immune system overresponds by producing antibodies, proteins manufactured by the body. It is this hypersensitivity that makes your nose run and sneeze; your eyes itch; and your skin swell, itch, and break out in a rash. In rare instances, a very severe form of allergy, called anaphylaxis, can occur. In the unlikely event that anaphylaxis occurs, the dentist should have drugs and instruments to maintain the cardiopulmonary system until emergency support arrives.

Allergies develop when there is a repeated exposure to an allergen or substance that induces the heightened immune response. If you have a history of allergy to one substance, you may be or become allergic to something else. If you tell your dentist that you are allergic to a drug or anesthetic used in a dental procedure, it will not be used. To determine whether your response was an allergy or a side effect of a drug, your dentist may ask you to describe the nature of your past reaction.

A great number of medications, anesthetics, and materials are used in dentistry. Listed below are some that have caused allergies in susceptible individuals.

Medications. The antibiotic penicillin, used in dental treatment in a variety of forms, induces a fairly high rate (between 1 and 10 percent) of allergies. Erythromycin often can be substituted successfully.

Anesthetics. Although rare, allergic reactions have occurred to local anesthetics used in dentistry. Most of these result from the preservative methylparaben (incorporated in lidocaine) and anesthetics containing sulfites, which particularly affect persons with allergic asthma.

Dental Materials. Allergies have been reported to the acrylics used in crowns, bridges, and dentures; composite resins used in fillings; nickel in chrome-cobalt prostheses; eugenol (used in liners for fillings); tooth-pastes; mouthrinses; and, rarely, to gold restorations and the mercury content of dental amalgam. If the soft tissues of your mouth become inflamed on contact with one of these materials, inform your dentist.

BLOOD DISORDERS

Drugs or diseases either can decrease the numbers of platelets in the blood (they are instrumental in its clotting) or disrupt their ability to aggregate. When this occurs, the blood takes longer to clot, cuts and bruises bleed longer and more profusely, and healing is retarded.

The following are some of the types and causes of bleeding disorders for which routine dental procedures can carry risks:

Thrombocytopenia. This disorder entails a reduction in the number of platelets. This can result from an immune reaction (the body develops antibodies to its own platelets); diseases, such as leukemia, lymphoma, and aplastic anemia; severe infections; and a variety of drugs, including quinidine, sulfonamides, heparin, and oral antidiabetics.

Hemophilia. This inherited bleeding disorder results from a deficiency in one of the clotting factors or proteins in the blood that are necessary for coagulation. Bleeding can be excessive and life threatening.

Von Willebrand's Disease. This most common inherited bleeding disorder is caused by a deficiency of one of the clotting factors.

Anticoagulant Medications. These include heparin, dicumarol, and warfarin, which commonly are given to prevent the blood from clotting inside blood vessels to avoid heart attacks or stroke, after surgery, or for kidney dialysis. These medications may cause severe bleeding following dental surgical procedures.

Aspirin. Taken frequently in high doses by persons with rheumatoid arthritis and chronic pain and as a prophylactic measure against heart attacks and strokes, aspirin reduces clot formation by interfering with the ability of platelets to aggregate.

Liver Diseases. These conditions, such as hepatitis and cirrhosis, result frequently in bleeding disorders because they damage the liver where many of the clotting factors are manufactured.

Dental Treatment

If you have a blood disorder and need dental surgery, your dentist will order the necessary tests to determine how long your blood takes to clot. Depending on the result, your dentist may consult with a hematologist before treating you. If your blood clots within an acceptable range, surgery is usually feasible. If it does not and you are taking anticoagulant medication, surgery may be performed provided a physician reduces the dosage at an appropriate time prior to surgery and your dentist takes measures to control bleeding (described subsequently).

To establish normal or near-normal coagulation for individuals who have congenital bleeding disorders (hemophilia, von Willebrand's, etc.), a hematologist needs to replace the missing clotting factor one to three days prior to dental treatment. Persons with thrombocytopenia who have a *significant* decrease in the numbers of their platelets resulting from drug use or an infection should have their condition brought under medical control before they undergo dental treatment. If you are taking aspirin regularly, your physician or dentist may advise you to stop taking it one week before treatment.

During and after treatment dentists can take the following measures to reduce bleeding:

- A local anesthetic can be injected into the submucosa layer of connective tissues in the mouth where there is less chance of contacting a blood vessel.
- The wound or incision can be sutured and / or packed with agents that aid clotting (microfibrillar collagen, thrombin, etc.).
- Occasionally, after a tooth is extracted, a plastic splint similar to a mouthguard can be placed over the soft tissues to assist clot formation.
- Acetaminophen with or without codeine can be recommended for pain instead of aspirin or aspirin-containing medications.

With proper management, many persons with bleeding disorders can be treated effectively on an outpatient basis in a dental office. Hemophiliacs and others with severe bleeding disorders may require hospitalization before dental treatments involving bleeding. In addition, hemophiliacs need to be careful when brushing and flossing their teeth to discourage bleeding.

Anemias

"Anemia" is the term used for a decrease in the numbers of red blood cells or in an abnormality in hemoglobin, a molecule responsible for the transport of oxygen to other parts of the body. Infection (which usually can be prevented with antibiotics) and slowed healing are the usual dental problems associated with anemia. If you have sickle cell trait or disease, you should consult your physician before any dental treatments. Hospitalization is advised if general anesthesia is anticipated.

White Blood Cell Disorders

A variety of white blood cell, whose function is to destroy harmful bacteria, is found in the blood. Therefore, disorders that decrease the numbers of white blood cells or cause abnormalities in them will hamper severely the body's ability to fight infection.

Leukemia. This is a group of cancers that affect the blood. Both the condition and the powerful chemicals and drugs used to treat it can cause oral changes, including swelling, inflammation, and bleeding of the gums, candidiasis, and lesions in the soft tissues of the mouth. Patients whose leukemia is in remission usually can receive dental treatment, although the clotting time of their blood should be tested before scaling or surgery. If the blood clots within the acceptable time, treatment can proceed; if not, it should be postponed. Only conservative emergency care is recommended for patients who have acute symptoms of the disease. To discourage infection, premedication with antibiotics before dental surgery may be recommended if the leukemia is severe.

Leukopenia. In this condition, which can result from drugs, radiation, or disease, there is an abnormal decrease in the numbers of one or all kinds of white blood cells. As a consequence, the individual is susceptible to infection (which may warrant premedication with antibiotics before certain procedures), periodontal disease, and oral ulcers.

CANCER THERAPIES

Radiation that is used to treat cancers of the head and neck can cause a number of acute and chronic dental problems. It can destroy the salivary glands so that the mouth is very dry, swallowing becomes difficult, and dental caries is rampant. Other oral side effects of radiation therapy include mucositis (the tissues of the mouth become sore, ulcerate, and bleed easily), candidiasis, sensitivity of the teeth, loss of taste, and damage to the bone caught in the radiation beam. The drugs used in chemotherapy can cause mucositis and suppress bone marrow production; the latter produces anemias and increases the individual's risk of excessive bleeding and infection.

You should have all needed dental work, such as fillings, root canal therapy, and oral prophylaxis, completed before starting radiation therapy or chemotherapy. If your teeth cannot be repaired or there is advanced periodontal disease, they may need to be removed prior to therapy. (Extraction after therapy can result in an infection in the jaw that is difficult for an immune system or bone compromised by radiation to combat). Antibiotics must be given prior to dental surgery. To maintain optimal dental health and prevent severe caries, you should establish a good regimen of oral hygiene including daily fluoride applications via toothpaste, gel applied in a tray, and a mouthrinse (some dentists may recommend chlorhexidine rinse). Throughout the cancer therapy a dentist should monitor your dental health and manage the oral complications that develop frequently. Your regular general dentist may not feel competent to treat the oral complications associated with cancer chemotherapy and may refer you to a dentist with more experience in this area.

CARDIOVASCULAR SYSTEM DISORDERS

Be sure to tell your dentist if you have any type of cardiovascular disease so that appropriate precautions may be taken when treating you. Only urgent dental treatment is recommended if you have a serious cardiovascular disorder, such as very high blood pressure, unstable angina, or congestive heart failure that is severe, unstable, or not well controlled. The same restriction applies if you have suffered a heart attack within the past six months.

Bacterial Endocarditis

One of the most serious complications of dental treatment for persons with some forms of cardiovascular disorders is the possibility of developing bacterial endocarditis, an infection of the heart valves and tissues. When bleeding in the mouth occurs, bacteria (most often *streptococci* and *staphylococci*), fungi, and other microorganisms can enter the bloodstream and travel to the heart valves where they lodge on valves scarred and roughened by previous disease or surgery. This may result in further damage and/or infection. Individuals with cardiovascular defects should consult their physicians about taking systemic antibiotics (and the use of antibacterial mouthrinses) before dental surgery, probing, professional cleaning, or other procedures that involve bleeding in the gums or mouth. The American Heart Association (AHA) has developed guidelines, which are endorsed by the American Dental Association (ADA), for patients who are at risk of developing endocarditis. The AHA recommends prophylactic antibiotics for certain dental procedures for persons with:

- Mitral valve prolapse with valvular regurgitation
- History of certain types of vascular surgery
- Artificial heart valves
- Rheumatic heart disease caused by rheumatic fever
- Presence or history of significant heart murmurs (caused by structural abnormalities in the heart)
- Unrepaired or persistent congenital heart defect or lesion
- History of bacterial endocarditis

If you have another cardiovascular or medical condition, you may be premedicated with antibiotics before dental treatment if your dentist and physician feel it is warranted. Consult with your dentist about your oral hygiene and what you should do to avoid unnecessary damage to oral structures that could cause bacteria to enter the bloodstream.

Stress-Related Problems

When faced with stress, the body reacts by releasing adrenaline, a hormone from the adrenal glands. Adrenaline causes the heart to beat faster and the blood vessels to narrow, and thereby raises the blood pressure.

Epinephrine, a synthetic form of adrenaline (and drugs with similar action, which are sometimes added to local anesthesia to prolong its effects) has pharmacologic effects similar to those of adrenaline. When used excessively or injected inadvertently into a blood vessel in patients with cardiovascular problems or a history of stroke, it can present some risks. Yet when epinephrine is used in local anesthesia in a low concentration of 1 part to 100,000 and not injected into a blood vessel, it should not have this effect. However, there are local anesthesias, which your dentist may choose if you have cardiovascular disease, that do not require the addition of epinephrine. Both the AHA and the ADA recommend that vasoconstrictors should be used in dentistry only if their use shortens the procedures and increases the pain relief. They also advise that local anesthetics containing vasoconstrictors should never be injected into a blood vessel and always be used in the smallest possible amounts.

If you feel the stress of a dental visit might put you at risk of some cardiovascular condition, consult your physician and ask your dentist for antianxiety medication or nitrous-oxide–oxygen inhalation to reduce anxiety. To further minimize stress, schedule dental appointments for the morning or early afternoon hours and keep them short (which may mean more visits).

Tendency to Bleed

Bleeding may be excessive after scaling and surgical dental procedures if your blood pressure is elevated significantly or if you are using anticoagulant medications (which are frequently given to prevent heart attacks or after heart surgery). The precautions listed in the section "Dental Treatment" under "Blood Disorders" should be taken.

Angina Pectoris

This brief, intense chest pain caused by a reduction in blood flow to a portion of heart muscle is a common symptom of coronary artery disease. Since the stress and anxiety of a dental visit may trigger an angina attack, dentists will take those measures that reduce stress and are listed in the section "Stress-Related Problems." If your angina is stable, routine dental care can be administered provided the appropriate precautions are taken. Vasoconstrictors used in local anesthetics (with the exception of epinephrine in low doses), in packing material for gum tissues, and to control local bleeding should be avoided. Substitutions for retraction cords used for crowns and bridges, which contain alum or zinc chloride, are available. You should bring your medication to the dentist with you. If you forget, your dentist probably will have nitroglycerin or amyl nitrite.

If you experience chest pain during the visit, your dentist may decide to terminate and reschedule the appointment. If you have the unstable form of angina, you should receive only dental care that is necessary to prevent or treat dental pain and/or infection. The previously stated precautions about vasoconstrictors and local anesthesia apply to patients with angina.

Hypertension

A dentist who knows you have hypertension (high blood pressure) will make every effort to make your dental appointment as relaxed and stress-free as possible (see the suggestions in "Stress-Related Problems"). To further reduce anxiety, the dentist may prescribe a low dose of a benzo-diazepine, such as diazepam (Valium), the night before and one hour prior to the appointment. The use of nitrous-oxide–oxygen inhalation as a sedative during the visit is another option.

Medications used to treat hypertension can cause oral side effects (decreased salivation, oral lesions, gingival hyperplasia), produce nausea and vomiting when the gag reflex is stimulated, or interact adversely with vasoconstrictors employed in dental procedures. For these reasons, it is important to tell your dentist what medications you are taking, so that he or she can take the necessary precautions. For example, to prevent your blood pressure from rising, a dentist will avoid or use judiciously local anesthetics containing epinephrine if you are on adrenergic inhibitors or other antihypertensive drugs. Likewise, to avoid a hypertensive crisis, a dentist will not administer phenylephrine to persons taking monoamine oxidase (MAO) inhibitors or tricyclic antidepressants. Gingival retraction cords used for crown and bridge procedures also contain a vasoconstrictor that should not be used on someone with high blood pressure; effective substitutes are available.

Many types of antihypertensive medications, among them diuretics and adrenergic blockers, can cause postural hypotension, a rapid drop in blood pressure that occurs on standing or sitting up after lying down. To prevent the loss of consciousness (fainting) that can result, the dentist should return the dental chair to a vertical position gradually and recommend that the patient rise slowly.

Outpatient general anesthesia, administered in the dental office, is recommended only for hypertensive persons who fit the American Society of Anesthesiologists classification as healthy and normal or who have mild systemic disease. It is not advised for patients whose blood pressure is controlled by drugs or is greater than 200/104. Most dentists will want to consult with a physician for patients whose blood pressure is high. No one who has severe uncontrolled hypertension should undergo an elective dental procedure because there is a risk of excessive bleeding following surgery.

Valve Disorders

For more detail regarding antibiotic prophylaxis before certain dental treatments for the following conditions, see the section "Bacterial Endocarditis."

Mitral Valve Prolapse. To avoid the possibility of infection, individuals with mitral valve prolapse need to be premedicated with antibiotics before dental treatments that are likely to cause bleeding.

Heart Murmurs. Antibiotics are not required before dental treatment for innocent or functional murmurs, as there is no cardiac abnormality. Examples of common innocent murmurs not requiring antibiotic prophylaxis include ones detected during childhood and pregnancy that disappear before adolescence and after birth, respectively. Organic murmurs are caused by a defect in the heart and do require antibiotics before dental treatment to discourage cardiac infection.

What type heart murmur you have should be determined by a physician and not your dentist. If you report a murmur in your medical history, your dentist most likely will want to consult with your physician or cardiologist before treating you.

Prosthetic Heart Valves. Individuals with artificial heart valves are at high risk for contracting bacterial endocarditis from dental procedures involving bleeding. Therefore, it is essential that they receive prophylactic antibiotics before dental treatments that carry a likelihood of bleeding.

HORMONAL DISORDERS

The endocrine system comprises a number of glands and tissues that secrete hormones, chemical substances that trigger a response in another organ or part of the body. Through signals from nerves and other organs, hormones regulate many bodily activities, including reproduction, growth, metabolism, and the balance of fluids.

Diabetes Mellitus

In diabetes there is some defect in the amount, use, or release of insulin, a hormone produced in the pancreas. Diabetes affects nearly all functions of the body.

When diabetes is not well controlled, the white blood cells, which destroy disease-causing microorganisms, do not function well. As a result, the body's resistance is impaired, and the diabetic is made vulnerable to infections and slow to heal. The mouth frequently mirrors the diabetic's susceptibility to infection, with the development of candidiasis, ulcers, and periodontal disease. If you have diabetes, tell your dentist and discuss whether there is a need to talk to your physician regarding the timing and length of dental visits.

Adrenal Insufficiency

The adrenal glands are located on top of each kidney. They consist of a cortex and medulla. The medulla secretes epinephrine and norepinephrine, called catecholamines, and other similar molecules that function as nerve transmitters. The cortex, or outer portion, of the adrenal glands secretes a number of hormones that help to regulate the metabolism of fat, carbohydrates, and protein and maintain fluid balance and blood pressure.

Adrenal insufficiency, or hypofunction, can be caused by disease (e.g., Addison's disease) or the use of adrenal corticosteroids, which suppress the natural secretory activity of the adrenal cortex. It increases the individual's susceptibility to infection and retards wound healing. The dentist should determine the cause of your adrenal insufficiency so that the appropriate precautions can be taken. These might include increasing the dosage of steroids before extensive dental treatment and/or taking measures to minimize stress during dental procedures.

Thyroid Disease

The thyroid gland, located in the neck near the trachea and the larynx, controls almost all metabolic processes in the body. It depends on iodine to produce its hormone, thyroxine.

Hyperthyroidism. An overactive thyroid produces excess thyroxine, which causes the metabolic processes to speed up and results in weight loss, rapid heart beat, prominent eyes, and nervousness. When the disorder is not well controlled, medical evaluation is recommended before treatment because infection, trauma, and the stress of dental treatment may pose problems.

Hypothyroidism. To stimulate an underactive thyroid, thyroid hormones are administered. Because untreated hypothyroid patients might encounter some serious problems during dental treatment, dentists will refer dental patients who are suspected of having the condition (and are not being treated) to a physician.

INFLAMMATORY JOINT DISORDERS

Arthritis

Arthritis, or inflammation of the joints, is a large group of disorders affecting the muscles, joints, and bones. Both rheumatoid arthritis and osteoarthritis, the two most common forms, can affect the temporomandibular joint and cause it to become stiff and painful. The problems can become so severe that they require therapy, which can include surgery. Aspirin and nonsteroidal anti-inflammatory drugs, taken to treat the joint pain and inflammation associated with these diseases, can cause bleeding, whereas therapy with gold salts and sulfasalazine can induce inflammation in the mouth.

The pain and immobility caused by these disorders may require accommodations during treatment and care. These include using supports while sitting in the dental chair, changing positions frequently, and modifying home dental care (see also Chapter 10).

Artificial Joints

The tissues surrounding the plastic or metal prostheses used to replace joints damaged by rheumatoid arthritis and injuries (most commonly the knees and hips; less commonly the shoulders, elbows, and wrists) are prone to bacterial infection. There is no firm evidence that bacteria from the mouth caused by dental treatment can infect these sites. However, persons who have severe type 1 diabetes, hemophilia, active rheumatoid arthritis, immune deficiency, a loose prosthesis, or a history of an infected one are at an increased risk for infections in general. Whether prophylactic antibiotics are needed for dental treatments should be determined on an individual basis in consultation with an orthopedic surgeon.

KIDNEY DISEASE

There are different kidney disorders that can progress to chronic renal failure and severely compromise the organ's functioning. The resulting deterioration affects many systems in the body and has the following repercussions for dental treatment:

Risk of Bleeding. This is increased from anticoagulants taken before dialysis and from the filtering of the blood by an artificial kidney. Individuals who are on dialysis should have the clotting time of their blood checked.

Risk of Anemia. This is increased because the factor that stimulates the formation of red blood cells is produced in the kidney.

Intolerance to Drugs Used in Dentistry. Many analgesics, nonsteroidal anti-inflammatory drugs, and antibiotics are eliminated in the kidneys. Because these medications can reach toxic levels when not promptly eliminated and damage an already impaired organ, they should not be taken by individuals who have kidney disorders.

LIVER DISORDERS

Cirrhosis (which usually results from chronic abuse of alcohol) and viral hepatitis are two of the most common liver disorders. Cirrhosis is a chronic liver disease in which the normal liver architecture is replaced by scar tissue and fat. Liver and kidney failure can ensue.

Many of the drugs used in dentistry, among them diazepam (Valium), local anesthetics, barbiturates, and some antibiotics, are metabolized in the liver. If liver function is deficient, substitutions or reductions in dosages may be required. Persons whose livers are scarred from cirrhosis tend to bleed and thus require the measures to control excess bleeding that are explained in the section "Blood Disorders."

NEUROLOGICAL DISORDERS

Individuals with disorders involving the central and peripheral nervous systems, such as epilepsy, Parkinson's disease, multiple sclerosis, stroke, and cerebral palsy frequently experience difficulty brushing and flossing their teeth. In addition, some medications taken for these disorders can cause xerostomia (dry mouth). (See also Chapter 10.)

Epilepsy

When treating patients known to be epileptic, especially those who experience the most severe symptoms, measures to alleviate stress should be taken. Many anticonvulsants interact with drugs used in dental treatments, such as opioid analgesics, anesthetics, and antianxiety medications.

Gingival hyperplasia, an overgrowth of the gums, is a common side effect of phenytoin (Dilantin), an anticonvulsant medication. If it becomes severe, surgery may be required to correct it. Studies indicate that practicing good oral hygiene can reduce its severity.

Most dentists recommend that stronger, less fracture-prone materials that are better able to withstand the damage sustained during a seizure be used to replace or restore teeth for persons with epilepsy. Thus, a removable prosthesis is preferred over a fixed prosthesis, and metal and acrylics usually are better choices than porcelain.

Stroke (Cerebrovascular Accident)

During a stroke, the blood supply to the brain is interrupted by a clot blocking an artery or by a rupture of a vessel. With the loss of its blood supply, brain tissue dies. Usually a stroke results from a chronic cardiovascular disease, such as atherosclerosis or high blood pressure. Survivors frequently are left with compromised motor function and sometimes reduced mental capacities, which make it difficult for them to care for their teeth and gums. The dentist should take measures to reduce stress during treatment and take precautions to stem bleeding for individuals who are on aspirin, coumadin, dipyridamole, and other medications with anticoagulant properties.

ORGAN TRANSPLANTS

Candidates for transplants of the kidney, pancreas, heart, liver, or bone marrow are in a severe end stage of disease. Hemodialysis can keep individuals with end-stage renal disease alive, but their quality of life improves with a kidney transplant. The severity of their medical situation requires that organ-transplant candidates and recipients consult with a physician before they receive dental treatment, both before and after transplantation.

Recipients of organ transplants heal poorly, can bleed excessively, are vulnerable to infection, and may not respond well to stress. The immunosuppressive drugs they must take for the rest of their lives can cause lymphoma, squamous cell carcinomas of the skin and lip, Kaposi's sarcoma, high blood pressure, candidiasis, gingival and periodontal disease, anemia, diabetes, and gingival overgrowth of gum tissue, all of which have an impact on their oral health. As a consequence, they require appropriate therapy for these problems and must adhere to an aggressive regimen of oral hygiene. Their dentists need to take suitable precautions and may consult with their physicians to avert complications that can arise during dental care.

RESPIRATORY AND LUNG DISORDERS

Persons who have asthma, chronic bronchitis, emphysema, cystic fibrosis, lung cancer, and other respiratory and lung disorders have difficulty breathing and delivering enough oxygen to their lungs and the rest of their body. Because some of the medications and anesthetics given for dental treatments further depress respiration and/or because individuals with these conditions frequently are on medications that interact with those used in dentistry, dentists need to consult with the physician in charge and modify the following aspects of dental care:

- Barbiturates and narcotics should not be used because they depress respiration.
- Antihistamines and anticholinergics should not be given to persons who have chronic bronchitis and emphysema. These medications cause the mouth to dry and make it more difficult to clear mucous from the throat and nasal passages.
- General anesthesia should be administered in a hospital only.
- The antibiotic erythromycin should not be given to individuals who are taking theophylline; it also decreases the sedative effect of diazepam.
- Patients taking corticosteroids may require supplementation of these drugs.
- Nitrous-oxide–oxygen inhalation for sedation is acceptable for most asthmatics, but it is not appropriate for persons who have emphysema, chronic bronchitis, or cystic fibrosis.
- Patients with severe chronic bronchitis or emphysema should remain upright in the dental chair to avoid compromising their breathing.
- A rubber dam (a thin piece of rubber used to isolate individual teeth during dental procedures, such as fillings, crowns, and root canal therapy) should not be used on persons with severe chronic bronchitis or emphysema.

- Asthmatics should bring their inhalers to every dental appointment.
- To avoid inciting an asthma attack, aspirin, nonsteroidal anti-inflammatory drugs, and local anesthetics that contain sulfites (see "Allergies") should not be administered. In addition, the dentist needs to take measures to alleviate stress.

THE PHYSICALLY AND MENTALLY CHALLENGED

People who are functionally impaired as a result of injuries, mental retardation, or congenital defects, including spinal cord injury, multiple sclerosis, blindness, Alzheimer's disease, arthritis, cerebral palsy, stroke, or Down syndrome, face obstacles concerning their dental care. They may have varying degrees of difficulty in performing routine dental hygiene; this increases their risk of periodontal disease and caries. Many require assistance in getting to and from the dentist's office. Because their handicap may affect their ability to earn a living, many will have difficulty paying for dental services or be on Medicaid, which has limited provisions for dental treatment. (Box 12.1 offers tips for caregivers who assist those who are impaired in performing home dental care; Box 12.2 lists organizations offering financial assistance and referrals of dentists. Chapter 10 offers suggestions on home care when manual dexterity is limited.)

BOX 12.1

TIPS FOR HELPING INDIVIDUALS WHO NEED ASSISTANCE WITH THEIR DENTAL HYGIENE

If you brush and floss the teeth for someone who is unable to or has difficulty doing so, you may find that the following suggestions make it easier. When he or she is:

Sitting in a Wheelchair. Stand behind the wheelchair and wrap your arm around the person's neck. Cup the chin with your hand. Use the chair or your body and a pillow to brace the person's head.

Lying Down. Sit on a sofa with the person's head in your lap or on a pillow. Bend over from behind the head.

Sitting in a Foam or Beanbag Chair. These are helpful for individuals who are unable to sit up straight. Stand next to or behind the chair and cradle the person's head with your arm.

A Child or a Small Person Sitting in a Wheelchair. Lock the wheels and tip the wheelchair back. Support the chair in your lap or against your body as you sit or stand behind it.

In preparation:

• Be sure there is good lighting.
• Explain what you are going to do before starting.
• Schedule sessions when the person is well rested and most cooperative.
• Have all positions for brushing and flossing approved by the individual's physician and dentist.

During care:

• Move in a calm and slow manner.
• Encourage the person to perform as much as he or she can alone.
• Use a mouth prop for individuals who are unable to keep their mouths open. Before using, ask their dentists whether it is appropriate and how to insert it without causing injury or anxiety.

When helping someone with Alzheimer's disease or another disorder that has resulted in disorientation and the loss of memory:

• Demonstrate the procedure and have the person follow your movements.
• Use visual aids, such as a picture of the step-by-step process of brushing and flossing.

BOX 12.2

RESOURCES

The following organizations offer varying amounts of assistance for disabled persons.

American Dental Association (for address see Appendix 1)

American Academy of Pediatric Dentistry (for address see Appendix 1)

National Foundation of Dentistry for the Handicapped
1800 Glenarm Place, Suite 500
Denver, CO 80202
800-366-3331
It operates a dental van program in New Jersey, Colorado, and Chicago, Illinois.

The Grottoes of North America
Dentistry for the Handicapped
1696 Brice Road
Reynoldsburg, OH 43068
614-860-9193
Fax# 614-860-9099
This fraternal organization, affiliated with the Masons, provides reduced-fee care for some dental services for children under the ages of 18 who have muscular dystrophy, cerebral palsy, mental retardation, and myasthenia gravis. Treatment can be administered at the Illinois Masonic Medical Center in Chicago and at the Medical College of Ohio in Toledo. In other parts of the country, children can be treated by individual dentists who submit a preauthorization claim to the group prior to treatment.

Choosing a Dentist

Although all dentists should have the requisite dental skills to treat patients who are physically or mentally challenged, the latter may prefer to be treated by dentists who are familiar and better equipped to deal with their special needs. Dentists and their staffs usually need to devote extra time and have more patience in dealing with special patients. In addition, dental offices must be designed to have space that is free of obstacles and large enough for a wheelchair to maneuver. Dentists, hygienists, and assistants who introduce an instrument or procedure slowly may be more successful in reducing a patient's anxiety. For recommendations of dentists, try the following sources:

- Your state dental society (see Appendix 3).
- A local chapter of an organization specializing in a disorder, for example, the Arthritis Foundation or National Down Syndrome Society. Their telephone numbers and addresses can be found in the white pages of the phone book or in the *Encyclopedia of Associations* available at a local library.
- A primary care physician if associated with a teaching hospital that has a dentist on its staff who is knowledgeable regarding the treatment of disabled patients.
- The organizations listed in Box 12.2.

Making Appointments

When making the appointment, be certain to:

- Ask whether the building is accessible for the disabled.
- Describe the restrictions or needs the patient has.
- Inquire about parking or public transportation to the office.
- Find out whether there is an elevator. If there is, ask whether it is self- or assistant-operated and (if applicable) whether the buttons can be reached from a wheelchair.

PART V

DENTAL PROBLEMS
AND
TREATMENTS

CHAPTER 13

Endodontics

If ever a reputation preceded a procedure in dentistry, it would be that of root canal therapy. The pain that many equate with it is attributable more frequently to the painful symptoms a tooth exhibits because it *needs* treatment than any discomfort involved with the procedure itself. For most people, the most uncomfortable part of root canal treatment is the injection of the anesthetic. The treatment itself hurts only for a small, and sometimes vocal, minority. In fact, many welcome endodontic treatment because it relieves the pain that has resulted from a diseased pulp. And finally, having a diseased tooth treated endodontically before the inflammation spreads beyond the root prevents far greater pain and dental destruction in the future.

WHAT IS ENDODONTICS?

Endodontics is the branch of dentistry that is concerned with preventing, diagnosing, and treating diseases and injuries to the dental pulp and the soft tissues and bone surrounding the tip of the root. An endodontist is the dental specialist trained in performing endodontic treatments.

THE DENTAL PULP

Dental pulp is the soft tissue inside the tooth that contains cells, nerves, blood, and lymph vessels. The area that contains the pulp tissue within the crown of the tooth is called the pulp chamber and the space within each root is called a root or pulp canal. (To help you visualize the anatomy, refer to Illustration 1.1.) Some teeth have more than one root and therefore have more than one root canal. Some roots also have more than one canal.

The pulp canal extends to the tip of the roots and the apical foramen, the opening at the tip of the root. At this opening, blood vessels enter and exit the tooth, supplying the oxygen and nutrients to maintain the pulp. The pulp contains a network of nerves that also gain entry at this opening. The nerves that come from branches of the trigeminal nerve (the fifth cranial nerve) are necessary for chewing and control of the face and are the ones that transmit pain from heat or cold or pressure on the tooth.

Both the pulp chamber and root canals are encased in dentin. Because of its close connection with dentin, the pulp and dentin should be thought of as a complex. Although hard, dentin is not solid. It consists of tubules that act as a sieve and are large enough to allow bacteria to pass through. They are filled with fluid that moves in response to temperature changes and pressure. When something cold, like ice cream, is eaten, the fluid contracts. Conversely, the fluid expands when something hot, such as coffee, touches the tooth. The movement of the fluid stimulates the sensory nerve fibers, and these sensations register as pain when the pulp is inflamed from decay (caries) or injury or when there are open dentinal tubules during cavity preparation.

The pulp also has a close connection to the periodontal ligament through the nerves and blood vessels that enter and exit at the apical foramen. Through this link, an infection in the pulp can spread to the soft tissues and bone in the periapical area surrounding the tip of the root and set the stage for potent destruction.

DAMAGE TO THE PULP

Damage by bacteria from caries is the most common cause of pulp disease. Whenever the pulp is exposed, it will be invaded quickly by bacteria. The bacteria can reach the pulp as a result of caries, inadequate cavity preparation, attrition (wear), erosion, abrasion, or a crack or fracture in the dentin in the crown or root of the tooth. Cracks or fractures may appear at the margin of or under a restoration or be created by caries or injury. Many microorganisms cause infection of the pulp, but *streptococci* and strains of anaerobic bacteria, for example, *Bacteroides,* are the ones cultured most often from infected pulps.

Although they are not as frequent causes of damage as bacterial invasion, dental pulp can also become injured by trauma, heat, and dental procedures. If a blow to a tooth is sudden and strong enough, it can sever

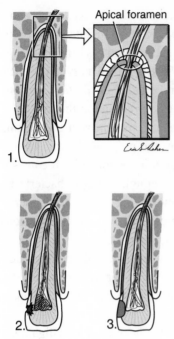

Apical foramen

1.

2.

3.

ILLUSTRATION 13.1.
AVOIDING ROOT CANAL THERAPY.
As this illustration shows, having caries, or decay, treated early often prevents damage to the tooth's pulp that requires root canal therapy. **1.** Nerves and blood vessels enter and exit through the apical foramen to keep the pulp of the tooth alive. **2.** When caries attacks the tooth, even though it does not invade the pulp, it can cause it to inflame. **3.** By having caries removed and treated with a filling before the caries invades the pulp, the inflammation can subside and the pulp can return to health.

the blood supply and the pulp will die without becoming inflamed. The pulp can be damaged whether or not the crown or the root of the tooth is fractured.

Various dental procedures, among them cavity or crown preparation, have the potential for damaging the pulp. Tooth wear from abrasion or attrition, including habits such as grinding the teeth or using them to hold pins, as a tool, or to bite fingernails or thread, can occasionally be so severe that they damage the pulp.

THE DISEASE PROCESS

When the bacteria first invade the pulp, they are confined to a small portion of it. With the pulp surrounded by rigid dentin, the inflammation has no place to swell. When it is severe, the inflammation *may* cause pain, yet most persons are still unaware of the infection. Why some people feel pain and others do not is not known.

Local areas of tissue death within the pulp can develop. The inflammation can be chronic and localized for quite some time, and then flare up or eventually cause the death of the pulp. Some but not all people feel pain.

When the pulp dies, the bacteria invade the dead tissue. The dead pulp supplies food for the bacteria, and so helps to perpetuate the infection. Bacterial by-products seep out via the apical foramen to the soft tissues and bone surrounding the tip of the root where they create an inflammation around the tip of the root. This may provoke pain, especially when the tooth is depressed slightly in its socket.

To create space for an expanding inflammation, the body resorbs or dissolves bone, in this case, the alveolar bone surrounding the tip of the root. When large numbers of bacteria escape through the apical foramen, a local pocket of pus can form in the periapical area and produce an *acute apical abscess,* a potentially serious infection. As the body mounts its defenses to fight infection, the area swells, the tooth feels raised in its socket, and some individuals develop a fever and feel weak. Fortunately, these symptoms are almost always dramatic enough to send the patient to visit a dentist. Yet even though someone may be experiencing extreme discomfort, the inflammation may not show on a radiograph until sufficient bone has been resorbed. An acute apical abscess has the potential to destroy the alveolar bone that supports and surrounds the affected tooth. If enough bone has been destroyed, the tooth may have to be extracted.

When the alveolar bone resorbs, the pressure is relieved along with the pain in many cases. If an acute apical abscess is not treated or is not localized and extends to other areas in the face, it can cause cellulitis. A danger of cellulitis is that the infection may spread through the lymph system and blood to the brain or spinal cord. A severe infection in the lower jaw can produce swelling that is so great that air passages are closed off. If this occurs and the infection is not treated correctly and rapidly, death may result.

An untreated periapical infection may also spread beyond the area immediately surrounding the affected root to infect other areas of the alveolar bone and cause osteomyelitis, a very dangerous infection that must be treated without delay. At this point, the pain is severe, the lymph nodes are swollen, the teeth are loose and uncomfortable, and the person has a fever.

Organisms that are not quite as virulent can produce a chronic abscess, usually without symptoms. If the inflammation drains through a sinus tract, the only symptom may be a gum boil or a bad taste.

DISEASES OF THE PULP

Listed here are some of the types of pulp diseases. Although which type disease you have is not as important as whether the pulp of your tooth is alive or dead, knowing which type helps your dentist determine whether you require endodontic therapy and, if you do, which treatment will be effective.

Pulpitis

Pulpitis, or inflammation of the pulp, can be chronic or acute, affect a portion or all of the pulp, may involve bacteria, and may cause pain, although frequently it does not. Not all damage or inflammation of the pulp results in its death.

When the pulpitis is reversible, the pulp will react to an irritant or injury by depositing an extra layer of dentin to protect the pulp. This allows it to recover and return to a noninflamed state. Pulpitis is deemed irreversible when the pulp is unable to recover and the irritant or injury leads ultimately to the death of the pulp. How the pulp reacts to irritation (e.g., physical injury, thermal injury from heat generated during cavity preparation, bacteria from caries, or dentin that is exposed at the neck of the tooth by abrasion) depends on the severity of the irritation, the individual, and the inherent resistance of the pulp to injury. The line between reversible and irreversible cannot always be predicted.

Hyperplastic Pulpitis. This type of irreversible pulpitis is sometimes called a pulp polyp. It usually develops only in children and young adults. It is a large, open cavity leading to the pulp chamber that is covered with granulated pulp tissue and caused by caries. Although it looks as if it should hurt, it seldom causes discomfort, except during chewing. Root canal therapy is required provided the tooth roots are fully developed.

Pulp Degeneration. This condition, which is most often present in older persons, takes various forms. Part of the pulp may be replaced with stones of calcified material. These most commonly develop in the pulp chamber, although they can also be present in the root canal. It is generally harmless and painless and may be part of the aging process.

Internal Root Resorption. In this disorder, cells digest the hard tissue of the dentin surrounding the pulp chamber and the root canals and the tooth is resorbed (dissolved) from within. It is caused by an infection in the dentin. Many people who have it remember having had a previous injury to the tooth. It has also been known to occur in teeth that have caries, have received orthodontic treatment, or have cracked. The process may develop slowly, over one or two years, or very quickly, and is always painless. Internal resorption may involve the root or the crown of the tooth or both. Although it can affect any tooth, it is most common in the upper front teeth.

Occasionally, when the resorption is advanced and occurs in the crown of the tooth, it may cause a pink spot. More commonly, it is detected through routine radiographs. Because it almost never corrects itself, teeth with it should receive root canal therapy. Treatment is usually successful if the resorption has not penetrated through the crown or the root. If the resorption continues, it can perforate the root of the tooth. When this occurs, it is difficult to seal the root during endodontic treatment.

Necrosis, or Death, of the Pulp

Dental pulp can die as a result of any of the causes of pulp disease just considered. It can also occur as a result of inflammation, an injury before inflammation occurs, and the harmful bacteria that cause periodontal disease.

A fully necrotic pulp produces no pain. For this reason and because it does not always show on a radiograph, pulp death can be difficult to diagnose. If only some of the pulp has died, the tooth may still be painful when exposed to heat or cold. The first sign that the pulp has died may be discoloration; the tooth may take on a gray cast and look dull.

DISEASES OF
THE PERIAPICAL AREA

Acute apical periodontitis and acute apical abscess are explained in the preceding section entitled "The Disease Process." When an apical periodontitis becomes chronic, it usually causes no or only a few mild symptoms, such as a little tenderness when the area over the root tip is touched or the tooth is tapped. A chronic apical periodontitis can become an acute abscess after a period of quiescence. It is then labeled a phoenix abscess, for the legendary and eponymous bird's ability to die and resurrect itself. A phoenix abscess may occur after endodontic treatment on a tooth with chronic apical periodontitis. During the treatment, bacteria may be spread forcibly to the periapical area or air may be introduced when the tooth is opened up, and thus cause a flare-up. Soon after, the person who had no symptoms develops pain and swelling.

In external root resorption, the dental hard tissues are eaten up, or resorbed, by osteoclasts, cells that destroy bones, as well as other tissues. With *surface resorption,* the resorption remains confined to the root surface. It can be caused by clenching the teeth, orthodontic treatment, or trauma.

External inflammatory resorption works from the outside of the root inward. If the pulp of the tooth is infected, the osteoclasts continue resorbing. Endodontic treatment is necessary to halt the destruction.

The resorption will continue if the stimulus, for example, orthodontic force, remains. The damage can become so great that it destroys the periodontal ligament, which separates the tooth from the bone. When this happens, the tooth and bone fuse; this causes *ankylosis* and *replacement resorption.*

WHO SHOULD PERFORM ENDODONTIC THERAPY?

Endodontists are the dentists who are most knowledgeable about the diseases of the dental pulp and their treatment. Yet many patients, especially those who live in parts of the country where they do not have ready access to dental specialists, go to general dentists for their endodontic therapy. Although many general dentists are competent to treat endodontic cases, your general dentist should refer you to an endodontist if you request one and/or your problem is beyond your dentist's capabilities or experience.

DIAGNOSIS

Dentists use a number of different tests to diagnose pulp and periapical diseases and to determine whether endodontic treatment is required. They also rely, sometimes to a great extent, on the symptoms their patients are experiencing.

Pain

Frequently the first sign of injury to the pulp that drives someone to the dentist is pain. An estimated 90 percent of all dental pain is endodontically related. And yet many times when the pulp is diseased or dead, there is no pain. Many people are surprised when their dentist, after a routine exam, tells them they need root canal treatment.

If your face or one of your teeth hurts, your dentist will listen carefully as you describe your pain, its location and duration. When the inflammation is confined to the pulp, it may be difficult for you to identify the specific tooth that is the source of pain. The pain may be spread over a number of teeth or be referred to other ones. When a back tooth is involved, you may feel the pain outside your mouth or in your sinuses, temple, or ear. The pain from an inflamed tooth seldom will be referred, however, across the midline to the other side of your face. When you can identify the tooth that hurts, it is usually an indication that the inflammation has spread beyond the tooth into the periodontal ligament.

Different people describe the pain of pulp disease differently. Some feel it occasionally, whereas others feel it continuously. To some, the pain is sharp or shooting, and severe; for others, it is only a mild ache.

How long the pain lingers frequently is an indication that the pulp is involved. A tooth that is painful for a short period and only when exposed to cold, *may* recover on its own or after having the irritant, such as caries, removed and a filling placed. (More frequently, however, caries produces a pulpitis that has no symptoms and will resolve once the lesion is treated.) These quick stabs of sometimes intense pain may last for weeks or months until the pulp either dies or recovers.

Pain that persists for minutes to hours after the stimulus (cold, heat, sweet) is removed or is present when there is no apparent cause frequently indicates pulp disease that needs to be endodontically treated. In general, a tooth that is painful when it is exposed to heat or when you chew or change the position of your head usually requires endodontic therapy. When the inflammation has extended to the periapical area, the pain can become so intense that it either awakens you or keeps you from sleeping altogether and may be accompanied by fever and nausea.

Examination

After asking you about the pain, the dentist examines the hard and soft tissues of the mouth for changes in color, contour, and consistency. For example, if inflammation is present in the oral mucosa, it may have reddened lesions or appear grayish and swollen instead of pink, and it may be spongy, rather than firm, to the touch. Likewise, teeth that are discolored or opaque may indicate that the pulp is inflamed, dead, or degenerated. (They can also be stained from old amalgam or root canal fillings or from tetracycline.) The dentist examines the teeth for cracks where bacteria might gain entry.

To determine whether the infection has spread to the periodontal ligament, the dentist will tap the tooth (or teeth if you cannot locate which tooth is bothering you) with a finger or an instrument to detect pain or sensitivity. Sensitivity or pain when a tooth is tapped can also be caused by other dental problems, among them rapid orthodontic movement of the teeth, a restoration that is too high, a periodontal abscess, or sinusitis. By pressing gently with a finger on the gums above the tooth and feeling whether the lymph nodes under the jaw are swollen, the dentist is feeling for areas of tenderness or swelling that indicate the pulp has died and the inflammation has spread to the periapical region.

The dentist tests the tooth for mobility (to find out whether it moves around in its socket) and depressibility (to determine whether it can be pressed into its socket) by using instruments and/or fingers. Mobility and depressibility are signs that the infection has spread beyond the tooth. As with the other tests, an acute apical abscess is not the only explanation for a loose tooth. Other causes include periodontal disease, habitual grinding or clenching of the teeth, and certain types of fractures of the tooth root.

Radiographs

Periapical radiographs are important aids for diagnosing pulp problems. Radiographs reveal the shape and structural anomalies of the tooth and surrounding areas, information that is of utmost importance for end-odontic treatment. They can also show calcifications and blockages within the pulp; the extent and depth of restorations and carious lesions; some periodontal and other problems, among them resorption, perforations, and fractures of the tooth roots; and degeneration of the pulp.

Radiographs, however, have limitations. They cannot reveal whether the pulp is healthy or dead or dying. They can show bone resorption but only in its later stages, after a considerable amount of destruction has already taken place.

Electric Pulp Testing

A tooth's response to an increasing amount of electric current is used to determine whether the pulp is vital (living). When there is a response, it indicates the pulp is still alive; when there is no response, it may indicate the pulp is dead. To conduct the test, the dentist dries and isolates the teeth. The electrode of the tester is placed on the tooth and the electric current is turned on and increased slowly until you first feel a sensation (tingling).

False readings may occur in teeth that have extensive fillings, have been recently injured, are recently erupted, have incomplete roots, or are undergoing orthodontic treatment or in patients who are on sedatives. The test should not be used on persons who have heart pacemakers.

Thermal Testing

These tests evaluate whether heat or cold causes pain and/or sensitivity, symptoms that can indicate an inflamed pulp. A tooth that does not respond to either extremes in temperature indicates a pulp that is not vital (or possibly a false negative response to the test). When a tooth does respond, how long the pain persists after the temperature is removed helps the dentist determine the extent of the pulpal inflammation and whether endodontic therapy is required.

A number of methods can be used. For all, the teeth are isolated and dried. A test for cold involves applying a cotton pellet that has been sprayed with ethyl chloride to the surface of the teeth. Alternatively, one of the simplest methods is to wash the tooth with either cold or warm water.

Test Cavity

This test is used infrequently and only when all other methods of diagnosis have failed. It is done most commonly for persons whose teeth have many porcelain-to-metal-fused crowns.

Using no anesthesia the dentist drills at slow speed through the crown into the dentin of the tooth. If the pulp is vital, the individual feels a sharp stab of pain. If no pain is felt, it may indicate that the pulp has died. The test cavity is then extended to open the pulp chamber for endodontic treatment.

Anesthetic Testing

This test is used as a last resort for persons who are in pain at the time of the exam and whose pain cannot be linked to a particular tooth by other tests. The dentist injects an anesthetic near the tooth that is suspected of being the painful one. If the pain persists after the tooth has been anesthetized, the dentist numbs the next one toward the front, and so forth, until the pain disappears. The diseased tooth is the tooth last anesthetized.

WHY IS ENDODONTIC TREATMENT NEEDED?

If the pulp is diseased and you do not have endodontic treatment, the tooth will have to be extracted at some point. Removing the diseased pulp prevents an infection from spreading to the surrounding tissues, where it can damage the periodontal tissues and the bone in the jaw that supports and secures the teeth.

In the past, teeth with diseased pulp were routinely extracted. This is still often done for poor people because endodontic therapy is viewed as an expensive solution. However, such thinking is shortsighted. Saving a tooth endodontically instead of removing it provides a number of benefits. When a tooth is extracted and not replaced, the teeth on either side of the space drift toward it. To fill the gap an extraction creates, a prosthesis is needed. Endodontic treatment almost always is less costly and less involved than replacing a tooth with an implant or a fixed partial denture (bridge), which involves doing extensive work on adjacent teeth. If a fixed partial denture is needed, an endodontically treated tooth can serve as an abutment.

TREATMENT

Treatment depends on the type and extent of the inflammation and on whether the diseased or injured pulp is dead or can repair itself.

Root Canal Treatment

Depending on how many roots the tooth has and how difficult it will be to treat, root canal treatment usually involves from one to three visits. The following is a typical scenario for three-visit therapy.

First Visit. If the pulp is still vital, local anesthesia is injected to anesthetize the affected tooth and area. A rubber dam is applied to isolate the tooth. Although some people object to rubber dams, finding them

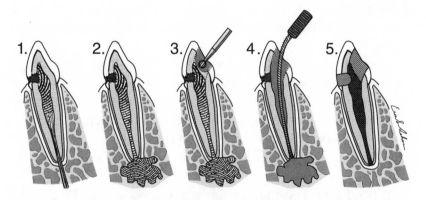

ILLUSTRATION 13.2. **THE PROCESS OF ROOT CANAL THERAPY.**
1. Caries invades all of tooth. **2.** Pulp inflammation extends into the bone and an abscess forms at the apical foramen. **3.** An opening is made in the tooth to gain access to the root canal system. **4.** Pulp tissue is removed from the pulp chamber and root canal. The root canal is cleaned and enlarged to receive a filling. **5.** Filling material is placed in the root canal and the bone heals in the apical foramen area.

uncomfortable and even claustrophobic, they are essential. Rubber dams prevent bacteria in saliva from contaminating the canal and make it easier for the dentist to see the area. In addition, their use prevents the possibility that the small instruments the dentist uses drop inadvertently into the esophagus or lungs, which would require emergency removal.

A cavity is prepared in the crown of the tooth to gain access to the root canal system. The pulp tissue is removed from both the pulp chamber and the root canal(s). The root canal(s) is cleaned to remove all bacteria, any particles of tooth structure, and pulp tissue. A solution of sodium hypochlorite (bleach) or other antiseptic is frequently used to kill bacteria. Next, the dentist enlarges the canal so it can receive a filling. Radiographs are taken throughout the procedure to be sure that the instruments the dentist is using have reached the proper length in the canal.

To destroy the harmful pathogens, medications, among them calcium hydroxide, sodium hypochlorite, or quaternary ammonium compounds, may be inserted into both the pulp chamber and the root canal(s) between appointments. Some of the medications can be irritating to the periapical tissues and cause the gingiva to itch. If you have a past history of an allergy to any dental medication or anesthetic, be certain to tell your dentist so that he or she can substitute something else.

The medication is sealed in with a temporary filling, usually of zinc-oxide-eugenol. This prevents the medication from leaking out into the mouth and food and bacteria in saliva from entering the root canal and infecting it.

If there is an acute periapical abscess, the dentist may keep the tooth open overnight to drain. Although some dentists routinely send all their patients home with a prescription for antibiotics, they are usually warranted only in patients who have signs of active infections, including fever or abscesses. Individuals with certain heart and other medical conditions, as described in Chapter 12, should be premedicated with antibiotics.

Second Visit. Local anesthesia usually is not needed for this visit. First, the dentist removes the temporary filling. Next, a permanent material (frequently gutta-percha, a rubberlike substance) is placed in the root canal and pulp chamber to seal off the apical foramina and any cracks in the canal. This should be done only when the canal is dry and shows no signs of inflammation and there is no pain. This step is essential to prevent bacteria from the oral cavity from reinfecting the tooth.

Third Visit. The last step in the process is to place a permanent restoration in the tooth. If the root canal treatment was done by an endodontist, he or she may send you back to your general dentist. Depending on the location of the tooth and the size of the opening, composite resin, gold, or other restorative material discussed in Chapter 6 may be used.

A crown is most likely to be required if the treated tooth already had a crown, if a significant amount of tooth structure was removed, or if the tooth must sustain a great amount of stress from chewing, and so is more susceptible to fracture. Teeth with little structure left that are to be crowned need a core to support the crown. This core usually is provided by a metallic post placed in the canal.

How Successful Is Treatment? In most instances, root canal treatment is successful. When treatment fails, retreatment or endodontic surgery (see the following section) may succeed. You must keep all follow-up appointments to ensure that the infection has not spread.

Discoloration. If root canal therapy has been performed correctly, a tooth should not discolor afterward. Dentists take the following measures during endodontic therapy to prevent discoloration: they thoroughly remove all pulp tissue and use only translucent filling materials in the crown. If you have teeth that were treated endodontically in the past, the filling materials that were used may have stained your teeth.

It is more likely that a tooth will discolor before endodontic treatment. Teeth that have been injured can take on a dark pink or reddish tinge right after the injury and turn pinkish grey a few days later. Even if the pulp is removed or recovers, the color may remain.

Some stains on teeth can be lightened effectively by bleaching, discussed in Chapter 14. The success of bleaching depends on what caused the stain and how long the stain has remained.

Pulpotomy

A pulpotomy is a modification of the root canal therapy just described that removes only the inflamed pulp within the crown and leaves intact the pulp within the root canals. A dressing, commonly calcium hydroxide, is applied to the remaining pulp to protect it and to promote healing. It is only performed on children and young adults to allow for an immature root to continue developing. A pulpotomy should be done only for mild to moderate inflammation that is restricted to the pulp within the crown of the tooth. It is not recommended if the pulp is inflamed severely.

Pulp capping differs from pulpotomy only in that less pulp tissue is removed before the medication is applied. Pulp capping should be done only if there is a traumatic pulp exposure. If caries and bacteria have reached the pulp, it will be too inflamed to heal. Regular root canal treatment is necessary in such a case.

ENDODONTIC SURGERY

Occasionally, endodontic treatment either fails or is not possible without surgery. Surgery is done most frequently when periapical inflammation cannot be relieved by nonsurgical treatment. For a small minority of individuals, surgery is also performed when it is not possible to seal the apical foramina through the root canals. This can result from anatomic abnormalities in the tooth, such as a curvature in its root, or because there are pulp stones or calcifications obstructing access to the root canals.

Flap Procedures

To obtain entry to the root or the periradicular area, the dentist makes an incision in the gingiva above the affected tooth to create a flap of oral mucosa. The flap is then raised to expose the bone, which may or may not be cut, depending on what needs to be done. Once the bone is exposed, various types of procedures, described here, can be performed. All are performed under local anesthesia (or general anesthesia or sedation, if the patient prefers).

Apicoectomy. In this procedure, the tip of the root is removed so that the root canal can be sealed. A filling is then placed in the canal and the flap is sutured back in place. An apicoectomy is necessary when the canal cannot be sealed with conventional root canal treatment. This occurs when the root apex has been resorbed or fractured; posts, cores, or restorations exist that cannot be removed; or large pulp stones and perforated roots prevent sealing the canal from within.

BOX 13.1

CARE AFTER ENDODONTIC SURGERY

For the first 24 hours after the surgery:

• To reduce swelling, apply ice to the face over the incision for ten minutes and then remove it for ten minutes.

• Avoid or restrict all activities involving the face, such as talking, laughing, or otherwise stretching your lips.

• Be aware that the incision may bleed or ooze gently for several hours.

Other recommendations:

• Follow the dentist's instructions.

• Although you may not need it, ask your dentist what you should take for pain after the procedure. Analgesics usually are recommended, unless you have a medical condition for which they are not advised.

• Keep your mouth clean by brushing your teeth frequently with a soft-bristled brush, taking care not to hurt the gums, and rinsing twice a day with a mouthwash containing chlorhexidine.

• Make and keep all recommended postoperative appointments with your dental surgeon and general dentist.

Call your dentist if:

• Bleeding is heavy or persists.

• You develop chills, fever, excessive swelling, or pain.

• Your sutures loosen or fall out before your appointment to have them removed.

• You continue to have pain after two days.

Root Resection. In this procedure, one root of a multirooted tooth is removed, while the other root or roots are left. Root resection is performed to address problems, such as deep carious lesions, fractures, severe resorption on one root, or unmanageable periodontal disease in the tissues between the teeth. To qualify for root resection, you must practice good oral hygiene and not have a high caries rate. In addition, the root (or roots), to be salvaged must be able to be treated endodontically and be able to anchor the remaining tooth.

First, root canal treatment is performed on the root or roots that are to be retained. The other root is then amputated.

Intentional Replantation

The same treatment used when a tooth is knocked out can also be used when it is not possible to perform flap surgery. In intentional replantation, the tooth is extracted, and the defect in the root is corrected while the tooth is out of the body. It is then replaced. This technique may also be appropriate when the root is fractured or perforated or when apical surgery would involve the removal of a major nerve or so much bone that the periodontal tissues would be damaged. Intentional replantation is indicated especially when a regular surgical procedure would damage surrounding structures.

CHAPTER 14

Cosmetic Dentistry

The impetus to undergo the procedures covered in this chapter is cosmetic. With veneering, bonding, and bleaching, darkened teeth can be lightened, gaps closed, chips and fractures repaired, short teeth lengthened, and twisted teeth made to appear even without the extensive invasion of tooth structure that crowns, once the only treatment, require. Reshaping teeth can also improve their appearance with minimal removal of tooth structure. Gingival surgery, used for cosmetic purposes, can redefine the gum line. These treatments can be performed on men and women of many ages, from their late teens on (even into their eighties), who have normal, healthy teeth and aesthetic concerns about them that were once considered too inconsequential to treat. (Other dental treatments, such as braces, orthognathic surgery, and implants, which are sometimes performed solely for cosmetic concerns, are covered in separate chapters. In general, these are less conservative and more invasive, involve greater expense, and, in the case of surgery, greater risks and a longer recuperation.)

Whatever your specific dental defects, the decision to do something about them depends more on how you perceive the image of your teeth than on the extent of the imperfections. How much someone is affected by a gap or a darkened tooth can vary markedly from one individual to another. A space between the upper front teeth that makes you self-conscious may be of little concern to someone else.

For some, the motivation to have cosmetic procedures is professional. Individuals who speak before groups are especially sensitive about the impression their smile and teeth make. For people in the entertainment industry, which puts a premium on "perfect" dentition or dental form and arrangement, bonded teeth have become *de rigueur.*

Whether the incentive is personal or professional, the goal of cosmetic dentistry for most is not always to enhance the smile but to minimize its defects. The effect most want is neutral, one in which the teeth no longer attract attention. When this is achieved, the reward is a sense of liberation, which allows you to smile and laugh freely without feeling inhibited.

WHAT ARE ATTRACTIVE TEETH?

The oft-used adage "beauty is in the eye of the beholder" summarizes accurately the subjectivity of attractiveness. What is pleasing aesthetically to you may not be to someone else. Indeed, norms of beauty vary from one culture to another and from one period of history to the next. In the United States, the standard for beauty has become more flexible than at any time before. The media reflect this by including actors and models of different nationalities and physical characteristics in movies, on television, and in magazines.

The norms for attractive teeth do not reflect such diversity. The "Hollywood smile," of even and straight white teeth with no gaps, still remains the ideal. It is this "Hollywood smile" many want replicated when they go to their dentist. This image may not always be appropriate for you, as the next section explains. Making teeth attractive is a complex process involving many considerations and, for the dentist, technical skills, as well as artistic judgment.

THE COLLABORATION BETWEEN DENTIST AND PATIENT

Cosmetic dental care involves an active dialogue between you and your dentist. The dentist relies on you to explain what it is about your teeth that dissatisfies you and how you want to change it. Your dentist then translates this desire into a realistic result.

In making aesthetic decisions, many factors need to be taken into consideration, among them the gender of the patient, the size of the teeth (relative to the surrounding ones), and their surface texture, contour, shape, and color. Many people have preconceived ideas, which may or may not be correct, about the treatment method they want or how their teeth should look.

One common misconception about teeth is that they are all white. In fact, teeth comprise other colors as well: yellows, blues, grays, greens, and oranges. Most people would not be happy with all-white teeth. With the exception of some people in show business who want their teeth to stand out, most want a natural look: teeth that are lighter but replicate enamel's subtle range of hues. Perfectly smooth teeth are not desirable either. If veneering material is not given texture, the teeth can end up looking like pieces of shiny chiclet gum.

Tooth shape is influenced by gender and ethnicity. Women have teeth with softer lines and rounded arches. When they smile, they show more of their teeth than men do. The teeth of men, on the other hand, have straighter lines, sharper angles, and squarer arches. Different ethnic groups can have specific dental characteristics. If these variations are not incorporated, the result is incongruent.

VISUALIZING THE CHANGES

If you are contemplating making changes in your smile, your initial visit with the dentist should be reserved for discussion and visualization only. Difficult cases may require more than one pretreatment visit and involve consultation with other specialists, among them orthodontists and oral surgeons.

Different Techniques

Your dentist may use a number of the following techniques, which run the gamut from low tech to state of the art, to help you visualize the changes a proposed treatment will make.

Evaluation Forms. A cosmetic evaluation form can help you highlight specific concerns you have about your teeth (e.g., their color, shape, or size) to determine which treatment is best. The form also identifies personal habits, like ice chewing or nail biting, that could compromise the longevity of some of the treatments.

Medical History. Certain medical conditions can contribute to dental problems or preclude a treatment. This information may be included on the evaluation forms or taken verbally by your dentist.

Photographs. Before and after photographs of other patients allow you to see what treatments have done for others, but they do not show you how you will look.

Temporary veneers. Your dentist can put a mock-up veneer on your teeth to approximate the look that the permanent ones will give you.

Computer Imaging. The most current imaging technique utilizes computer technology. With a video camera linked to a computer, the dentist can record your face and freeze it on a monitor screen. The frozen image can be altered to reflect changes in the color and shape of the teeth. These can be adjusted to arrive at the most appealing picture. You can view the present and future images simultaneously and even have instant photos to take home.

Computer imaging has been hailed as the best tool for projecting what the outcome of cosmetic dental work will be for an individual. This technology, however, often has fallen short of its expectations. It is seldom sensitive enough to discriminate between subtle shades of color, nor can it replicate the minute fractions of an inch required to get a precise sense of the contour and shape of the final outcome.

Discussion

Although these tools help give you an idea of how you will look if a gap is closed or a chip repaired, none of them allow you to gaze into a crystal ball and precisely envision beforehand what the result will be. To avoid any dissatisfaction and to understand realistically what the procedures can and cannot do for you and your teeth, you should discuss thoroughly all aspects of the treatment with your dentist: how long it will take, how much it will cost, how long it will last, how it will change your appearance, and how you can maintain it. To protect themselves from possible misunderstandings, some dentists have their patients sign informed consent forms (see Chapter 4).

EXAMINATION

In general, before teeth are bonded, veneered, or bleached, they need to be examined, radiographed, and cleaned to remove superficial stains. If there is evidence of caries, periodontal disease, or defective fillings or other restorations, these need to be taken care of before treatment begins.

Your gums should be checked for signs of recession and to determine whether any enamel has worn off. Periodontal disease is usually not a problem on the front teeth on which these procedures are done. If necessary, you will be referred to a periodontist before treatment.

BLEACHING

Until recently, bleaching was confined to nonvital teeth (those in which the pulp has died). During the last decade there has been a dramatic increase in the frequency with which people are having their healthy teeth bleached.

Bleaching is done to lighten teeth. It will not give them the "Hollywood" white. If this is what you want, bonding or veneering, alone or in conjunction with bleaching, will be a better alternative. Bleaching will not change the color of an existing crown or resin filling, so there may be a noticeable discrepancy in shading between the restoration and the newly bleached teeth. With this in mind, if you are having your teeth bleached, you may want new restorations; if you are contemplating veneering, bonding, or crowning your teeth, you may want to consider bleaching first.

Teeth can be stained for many reasons, among them aging; trauma; illnesses; dental materials; improper dental treatment; use of tobacco, tetracycline, or excessive fluoride; and consumption of coffee, tea, and colas. Genetics also plays a role in how white your teeth are and how rapidly and how much they discolor.

Whether and to what extent bleaching is effective depends on the cause and the severity of the stains. Although there are no guarantees or absolute predictions, in general, the darker the teeth, the more difficult the discoloration will be to remove. Which bleaching process is used depends on whether the tooth is vital (alive) or nonvital (dead).

Bleaching usually is not recommended if the teeth are darkened severely, have deep pits or loss of enamel, are extremely sensitive, or have large pulp chambers. Pregnant women should postpone the process until after delivery, as the effects of peroxides on the developing fetus are not known. Although individuals with certain medical conditions, among them serious renal damage, nutritional deficiencies during tooth formation, and cerebral palsy, may respond to bleaching, bonding, crowning, or veneering are better alternatives for most.

Before teeth are bleached, caries should be filled and metal amalgam fillings replaced with composite resins to see whether this will not lighten them sufficiently. Teeth should be checked for hypersensitivity and radiographed to reveal the size of the pulp chambers.

Concerns over Safety and Efficacy

The Federal Drug Administration (FDA) recently has raised concerns about the long-term safety of bleaching solutions, in particular those containing hydrogen peroxide, and about the claims made for the efficacy of home bleaching kits. Since hydrogen peroxide causes a chemical reaction, the agency has declared it a drug. As a result, each manufacturer must submit studies proving the safety and efficacy of its products in order for them to enter or remain on the market. At present, the products are in a regulatory limbo, with insufficient research on their long-term effects to deem them hazardous or, conversely, to prove them safe.

Despite these concerns, bleaching vital and nonvital teeth, either directly by a dentist or under his or her professional supervision, has been performed satisfactorily for years. The FDA questions the use of hydrogen peroxide as a bleaching agent, regardless of whether it is applied by a dentist or controlled solely by the consumer. As will be explained in the section "Over-the-Counter Bleaching Kits," the manner in which the solutions are applied and monitored and the dosages used vary. As with all elective dental decisions and procedures, individuals contemplating these treatments need to have current and accurate information to weigh the benefits against the possible risks.

Bleaching Vital Teeth

The stains on healthy teeth that are easiest to remove by bleaching are those caused by food and beverages, fluorosis, and the normal aging process. The discoloration from tea and coffee will return if consumption is not reduced. Removing stains caused by tetracycline can be more difficult. The darker the staining and the striation caused by sporadic and repetitive use of the antibiotic, the poorer the prognosis. Conversely, lighter stains respond more favorably.

There are currently two effective methods for bleaching vital teeth.

The Chairside Method. This is done in a dentist's office by a dentist or dental hygienist or assistant under a dentist's supervision. The preparation is time consuming; each session takes from 45 to 90 minutes.

Prior to bleaching, the gums are coated with a protective gel and a rubber dam is stretched over the teeth to protect the soft tissues. Dental floss is tied on each tooth at the gum line. The teeth are cleaned and etched (to roughen the enamel) with phosphoric acid.

A solution of hydrogen peroxide is applied to the teeth through a gauze. Fresh solution is applied every 4 minutes for 30 minutes, during which a heat light is shined on the teeth to hasten the bleaching action. You are given protective eyeglasses and covers for your clothing and hands.

Because the dentist needs to know the degree of discomfort the heat or chemicals are causing to prevent potential damage to the soft tissues and pulp, anesthesia is not used unless the teeth are extremely sensitive. Teeth should be bleached whiter than the intended shade because they will darken in the 24 hours following treatment.

For a day or two afterward you may experience mild inflammation and irritation of your gums and your teeth may be unusually sensitive to extremes in temperature. If needed, your dentist can prescribe analgesics or anti-inflammatory medications.

Up to ten treatments may be necessary. Tetracycline-stained teeth usually require between five and ten sessions; teeth discolored from fluoride, one or two sessions. The teeth usually remain whiter for between one and three years, after which time the process may need to be repeated, but with fewer applications.

Costs vary. Some dentists charge per session (from $80 to $225); others charge one fee ($300 and beyond) for up to ten sessions, depending on the response.

Nightguard or Dentist-Prescribed Method. This is a recently introduced bleaching method that is growing in popularity. Progress is checked weekly by the dentist, but the work is performed and controlled daily by the patient.

There are differences and similarities between this and the chairside method. Nightguard bleaching uses a weaker concentration of chemicals (either carbamide peroxide or hydrogen peroxide) for a longer duration. It effectively removes stains from the same sources as the dentist-performed method, with the same degree of relative permanence. It is not recommended for pregnant women; people with a history of alcoholism, ulcers, hiatal hernia, or allergies to peroxides or glycerin; and children under the age of 13.

As with chairside and over-the-counter bleaching, you need to be informed of the questions that have been raised about this method and the lack of definitive clinical and laboratory studies. Your dentist may ask you to sign an informed consent form which, in addition to detailing the known and questioned risks, may set out the number of follow-up visits to the dentist you agree to make. Photographs may be taken to chart the response rate and to document any alleged damage.

After these preliminaries, impressions of the teeth are taken, from which a transparent resin tray is custom made. In the office, the dentist shows you how to use the device at home. The fastest results are obtained when the whitening gel, which is put into each tooth space, is replaced every hour. You can wear the tray from two to six hours a day but should remove it when you eat or drink or go to bed or if irritation occurs.

As with the chairside method, temporary irritation of the gums and sensitivity to extreme temperatures may occur. These are monitored weekly by your dentist to prevent possible problems, such as tooth hypersensitivity, sores on the gums, nausea, temporomandibular disorders, and sore throats.

Only one dental arch (six to eight teeth) at a time should be bleached so that the progress can be determined by comparison with the non-bleached teeth. Although the outcome cannot be predicted, most people begin to see results in two to three weeks of consistent use. The cost for bleaching one arch varies between $300 and $600.

Bleaching Nonvital Teeth

For bleaching to work on nonvital teeth, they must have had proper root canal therapy. Bleaching is not appropriate for nonvital teeth that have insufficient or damaged enamel, deep cracks, or dental tubules that have become filled with metallic amalgams used in fillings.

There are two methods of bleaching nonvital teeth, both performed by a dentist. The method used usually depends on the severity of the stain, which is determined most often by how long the material that caused the discoloration has remained in the pulp chamber.

The preparation for each is the same. First, the teeth are cleaned and anesthetized. Then the dentist opens the tooth from the back to expose the pulp. Some of the root canal filling material and dentin are removed and cotton is placed in the chambers. From here, the procedure varies, depending on the method used.

Chairside Method. After cotton is placed in the pulp chamber, it is filled with bleaching solution. Heat is applied for five minutes. The cotton is replaced and the process is repeated four to six times for a total of 20 to 30 minutes.

After this, the bleach and cotton are removed and the chamber is flushed with water and wiped with chloroform. The walls of the chamber are etched and air dried. The cavity is then filled with tooth-colored composite resin material.

The "Walking" Method. In this method, which usually is reserved for difficult stains, the bleaching solution is sealed into the chamber and the patient is sent home. The solution can remain in the chamber for up to a week, although the usual duration is from three to five days. The patient returns to the office to have the seal reopened, the bleach removed, and the chamber resealed, in the manner indicated for the chairside method.

Over-the-Counter Bleaching Kits

The newest techniques for bleaching teeth are kits sold directly to the consumer. Most of these employ a three-step process. The teeth are first rinsed with acetic acid. Next, hydrogen peroxide is applied in a gel form for one to two minutes to the front of the teeth with a cotton swab. Finally a tooth-whitening pigment is applied.

One of the concerns about home bleaching kits is that it is the patient and not the dentist diagnosing the reason for the stain. A salient difference between the over-the-counter kits and the bleaching done by or directly under the supervision of the dentist is that there is no professional control or monitoring of the process. At the time of this writing, the American Dental Association Council on Scientific Affairs has determined that sufficient information on the long-term use and safety of these products does not exist to consider any of them for approval. Until the issues of safety and efficacy can be resolved, we cannot recommend over-the-counter bleaching kits.

BONDING

The bonding process is a jack-of-many-trades for the dental profession. It has various uses, which are covered in other chapters: pit and fissure sealing for the surfaces of caries-prone teeth; an aesthetic alternative for amalgam fillings; capping, or crowning, a tooth; and the repair of injured teeth.

Bonding in dentistry refers to the sticking together of two surfaces: the tooth enamel (and sometimes the dentin) with the bonding material. For cosmetic dentistry, the process is used as a method of changing the shape and color of teeth to effect a more pleasing appearance. In this use, bonding can be used to close the space between front teeth, to cover stains, and to repair chips.

Bonding is considered a direct technique of veneering. In bonding, the composite resin is painted onto the tooth directly by the dentist, much as polish is applied to a fingernail. To enhance the adhesion of the composite resin, the enamel of the tooth needs to be etched with phosphoric acid to create a rough surface to which the material can bond more easily.

After this, the dentist applies the first coat of resin material on the tooth and cures it with light to set or seal it. Subsequent layers can be added to increase the length of the tooth or to fill a gap between the front teeth.

Direct veneering with composite resin may not have as many advantages as porcelain laminates, the cadillac of veneers. In many instances, however, composite resin is a wise choice economically. It is less expensive and requires one less office visit. Even though the material can fracture, it is repaired or replaced easily by a dentist. Although fees vary from one region to another, a good rule of thumb is that the price to bond a tooth directly should cost between one-third and one-half the price of a crown in the same area.

The longevity of composite resin bonds originally was estimated to be five or six years. Yet many are 12 to 15 years old and still wearing well. Eventually all bonds need to be replaced because the material rubs off. If the bond was placed to cover a stain, the tooth gradually will appear darker—a sign that it is abrading.

VENEERING

The terms "bonding" and "veneering" in dentistry can be confusing. "Bonding" refers both to the mechanical process of adhesion involving chemicals and the surface veneer that is created when the bonding material covers the tooth and improves its appearance. Bonding is a direct method of veneering because the material (the composite resin) is placed directly on the tooth by the dentist.

When the term "veneer" is used generically in dentistry, it refers to indirect veneers that are prefabricated at a laboratory and placed onto the tooth by the dentist, using the mechanical process of bonding to make them adhere.

A number of dental imperfections can be corrected effectively or camouflaged by indirect veneers, among them: defects in the enamel; gaps and other spaces; discoloration from aging, tetracycline, and fluorosis; and fractures. In addition, porcelain veneers can be used to lengthen a tooth and to give the illusion that malpositioned (i.e., rotated) teeth are straighter without orthodontics.

Although veneers can be composed of acrylic resin, microfill resin, or porcelain, the only material we recommend is porcelain because of its superiority in aesthetic qualities, strength, durability, and resistance to fluid absorption and discoloration. In addition, because a thin and smooth transition can be achieved between the porcelain veneers and the tooth near the gumline causing very little plaque accumulation, they may be better for your periodontal health than the composite resin material used in direct veneering.

Teeth must meet certain requirements to wear *porcelain laminate veneers* successfully. They must have enough sound tooth structure to support them. Teeth that have lost more than one-third their surfaces to caries are not good candidates and may indicate that the patient does not devote enough time to adequate oral hygiene. In addition, oral habits need to be evaluated. Individuals who chew ice habitually or bite their nails may be better off with direct veneers or crowns.

Having porcelain veneers requires three office visits. As with the other procedures described, the first should be spent in discussion and on imaging. During the second visit the teeth are prepared and the impressions made. The veneers are placed at the third visit.

To allow space for the veneer and the composite resin material, a small amount (⅟₃₂ inch or less) of the enamel needs to be removed. After this, an impression of the teeth is made. This, along with any photos, computer imaging, and shade selection, is sent to a lab where a ceramist fabricates the veneers. In shape and thickness, they resemble fake fingernails. If dentin has been exposed, temporary acrylic veneers, which will be removed at the third visit, may be applied.

Before placement, your teeth are cleaned with pumice and water and isolated. You will be asked to breathe through your nose to reduce possible contamination of the tooth surfaces from vapor escaping your lungs. A local anesthetic is usually used to minimize the discomfort involved in finishing the margins of the veneer near the gum.

The surfaces of the teeth are conditioned with a solution of 37 percent phosphoric acid, which when left on the enamel causes an irregular surface. The conditioner is thoroughly washed after 15 to 20 seconds and the teeth dried until the surface exhibits a fresh appearance.

To make them adhere, a fine coat of composite resin luting agent is applied to the tooth and on the backside of the veneer. Because the thickness of the resin or bonding cement influences the color, this final placement depends on the skill of the dentist. If too much pressure is applied, more cement will seep out; this results in a different shade. Finally, light is shone on the tooth to seal, or cure, the resin.

Although porcelain veneers excel in desirable qualities, they have some disadvantages. They are more expensive than having the teeth bonded because they require an extra office visit and laboratory and impression fees. The material also has a propensity to chip. Once in place, if a porcelain veneer is damaged, it is almost impossible to repair. If, however, the entire laminate debonds without breaking, your dentist can reattach it. If you follow good oral hygiene and avoid chomping, biting, and other fracture-prone activities (see Box 14.1), porcelain laminate veneers can last ten years or even longer.

Fees vary, depending on the challenge of the dental problem and your geographical area. In general, you should expect to pay between $750 to $1,050.

BOX 14.1

HOME CARE FOR
YOUR COSMETIC DENTAL WORK

How long your cosmetic dental work lasts depends, to a large extent, on how diligent you are in sticking to a home care regimen. To combat plaque accumulation and prevent fractures and discoloration, the following are recommended:

- At least once a day, floss and use a rotary cleaning device. Brush properly with a toothbrush for the other cleanings.
- Do not chew ice, hard candies, popcorn kernels, or sticky and sugary foods.
- Do not bite your nails or use your teeth for jobs better performed by a screw driver, scissors, or pair of pliers.
- Reduce or preferably avoid coffee, soy sauce, tea, curry, colas, blueberries, grape juice, and red wine.
- Wear a custom biteguard if you clench or grind your teeth.
- Do not brush your teeth with baking soda or use abrasive toothpastes.
- Do not use mouthwashes with a high alcohol content.
- Do not use toothpastes with stannous or acidulated phosphate fluorides. Sodium fluoride is the only active ingredient recommended.
- Avoid picking, scratching, or pulling at your veneers. Have all rough edges smoothed professionally.
- When engaging in contact sports, use a soft acrylic mouthguard.
- Adhere to your dentist's recommendations for professional cleanings. Three or four times a year are the usual recommendations. Ultrasonic scaling and air abrasive polishing systems might damage veneers. Your dentist or dental hygienist should use hand scaling and polishing for in-office cleanings.

In addition to the above guidelines for routine maintenance, the following are special precautions you need to take in the three days after bleaching or placement of veneers:

- Eat soft foods.
- Avoid ingesting very hot or very cold beverages or foods.

TOOTH RESHAPING

By removing small amounts of enamel, teeth can be reshaped to eliminate or minimize a number of imperfections. For example, upper canine teeth that are pointed can be made to appear less fanglike. Tooth reshaping (also referred to as enamel recontouring) can alter the shape, length, contour, or position of a tooth and its relationship to adjacent teeth to improve the appearance of the smile. It does so without removing substantial amounts of tooth structure, as is required for crowns. Among other cosmetic improvements, tooth reshaping can:

- Reshape chipped, overlapped, or fractured teeth.
- Minimize the appearance of crowding.
- Correct developmental imperfections and abnormalities, such as pitting and grooves in the enamel.
- Adjust the edges of the biting surfaces that have been worn from grinding the teeth.
- Correct small imperfections created after orthodontic treatment.
- Reduce shadows caused from overcrowding.

Although teeth usually are reshaped to improve their appearance, the procedure can also be performed to improve dental health. For example, areas that encourage the accumulation of plaque and tartar can be reshaped to make them easier to clean (and therefore less prone to developing caries or periodontal disease). Reshaping a tooth that has lost its bone support as a result of periodontal disease can reduce the amount of force from chewing that is transmitted to the jaw bone. Reshaping can also correct small problems with occlusion and function. For instance, for some people it improves the functioning of the teeth because it reduces the contact where they would wear down.

Teeth that do not qualify for reshaping include those which have thin enamel or large restorations, have recently erupted, have lost a significant amount of structure, or have gingival tissues between them that would be compromised by the procedure. In addition, individuals who have high rates of caries are not good candidates for reshaping.

As with all other cosmetic dental procedures, if you are considering having your teeth reshaped, you should have a thorough consultation with your dentist, in which you describe the changes you would like made. After this, the dentist examines your teeth and periodontal tissues. Radiographs are made to evaluate the size and location of the dental pulp and to determine whether there is sufficient bone between the teeth. Some dentists will make study models of the teeth (see Chapter 16 for a description). The dentist then looks at your teeth when you are sitting up, with your lips relaxed and smiling, to help determine what corrections need to be made.

It is helpful if the dentist takes photographs of your teeth before the reshaping so that you can see the improvements that have been made. Since many of the changes are subtle, it can be difficult to remember what your teeth looked like before treatment.

The dentist will mark your teeth with a pencil to indicate areas to be removed. Enamel is removed from the surfaces of the tooth using high- or low-speed hand pieces and from the sides between the teeth with abrasive strips that are moved back and forth, much the same way sandpaper is used. The teeth are then smoothed and polished. After the reshaping is completed, a chip from a tooth can be repaired with a bonding material. Because the procedure involves little, if any, discomfort it can be done without using anesthetic.

Treatment usually takes between one to three visits, depending on the amount of reshaping involved. Your dentist may ask to see you in seven to ten days after your teeth have been reshaped for additional therapy. For example, patients whose reshaped teeth were moderately crowded may need to wear an active removable appliance or apply pressure with their fingers for a set amount of time to help move the teeth if repositioning the teeth is one of the goals of the reshaping procedure. If teeth are to be bleached, it should be postponed until after the reshaping.

The cost of the procedure depends on how involved it is. In general it costs $150 to $350 or more per tooth.

GINGIVAL SURGERY

Surgery on the gums traditionally has been done to counteract the problems associated with chronic and advanced cases of periodontal disease. Recently, gingivectomies (described in Chapter 7) have been performed for cosmetic reasons, to make front teeth longer and to equalize those that

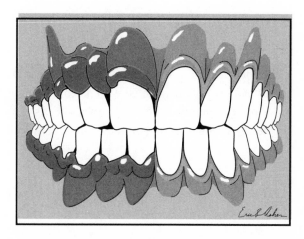

ILLUSTRATION 14.1. **THE COSMETIC EFFECTS OF A GINGIVECTOMY.**
The left side of the illustration shows gums swollen from chronic gingivitis. The right side shows that after receiving a gingivectomy, the swelling has subsided and the margins of the gums have been made more even. Gingivectomies are performed to improve the health of the gums, and by the removal of swollen gums, the smile is made more attractive.

appear to be of different lengths due to the unevenness of their gingival margins. These problems occur as a result of genetics and of techniques used in some orthodontic treatments.

The procedure usually is performed by a periodontist, often in consultation with a general dentist and orthodontist. The process for evaluation is similar to that for the cosmetic procedures described previously. As with any surgery, problems can arise. For this reason and because the results are irreversible and very visible, this surgical correction should not be undertaken casually.

PAYING FOR IT

Few insurance policies cover the procedures discussed in this chapter. (There may be exceptions made for veneering or bonding to correct fractured or chipped teeth.) It is not unusual for dentists to request full payment in advance of cosmetic treatments.

LOCATING A DENTIST

Since there is no specialty in cosmetic dentistry, many general dentists practice it. The best way to locate a dentist who performs these procedures is by asking your regular dentist whether he or she does the procedures and, if not, whether he or she can recommend someone who does.

CHAPTER 15

Orthodontics—More than Braces

Many adults who had orthodontic treatment when they were young can still recall the monikers of "metal mouth" or "tin grin" they were given. Fortunately, the stigma of wearing fixed orthodontic appliances has vanished. For most children today, wearing braces is acceptable among their peers and, for some, has even become fashionable. Patients today can choose brackets that are clear or tooth colored rather than those made of metal. Gum-colored acrylic retainers, at one time tucked away in dresser drawers, now can be embellished with personalized designs, including tiger stripes, teddy bears, animal faces, surfers, and the American flag. Adults, too, have jumped on the orthodontic bandwagon. Once representing only a small percentage, individuals over the age of 18 now make up almost 30 percent of orthodontic patients.

WHAT IS ORTHODONTICS?

The manner in which the biting (occlusal) surfaces of the teeth come into contact with each other is called occlusion. Occlusion involves the entire masticatory system, including the teeth and jaws, periodontal tissues, temporomandibular joint, facial muscles, and nervous system.

Orthodontics is the branch of dentistry that diagnoses, prevents, and treats problems with the spacing and positioning of teeth and with malocclusions, irregularities in how the teeth in the upper jaw occlude, or come together, with the teeth of the lower jaw. "Orthodontics" is a combination of two Greek words: *orthos*, meaning "to correct or right," and *odontos*, "tooth."

To realign and reposition teeth, orthodontists utilize corrective devices, referred to as appliances. Irregularities commonly treated with orthodontic appliances include teeth that are crooked, crowded, or too far apart or that protrude, or stick out. Surgery, alone or in conjunction with the use of orthodontic appliances, may be necessary to correct severe malrelationships of the jaws, such as protruding or receding upper and/ or lower jaws, and facial deformities, such as clefting.

ORTHODONTIC PROBLEMS

Most orthodontic problems are inherited. Examples include crowding of or excessive space between teeth, missing or extra teeth, teeth that are abnormal in shape or size or erupt in the wrong places, and protrusive or recessive upper and lower jaws.

Many inherited orthodontic problems relate to evolutionary patterns. The jawbones of prehistoric adults were larger than ours are today. As the size of the brain and the skull increased, the size of the jaws decreased. The size and number of the teeth, however, remained the same; this often resulted in crowding. Although the sizes of the teeth and of the jaws are inherited, genetically the traits may be controlled separately. As a consequence, individuals can have discrepancies between them, with small jaws and large teeth and, less commonly, the reverse.

Some orthodontic problems are acquired from medical problems or local factors. They may be due to habits like finger, thumb, or pacifier sucking; tongue thrusting; and mouth breathing that results from enlarged tonsils and / or adenoids, a deviated septum, allergies, diseases that cause a malfunction of oral and facial muscles, injuries to the face and teeth, dental diseases, and premature loss of primary or permanent teeth. Children are especially sensitive to dental and facial changes that can result from habitual mouth breathing. These include an increased distance between the nose and chin called long face syndrome and lip incompetence and a smile that reveals too much gum tissue. A malocclusion that has occurred recently may indicate a fracture of a jaw, a cyst or tumor, or inflammation.

HOW ORTHODONTICS WORKS

Fixed or removable orthodontic appliances exert gentle pressure on a tooth or group of teeth. This forces the root of the tooth to press against

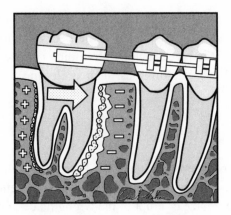

ILLUSTRATION 15.1. **ORTHODONTIC TOOTH MOVEMENT WITH BRACES.**
Gentle pressure exerted from the braces pushes the root of the tooth against the
alveolar bone. The pressure dissolves some of the bone. This creates space for
the tooth to move. (This movement is indicated by the − signs.) The space on
the other side of the tooth (indicated by the + signs) fills in with new bone
growth.

the alveolar bone surrounding it. The continual gentle force gradually
dissolves the bone on the pressure side, and so creates a space for the
tooth to advance. New bone grows to fill in the space left on the other side
of the tooth and helps secure the tooth in its new position. The process of
bone dissolving on one side and growing on the other is called bone
remodeling. During treatment the wires on braces are adjusted numerous
times to maintain the desired direction and amount of force on the teeth.
Thumbsucking and tongue thrusting also can move teeth, usually into
unfavorable positions, using the same mechanisms. Retainers help secure
the new tooth position until the recently formed bone solidifies.

How far the teeth can be moved depends on the character and the
amount of underlying bone. Bone remodeling occurs more quickly in
younger persons than it does in adults because the bone is less dense and
has a greater blood supply and more cells available for remodeling.

For most but not all people, facial and skeletal growth follows a
predictable pattern. By the age of two years, the face has reached 75
percent of its adult size; by the age of nine years, it has achieved 85
percent of its adult size. Orthodontists sometimes take advantage of
growth spurts that occur around puberty when repositioning teeth. The

average age for the peak of the pubertal growth spurt for girls is 12 years; for boys, it is 14 years.

The Age Factor

Until recently, the general belief was that adults did not make good candidates for orthodontic treatment because their jaws were no longer actively growing and their alveolar bone was too dense. Orthodontists now know otherwise. Although at certain times during childhood more extensive orthodontic therapy can be accomplished and in a shorter time, orthodontics can be successful for many adults. Some corrections, for example, expanding the palate, may not be possible or may be more difficult for an adult through appliances alone. To accomplish the more dramatic facial changes, surgery, combined with orthodontics, may be necessary. Adults may also require the care of other dental specialists during orthodontic therapy if they experience periodontal disease and/or loss of teeth that can change the occlusion.

When to Start

When children have their teeth treated orthodontically at the "right" time, therapy can be done more easily and quickly than when it is delayed until adulthood. It also may be less expensive and the outcome may be more successful. Ideally, an orthodontic assessment should be part of every child's (and adult's) comprehensive dental examination. This assures that children will be referred to an orthodontist at an early enough age for them to receive the optimal treatment. If this has not been part of your children's routine exams, you should be sure that well before puberty, when they have both primary and permanent teeth, a general or pediatric dentist evaluates their occlusion to make certain all teeth are present and positioned normally.

In general, for malocclusions that are severe, particularly those caused by skeletal discrepancies, such as mandibular retrognathism and prognathism, crossbites, and severe crowding of the teeth, children should visit an orthodontist when they have only primary teeth or primary teeth and a few permanent teeth. Children with cleft palates and lips or other craniofacial syndromes that require early intervention should be monitored from birth.

Patients with lesser problems also may benefit from early orthodontic therapy. These include congenitally missing or ankylosed (fused) teeth; teeth that may need help erupting in proper alignment; and possibly some habits, such as mouth breathing and digit or pacifier sucking, that continue after the permanent teeth erupt. Primary molars that are lost prematurely need to have their space maintained (see Chapter 8). Correcting the protrusion of a child's front teeth before the age of ten usually reduces the risk of their being fractured, chipped, or knocked out from sports or other activities.

Even if an orthodontist identifies a problem with your child at an early age, it does not necessarily mean that treatment will begin then. The orthodontist may decide to observe the dental development so that treatment can begin at the most desirable time, which is frequently when the child is losing the last primary teeth. For some malocclusions, early treatment that involves extractions of primary teeth or limited orthodontic therapy with fixed or removable appliances may be sufficient. For others, two phases of treatment may be required: one when the primary teeth or the primary and some permanent teeth are present and a second after all the permanent teeth have erupted.

In some instances, a compelling reason to start orthodontic treatment early is to prevent or minimize the emotional and psychological toll that dental irregularities can exact. Children with protruding teeth or misaligned jaws are too often the butt of classmates' teasing, which can affect their self-esteem.

WHO SHOULD TREAT ORTHODONTIC PROBLEMS?

Some general and pediatric dentists are trained to handle some orthodontic problems. A general or pediatric dentist will refer your child to an orthodontist if your child's malocclusion is beyond his or her scope of orthodontic training or would be better treated by a specialist. At times, orthodontic treatment may involve a team effort between a general dentist, an orthodontist, and other dental specialists, such as a prosthodontist, periodontist, and/or oral surgeon.

ORTHODONTIC EVALUATION

A full orthodontic assessment by an orthodontist usually involves a clinical exam and includes tests, study models, photographs, and radiographs. It may take one or two office visits.

Patient's History

At the first visit the dentist records the patient's dental and medical history. This includes the patient's complaints (physical and psychological) about the teeth and gums, family history of problems and habits, and personal history (e.g., dental habits, head and neck injuries, and medical and dental conditions).

Few medical conditions preclude the wearing of orthodontic appliances. Patients with blood dyscrasias or disorders, such as leukemia or hemophilia, in which the elements of the blood are abnormal require special management for extractions, and individuals with recurrent aphthous ulcers (canker sores) may be unable to wear their appliances consistently.

Examination

This is usually divided into two parts:

Extraoral. While your child (or you) is seated and looking straight ahead, the orthodontist examines the profile and face full on, looking at the underlying bone structure and the muscles covering it to note the presence of acquired or inherited defects. The orthodontist will:

- Assess the relationship of the jaws, the height of the lower face, and the overall symmetry of the face.
- Evaluate the positions of the lips and tongue at rest and when swallowing.
- Check the temporomandibular joints for restriction of movements, clicking, or defects and for muscle tenderness surrounding them.
- Note speech defects and habits, such as tongue thrusting.
- Check whether breathing is through the mouth. If it appears to

be, the orthodontist will look to see if the adenoids or tonsils are obstructing the nasal passages. If they are, the dentist may refer your child to another specialist for further evaluation.

Cephalometric analysis serves an essential function in formulating a treatment plan, especially for patients whose malocclusions involve a skeletal discrepancy. To make a cephalometric analysis, the orthodontist compares the coordinates of anatomical landmarks of the skull and jaw, taken from the lateral skull radiographs or cephalographs, with standardized measurements. (These measurements help to evaluate the relationship of the upper and lower dental arches with each other and the relation of the alveolar bone and the incisors in both jaws.) To obtain an average facial growth rate, the mean of the same skull coordinates are taken from a varying number of individuals at each year between the ages of 1 and 18. Comparing your child's measurements with these growth standards helps the orthodontist predict the size and shape of your child's face at a time in the future. Cephalometric analysis is made usually before and sometimes after orthodontic treatment to assess the effects growth and treatment have had on the occlusion. Although cephalometric analysis proves useful in projecting the size and shape of the skull and jaws of patients who fall within these average growth patterns, it is not as helpful for individuals whose growth patterns fall outside them.

The coordinates from a patient's lateral skull radiographs can be fed directly into a computer, which digitizes them and performs the analysis. The measurements can be stored and printed out later and superimposed on the posttreatment measurements for a record of your child's progress.

Intraoral. In this portion of the exam, the orthodontist assesses the health and condition of the mouth, the soft tissues, alveolar bone, and the teeth and their supporting structures and detects dental defects and periodontal and other dental diseases using photographs, radiographs, and diagnostic tests. The orthodontist records the angle, spacing, crowding, rotation, displacement, or impaction of the different teeth, the relationship of the upper and lower incisors to determine whether overbite and overjet are within normal limits, and the relationships of the cusps of the teeth on one dental arch with those of the other arch. Factors that may make orthodontic treatment less successful, such as poor oral hygiene, enamel defects, and caries, also are noted.

Usually full-mouth, or preferably panoramic, radiographs are taken to show the presence or absence of teeth, their stages of development, and positions. If there is a problem with one or several teeth, the orthodontist will make more detailed radiographs, such as bitewings and periapicals.

Study models that show the teeth, dental arches, and alveolar process further aid the orthodontist in planning treatment. They also help patients to visualize their orthodontic problems and the proposed corrections. To make them, the dentist takes impressions of the teeth using a soft material. The dentist also measures the movements the jaw makes by having your child move his or her lower jaw forward and backward and to the right and left. Tracings of these measurements can be made and recorded. The impressions are sent to a laboratory where stone is poured into them to create the casts, or study models. When necessary, the dentist may mount the casts on an instrument called an articulator and adjust them to reflect the measurements of the jaw movements to make an accurate model of the relationship of the dental arches and teeth.

TREATMENT PLANNING

Using the information gathered from the radiographs and other tests, the orthodontist diagnoses the dental irregularity on the basis of the position of the teeth and skeletal pattern. For their own purposes, most orthodontists use a modification of a classification system devised by Edward H. Angle in 1880. In describing the malocclusion to you or to your child, however, it is more likely your orthodontist will use the terms listed in Box 15.1.

Next, the orthodontist describes what needs to be done to correct the problem, how long it will take, how much it will cost, and what outcome to expect. On average, comprehensive treatment lasts 18 to 30 months, depending on the severity of the malocclusion or facial irregularity, the patient's age, and the amount of tooth movement that is necessary. The fee for comprehensive treatment performed in a private office usually ranges from $3,000 to $6,000. Costs vary widely depending on the region of the country and the severity of the orthodontic problem and tend to be higher in larger cities than in suburban and rural areas.

B O X   15.1

SOME COMMON TYPES OF MALOCCLUSIONS

Anterior Open Bite. The back teeth are in contact with each other, but there is no overlapping of the front teeth. This often leaves a space between the upper and lower incisors.

Cross bite. The cusps of either the lower or upper molars do not fit properly into the fossa of the same tooth on the opposing dental arch.

Crowding. There is not enough space within a dental arch or a segment of it to accommodate the widths of the teeth.

Diastema. This space between two teeth often occurs between the upper central incisors (and sometimes between the lower central incisors where it is called a midline diastema).

Ectopia. A tooth erupts in an unusual, abnormal position in the mouth.

Impaction. A tooth is prevented from erupting by another tooth next to it, generally because of lack of adequate space.

Lip Incompetence. When the lower jaw is in a relaxed position, the lips are separated and do not form a seal (see lip seal).

Lip Seal. When the lower jaw is in a relaxed position, the lips come into contact naturally or form a seal.

Overbite. In the ideal occlusion, the upper incisors should overlap the height of the lower incisors by 1 or 2 millimeters. When the upper incisors overlap the lower ones more than a third, it is called a *deep overbite.* In a *complete overbite,* the edges of the lower incisors may touch the soft tissues of the palate. When the edges of the lower incisors dig into the soft tissues to such an extent that they cause sores or inflammations, the overbite is called *traumatic* or *impinging* and may cause damage to palatal soft tissue or bone. In a *reduced overbite* the upper incisors overlap the lower incisors less than one-third their height.

Overjet. When the teeth are occluded, the horizontal space between the lower and upper incisors is excessive. (You can test for it by trying to insert your little finger in the space between your lower and upper incisors.)

Rotation. A tooth is turned or rotated within its socket and appears twisted.

Transposition. The normal positions of two teeth are exchanged, for example, the first premolar is in the position of the maxillary canine and vice versa.

REASONS FOR TREATMENT

The majority of people today who undergo orthodontic treatment do so to improve the appearance of their smile and face. There are, however, some orthodontic problems that can affect aspects of dental health. Teeth that are crooked or crowded can be more difficult to clean; this makes them more susceptible to caries and periodontal disease. Some types of overjets or open bites may cause mouth breathing, which makes the teeth more prone to accumulating plaque and the individual more susceptible to periodontal diseases and caries. Other orthodontic problems can cause the teeth to wear down unevenly. This may place stress on the tissues, periodontal ligament, bones, and joints of the jaw, which may result in headaches and facial pain. Open bites, deep bites, and cross bites have been implicated in temporomandibular disorders (TMDs). (Although TMDs are sometimes treated orthodontically and sometimes successfully, there is no scientific proof that any one treatment will alleviate these problems for an individual.)

For most children orthodontic problems have little effect on speaking. An exception is lisping which can result from an anterior open bite or very wide spacing between front teeth.

TREATMENT

If the space required to bring the teeth into their corrected positions is insufficient, the orthodontist will decide the best way to create it.

Extraction

This common way of gaining space is necessary most often for patients who have crowding in one or both of their dental arches. Usually the same type teeth on one dental arch are removed to retain an aesthetic and functional balance.

After extraction, teeth adjacent to the one extracted will tend to drift toward the space. To prevent this and to maintain the space while teeth are uncrowded or retracted (moved back), different devices are used:

Headgear Worn at Night. This consists of a facebow and an elastic and cloth strap that circles the head and fits into bands on the upper first permanent molars.

Fixed Palatal Arch. A wire crosses the palate and is soldered to the upper first permanent molars.

A Removable Appliance. This consists of an acrylic base with clasps, usually on the upper first permanent molars.

Fixed Lingual Arch. An archwire runs along the inside of the lower teeth facing the tongue and is attached to bands on the molars.

Without Extractions

When just a little space is needed, the palate can be expanded and/or the shape of the dental arch changed to provide space to accommodate crowded teeth by using fixed, functional, and/or removable appli-

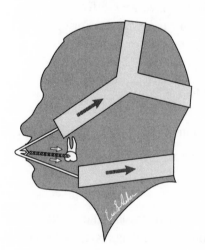

ILLUSTRATION 15.2.
ORTHODONTIC HEADGEAR.

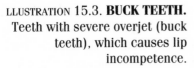
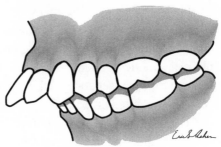

ILLUSTRATION 15.3. **BUCK TEETH.** Teeth with severe overjet (buck teeth), which causes lip incompetence.

ances. The type appliance used depends on the type of tooth movement desired.

TYPES OF ORTHODONTIC APPLIANCES

The type orthodontic appliance an orthodontist chooses for a patient and how long it needs to be worn depends on the type tooth movement(s) to be made and the patient's age, dental condition, and health. Frequent visits to the orthodontist are required throughout the duration of treatment so the orthodontist can monitor progress and make adjustments. For example, braces usually need to be adjusted every four to six weeks.

Fixed Appliances (Braces)

The wide variety of fixed appliances all use the same principle to reposition teeth: brackets bonded to the tooth crown act as a handle through which a force is applied to the tooth from archwires. Operating in this manner, a tooth can be moved within three planes of space: the root and crown can be moved in the same direction, they can be moved in opposite directions, and the tooth can be pushed in or pulled out. This ability to move both crowns and roots makes fixed appliances very efficient for moving teeth into the space left from an extraction or for creating spaces for prostheses. Teeth that are rotated can be derotated, and mild to moderate overjets can be reduced.

Fixed appliances offer many advantages. They are the most versatile and common of orthodontic appliances and can accomplish the greatest amount of repositioning for the greatest number of teeth. They are the only orthodontic appliance that can achieve the different movements at the same time, for separate teeth or different groups of teeth. Fixed appliances also require less patient cooperation than do removable appliances.

The design of the different types of fixed appliances varies, but each consists of similar components. Brackets of varying widths are bonded to the tooth with composite resin. The archwires may extend from molar to molar or be inserted into the brackets in sections. Different bends and loops may be incorporated into the archwires to make them more flexible and to achieve a specific type force or tooth movement. Elastics, in the form of rubber bands, threads, or coil springs can be attached to the arch wire to further aid tooth movement or to anchor teeth in their corrected position.

Braces may also be attached to headgear to help move teeth or secure them to their new position. Headgear usually is recommended for bedtime or at-home wear for 12 to 14 hours a day or as otherwise prescribed by the orthodontist. Although it should not cause severe pain, the teeth may become slightly sore and sensitive with initial wear and for an hour or two after the headgear is removed.

Several innovations have been made in recent years to make braces less noticeable and more appealing. Instead of metal, brackets can be clear or tooth colored. Minibrackets are smaller and impart a more delicate appearance to the braces. Nickel-titanium wires cause less discomfort than the conventional stainless steel and in some cases may shorten the overall treatment time. Elastics are available in tan, white, or, for the more adventuresome patient, vibrant colors. With lingual braces (also called invisible), the wires and brackets attach to the insides of the teeth (facing the tongue) so that they do not show.

Lingual appliances are not appropriate for all patients and present problems not encountered with traditional braces. Because of their location, they can irritate the tongue and interfere with speech. They are more difficult to place, more expensive, and require more frequent adjustments. Yet for adults who qualify for and want lingual braces, they may make the difference between seeking orthodontic treatment and forgoing it.

Removable Appliances

Although functional appliances, described later, also can be removed by the patient, the term "removable" is used to describe an orthodontic appliance that consists of a thin acrylic base that is held in the mouth with stainless steel clasps. It may also contain springs or occasionally expansion screws. To keep the appliance in position at the back of the mouth, clasps usually grasp the molars or premolars. To secure the appliance to the front teeth, a labial bow (a long arched wire that usually spans the front six teeth) is attached to the base plate, usually at the second premolar area.

Removable appliances are used most often to make simple tooth movements of one tooth or a group of teeth. They are not efficient in making rotational movements and are limited usually to tipping movements in which the tooth leans in the desired direction. To be effective, they must be worn as directed by the orthodontist. Most often they are worn full time and removed only during meals and when brushing.

Removable or Fixed Appliance?

A fixed appliance is required for most orthodontic treatment, especially comprehensive therapy involving moving both the root and crown of a number of teeth, derotating teeth, or pulling them in or pushing them out. When teeth require only minimal tipping movements, either a removable or fixed appliance can be used.

When deciding which appliance to use, the dentist will consider several factors. In general, a removable appliance is less costly than a fixed appliance because it does not require as much of the dentist's time. Since fixed appliances cannot be removed, they may be more successful for individuals, especially some children, who will not wear a removable appliance consistently. Braces do not need to be removed for cleaning or athletic activities and interfere less with speech than do removable appliances.

Functional Appliances

These appliances can be used alone or before and after treatment with a fixed appliance. When worn prior to fixed appliance therapy, they are used to change the relationship of the jaws and dental arches.

There are different types of functional appliances. Although they vary in design, all usually have a labial bow across the top incisors, which is inserted into an acrylic base.

Functional appliances offer advantages, as well as disadvantages. Because they are removable, they demand cooperation from the patient. Unlike fixed appliances, they do not trap food and therefore do not result in decalcification of the enamel or gingival hyperplasia.

BOX 15.2

KEEPING YOUR TEETH HEALTHY
WHILE WEARING ORTHODONTIC APPLIANCES

The following tips will help prevent or minimize caries from developing, reduce damage to your appliance, and maximize the effectiveness of orthodontic therapy.

- Brush after every meal or snack.
- Clean between your teeth at least once a day. Consult with your dentist or orthodontist for the correct way to floss around appliances.
- Use a fluoride mouthrinse every night before bed and after brushing or at the direction of the dentist.
- Ask your dentist about using an oral irrigator.
- Keep all appointments with your general dentist for regular cleanings and exams.
- Keep all appointments with your orthodontist.
- Wear all removable and functional appliances for the recommended time.
- Do not eat sticky foods, like taffy, caramel, or gum.
- Do not eat hard and crunchy foods, such as popcorn, nuts, peanut brittle, corn chips, corn on the cob, raw apples, or carrots.
- Cut hard foods, such as carrots, apples, meats, and bread crusts, into small pieces.

They may be difficult to wear, especially during the first few weeks. Occasionally they can cause abrasion, soreness, and ulceration of the oral mucosa, tenderness of the teeth, and temporary discomfort of the temporomandibular joint, especially on waking.

A functional appliance is worn for short periods for the first few days, then progressively for longer periods, until it can be worn round-the-clock, except for mealtimes. When introduced in this manner, the tissues of the mouth become accustomed to it. Rinsing with a saline mouthrinse during the first week helps reduce some of the initial soreness of the oral tissues. If discomfort persists, the patient should return to the orthodontist for possible adjustment of the appliance.

RETENTION

After orthodontic treatment, repositioned teeth have a tendency to return to their original position. To maintain the corrected tooth position until the bone and tissues can reorganize, removable or fixed retainers are used. Removable retainers are worn for varying lengths of time each day and in toto (from as little as three months to two years or more).

Of the three most common types of retention devices, the Hawley retainer is used most often. It is removable and usually passive (meaning it only holds the teeth in position). It consists of wires on the outside of the teeth, which are attached to a resin base. Hawley retainers are usually made for both the upper and lower dental arches and are worn full time except during meals for the first several months. After this, the wearing time is reduced, depending on the patient.

Some dentists use tooth positioners, which resemble removable mouthguards, made from synthetic rubber or another synthetic material. These are held in place by biting into them and sometimes by metal clasps.

For teeth that were severely crowded or rotated, a fixed retainer that is bonded on the lingual (tongue side) of the lower teeth can be used. Because sometimes it is left on for two years or longer, the dentist needs to inspect it frequently to be sure plaque is not accumulating beneath it.

TREATMENT RISKS

There are risks and benefits to orthodontic treatment as there are with all dental treatments and procedures. To justify undergoing it, the benefits (listed in the section "Reasons for Treatment") should outweigh the risks. The following are some risks that are involved during and persist occasionally after treatment for some but not all patients:

Caries and Periodontal Disease. The potential for these increases when oral hygiene is lax during treatment and too many foods with sugar are eaten.

Root Resorption. When this occurs excessively, the support of the affected teeth may be jeopardized and early tooth loss may result.

Tissue Damage and Bone Loss. In some individuals, when plaque is not removed consistently and thoroughly, inflammation of the gum tissues and loss of the alveolar bone may occur.

Change in Tooth Positions. After treatment, teeth may shift for a number of reasons including the eruption of the third molars, growth and maturation, mouth breathing, playing a musical instrument, or other oral habits. This can be minimized by wearing a retainer conscientiously.

Temporomandibular Disorders. These occur occasionally with or without orthodontic treatment.

Damage to a Tooth Previously Injured by Trauma or a Large Filling. Root canal therapy may be necessary.

Damage to The Teeth. Permanent decalcification of the enamel on the teeth, especially around the brackets and under loose bands, can occur when sugary foods are eaten and the teeth are not well brushed and flossed. Decalcification (the beginning of the decay process) appears as bands and spots of white where the brackets were when the braces are removed. Clear and tooth-colored brackets may cause attrition of the teeth, flaking of the enamel, and fracturing (when they are removed).

Irritation or damage to the oral tissues. This may result from loose or broken appliances and dental instruments.

Accidental Swallowing or Aspiration of Broken Appliances.

Headgear Injuries to the Face and Eyes, including Blindness. Although uncommon, these risks are greatest when the headgear is worn (when it should not be) during a sport activity or rough play. Some headgear is equipped with safety devices to prevent these injuries.

Growth During or After Treatment. This may require additional orthodontic treatment or oral surgery.

Longer Treatment Time than Estimated. This may be due to different rates of bone growth, broken appliances, or little cooperation by the patient (e.g., poor oral hygiene, not wearing appliances as instructed, and missing appointments).

Risks Involved in Treatments Done in Conjunction with Orthodontic Treatments. These include orthognathic surgery, extractions, and restorative and periodontal therapies.

SURGICAL ORTHODONTICS

The use of orthodontic and/or orthopedic appliances can make changes in skeletal relationships only if used during a child's growth period. For severe jaw malformations, such as mandibular and maxillary prognathism, orthognathic surgery, usually with fixed appliance therapy before and after, may be required. To prevent growth from undoing the surgical corrections, surgery is seldom performed until after puberty when additional skeletal growth will be minimal. Surgery may be performed earlier if the facial irregularity causes severe psychological distress or problems with function. Orthognathic surgery involves a team effort by an oral surgeon and an orthodontist. (See Chapter 18 for more information.)

CHAPTER 16

———

Prosthodontics

LOST TEETH

Throughout history individuals have tried different tactics to replace or conceal their lost teeth. Over 2,000 years ago, the Etruscans made gold appliances and attached them to natural teeth with gold wire. Queen Elizabeth I used rolls of cloth to puff out her lips that had sunk from missing teeth. Toward the end of the nineteenth century, when the stability of dentures in the mouth was so precarious that they had to be removed for eating, many denture-wearing ladies forswore dining in public, supping alone in their bedrooms.

We may smile at these quaint stories from the past. Yet, even today, with the availability of resin materials for denture bases and bone-integrated implants, replacing natural teeth with artificial teeth that can function well and withstand the wet and bacteria-laden environment of the mouth remains a complex challenge.

Why They Are Lost

Teeth most frequently are lost as a result of dental caries and periodontal disease. Less common reasons include injury, congenital problems, and benign and malignant tumors.

Why You Should Replace Lost Teeth

Each tooth depends for its stability on forces exerted on it by the teeth next to and opposing it in the other jaw. When a tooth is lost, the teeth next to the space or in the other jaw tend to drift, tilt, or move up or down toward it. This can change the alignment of the teeth and cause problems including:

Less Effective Chewing.

Tendency to Brux (Grind the Teeth). This may create periodontal problems and cause pain in the teeth and the temporomandibular joint.

Alveolar Bone Loss. When a tooth is lost, the bone surrounding the root (alveolar bone) is usually resorbed. Such loss of bone is minimal if only one tooth is lost but increases as more teeth are missing.

Loss of Aesthetics. Being entirely toothless causes the face to "collapse" as the space between the nose and chin diminishes. In addition, to function naturally, the muscles of the face that control facial expression require the support of either natural or artificial teeth.

Speech Problems. These include in particular problems with the pronunciation of the sounds D, F, S, T, V, and Z.

Erosion of the Quality of Life. Missing teeth are socially unacceptable and may affect one's self-esteem, as well as employability.

Difficulties Playing Wind Instruments. To prevent any of these problems, it is usually important to have missing teeth replaced as soon as possible by one or a combination of the treatments outlined in this chapter. Delaying their replacement may necessitate more involved treatment, including orthodontic and surgical therapies.

Yet, whether to replace a lost tooth or teeth (especially molars) with a prosthesis can be a complex decision involving the guidance of the dentist and the consideration of many factors. In general, the greater the number of teeth that are lost, the more difficult it is to decide which prosthesis to use in replacement and whether the benefits derived from replacement outweigh the costs and commitment of time replacement requires.

Who Should Replace Them?

General dentists are trained to and capable of making crowns, fixed partial dentures (bridges), and dentures. Most often, general dentists only refer patients who have complex prosthodontic needs, such as long and complicated spans of fixed partial dentures, to prosthodontists. (As explained in Chapter 3, a prosthodontist is the dental specialist who has received postdoctoral training in prosthodontics in a program accredited by the American Dental Association.) If you prefer to be treated by a prosthodontist, ask your general dentist to refer you to one. Be prepared, however, to pay more for the additional training and expertise the prosthodontist has received.

EVALUATION AND PREPARATION

If you have lost or had one or more teeth removed, your dentist can help you determine what the best option for replacing them is. Which type prothesis you choose depends on the number of teeth you have lost, your dental and overall health, the amount of supporting alveolar bone you have, your preferences, and how much you can afford to spend.

Before placing any prothesis, your dentist examines you to assess your periodontal condition, teeth, bone support, occlusion, and temporomandibular joints. Radiographs are made and a complete medical and dental history taken.

The dentist makes a (negative) impression of your teeth and/or supporting tissues in your mouth. In the laboratory a positive reproduction (a cast and die) is made from this to serve as a working cast model for your prosthesis. Your dentist uses a facebow (an instrument with calipers that orients your maxilla, the upper jaw, to the temporomandibular joints) to record the relationship of the jaws and the position of the teeth in one dental arch with the ones in the other. After making these measurements, the dentist mounts the cast of the teeth and supporting tissues on an articulator. This is an apparatus that simulates the manner in which the teeth come together during function.

FIXED PROSTHESES
(CROWNS AND BRIDGES)

Crowns

As the name implies, a crown is a restoration that replaces tooth structure lost from the crown of a tooth. The crown of a tooth can be damaged as a result of injury to the tooth and pulp; wear from erosion, attrition, or abrasion; a broken tooth (often one that has been restored before and has developed either secondary caries or a broken piece); and congenital conditions, such as amelogenesis and dentinogenesis imperfecta (described in Chapter 2).

Crowns are placed for different reasons:

- Aesthetic, to change the shape, size, or angle of the tooth or disguise a stained or misshapen tooth
- Function
- To alter the occlusion
- To provide support for a fixed partial denture (bridge)
- To prevent a tooth from fracturing

Crowns can be made of different materials, used alone or in combination. These include gold alloys; precious, semiprecious, or nonprecious alloys; porcelain; and composite resins. Crowns most commonly are constructed of porcelain over metal. Fusing porcelain to a metal alloy (palladium and gold, silver and palladium, or nickel and chromium) gives strength to the porcelain. A porcelain jacket crown may have a thin layer of platinum foil underneath the porcelain. Because of its propensity to fracture, all-porcelain crowns usually are used only on front teeth where aesthetics are paramount. Crowns of all metal may be used on back teeth for someone who has an extremely strong bite. To be restored with a gold or porcelain-fused-to-metal crown, the root of the tooth must be intact and firmly embedded in the alveolus (the tooth socket) and there must be sufficient dentin remaining to which the restorative material can adhere.

A crown restoration may cover, or cap, the entire crown of the tooth or a portion of it. Depending on what portion is covered, it is referred to as a partial or quarter, half, three-quarters, or seven-eighths crown.

Because a significant amount of tooth structure must be removed to place a crown, you should consider the alternatives. Before having one placed on a front tooth, ask your dentist whether the tooth could be bleached or have a porcelain laminate veneer or porcelain inlay instead. Depending on where you live, the materials used, and whether it is placed by a general dentist or prosthodontist, a crown can cost between $600 and $1,600.

Procedure. Placing a crown involves several visits to your dentist. First, the enamel and some dentin are removed from the tooth to make room for the restorative material. If you have an acceptable filling, some of the material may be left or removed and replaced for support in lieu of the natural tooth structure. Teeth that have had root canal treatment will almost always need to have the filling material removed and the canal enlarged to receive a cast metal post, unless there is already a post. Pre-fabricated posts are sometimes used and a core of amalgam or resin material added to provide support for the foundation of the crown.

Next, the dentist makes an impression of the prepared tooth structure or core. You are sent home with a temporary crown (usually made from acrylic resin). In the meantime, the impression is sent to a lab where the crown is made from the die of the master cast.

At your next visit, your dentist checks the fit of the crown. When you and your dentist are satisfied, the crown is cemented permanently in place after cleaning and isolating the tooth.

Care. Brush and floss your crown to keep it clean and free of plaque. To prevent chipping or fracturing of porcelain, do not eat hard candy or chew on ice or other hard objects.

Fixed Partial Dentures (Bridges)

Operating like a bridge, which is the common and descriptive term for this type of dental prosthesis, a fixed partial denture spans the space created by one or more lost teeth. Although it usually cannot replace more than two missing teeth in a row without increasing the number of abutment teeth, it can replace a number of teeth. If, for example, every other tooth in an arch were lost, a fixed partial denture could be used to replace these multiple teeth.

A conventional bridge requires either implants or natural teeth with crowns to serve as abutment teeth on either side of it. An artificial tooth called a *pontic* is attached by metal connectors that are soldered or welded to the metal restorations or crowns on the abutment teeth. When porcelain is used, it is bonded to the metals.

Most pontics are made with metal and porcelain. The porcelain is veneered onto the metal on the tooth surfaces that are visible. When aesthetics are important, porcelain may also be used on the biting surfaces.

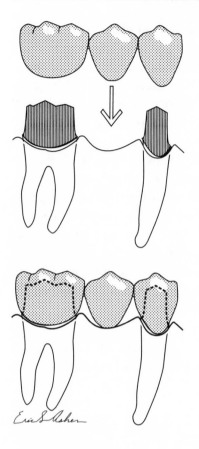

ILLUSTRATION 16.1.
FIXED PARTIAL DENTURE.
The fixed partial denture (commonly called a bridge) in this illustration consists of an artificial tooth called a pontic (in the middle) connected to crowns on either side. The crowns fit over the natural teeth that have been prepared to hold the fixed partial denture in place.

All metal is sometimes used on the back teeth where it is not noticeable and where the forces from grinding are intense. Pontics composed of composite resins with metal substructure supports are easy for a dentist to manipulate and repair. They will, however, wear and change size with temperature fluctuations and water absorption. At present, they are used most often for provisional prostheses, although some dentists use them for permanent prostheses when biting forces are heavy.

There are alternative designs, which are not as strong as the traditional type, but, in some instances, may be appropriate. On a *cantilever bridge,* only one side of the pontic is attached to a crown on an abutment tooth. Cantilever bridges usually are used on front teeth to avoid reducing the tooth structure of an intact healthy central or lateral incisor. In addition to being weaker than the conventional design, cantilever bridges can harm the periodontal tissues and cause the abutment tooth to tilt or drift. A *resin-bonded bridge* does not require crowns or much tooth preparation. Metal wings that extend from the pontic are bonded to the adjacent teeth. It, too, is not as strong as the traditional type and the long-term prognosis is usually not as predictable.

Teeth that are to serve as abutments must be evaluated carefully. Although the ideal candidate is a healthy and unrestored tooth, many people are reluctant to have healthy tooth structure removed. The health of the pulp of a prospective abutment tooth is evaluated using the tests described in Chapter 13. If it is questionable, the dentist may advise that the tooth first receive root canal therapy. Endodontically treated teeth can serve as abutments, although posts and cores are added to increase retention for the crown. Their roots must be of sufficient length and must not be so compromised from an apicoectomy as to erode bone support. Caries and restorations should be removed.

A tooth with bone loss needs to be carefully assessed before serving as an abutment. If bone loss is minimal, there may be little risk in using such a tooth as an abutment. In general, the greater the bone loss, the greater the risk of the tooth serving as an abutment. To compensate for the use of a tooth with bone loss, it may be advisable to use more than one tooth as an abutment. In all instances, however, the reasons for the bone loss must be diagnosed and corrective action taken to minimize future bone loss. Frequently, this requires periodontal treatment and close attention by the patient to maintaining excellent hygiene.

Problems increase when there are several teeth to be replaced using one long-span prosthesis. When a number of teeth need to be replaced, the natural teeth serving as abutments have greater forces placed on them from normal function and from habits, such as clenching and grinding. If the span of space to be replaced is too great for the number of abutment teeth remaining and / or the quality of the bone support on the abutments is compromised severely, it may be undesirable to replace the missing teeth with a fixed partial denture. In such situations, an alternative treatment might be a removable partial denture.

A fixed partial denture may also not be appropriate when there has been a loss of gum (gingival) tissue, which sometimes occurs when teeth are lost. The reason for this is that a fixed partial denture replaces tooth structure only. Therefore, when gum tissue has been lost, a better alternative may be the removable partial denture, which replaces both gum tissue and tooth structure.

Prices vary according to geographical area but generally are $800 to $1,500 per tooth unit.

Preplanning. All dental problems need to be remedied. Caries should be removed and restored, defective restorations replaced, and teeth that require it should be extracted or receive root canal or periodontal therapies. An analysis of the occlusion is necessary. Minor orthodontic movement of abutment teeth may be required to upright a tooth or alter its position.

Care. Whether a fixed partial denture remains secure depends on the health of the abutment teeth and the bone and gingiva that support it. The areas under and between the prosthesis and the natural teeth need to be kept clean and free of plaque. Dental floss threaders and interproximal brushes are helpful aids for this.

COMPLETE REMOVABLE PROSTHESES (DENTURES)

Conventional complete dentures are used when all the teeth in an arch are missing. The artificial teeth are affixed to an acrylic base.

Most people find it easier to wear the upper denture than the lower one. One reason is that the area supporting it is larger; this makes it more secure. The upper denture is supported by the maxillae (upper jaw). It is held in position by interfacial surface tension (the force that keeps two wet pieces of glass or plastic together) and a seal between the prosthesis and the movable oral mucosa of the lips and cheeks. When this contact is lost, the denture feels loose. The lower denture is supported by the mandible (lower jaw) bone and also is held in position by interfacial surface tension and a peripheral seal. However, the muscle movements of the tongue make the seal more difficult to achieve.

Because complete dentures depend on a combination of factors (including the facial musculature, the alveolar bones, the position of the tongue, and the quantity of saliva) for their success, not everyone is suited to wear them. For example, about 35 percent of the population has a tongue that is abnormal in size, function, or position, and so makes wearing a lower denture difficult and sometimes impossible. The following medical conditions and others may pose problems for wearing complete dentures:

- Cardiovascular diseases
- Xerostomia (dry mouth)
- Some skin diseases, such as pemphigus and erosive lichen planus
- Neurologic disorders, such as Bell's palsy and Parkinson's disease
- Osteoarthritis, especially of the temporomandibular joints
- Diabetes
- Blood dyscrasias
- Oral malignancies

Complete dentures cost between $500 to $2,500 per arch when made by a prosthodontist and between $300 and $1,200 per arch when made by a general dentist. There are reasons that the fee charged by prosthodontists tends to be higher. One reason is that prosthodontists have additional training and expertise in the art and science of placing and creating complete dentures. Another is that prosthodontists are often referred the most-complicated cases, such as when a patient has special needs or little to no bone remaining in the jaws to support dentures.

Preparation and Fitting

Before you can wear dentures, the dentist will examine your mouth to determine whether your oral tissues have been injured or damaged by other prostheses. If they have, removing the existing dentures for a period of time and using a tissue conditioner may be sufficient to allow the soft tissues to heal. To prepare the mouth for dentures, some teeth, especially if impacted, may need to be extracted.

If the bony (alveolar) ridges the dentures rest on have undercuts or are not broad or square enough, surgery may be performed to augment and / or recontour them. If there are bony lesions, including certain cysts, tumors, and soft tissue masses, they may need to be removed and biopsied. A frenectomy (see Chapter 8) may be required if the lingual frenum (the fleshy strip of tissue connecting the tongue to the floor of the mouth) is attached abnormally and would interfere with wearing dentures and prevent an adequate seal between the border of the denture and the tissues of the mouth.

To assist the dentist in selecting the size, shape, and shade of the artificial teeth, it is helpful if you have a photograph of yourself with your natural teeth. Replicating the small spaces or rotations they had will make your dentures appear more natural than if the denture teeth are evenly spaced, pearly white, and straight. In general, front teeth are chosen more for aesthetics and back teeth for their chewing ability. Artificial teeth are made from porcelain, which more nearly resembles natural teeth, or, more commonly, from acrylic resin. Porcelain is less resistant to abrasion caused by foods and toothbrushing, but is brittle and fractures more easily than acrylic resins. Porcelain teeth are attached to the denture base with pins, usually of gold; acrylic resin teeth are secured by bonding.

When arranging the artificial teeth on the denture base, the dentist takes into consideration the forces, leverage, relationships between the upper and lower jaws, shape of the underlying bony ridges, and occlusion, as well as aesthetic differences. All these vary with the individual. Because the teeth act as a unit, if any of these factors is out of balance, the comfort and fit of the entire denture will be affected, as can the health of the tissues, alveolar bone, and temporomandibular joints. For these reasons, it is very important to be treated only by a highly trained general dentist or prosthodontist for the diagnosis and fabrication of your dentures.

The dentist takes an impression of your dental ridges and surrounding tissues, from which a dental stone cast is made. This cast is put on an articulator to record the relationship between your upper and lower dental arches.

The dentist will set the teeth first in a wax base where they can be moved around or adjusted. When you are trying on your trial denture, be sure you are pleased with its look and fit before you approve it. You should be able to use your facial muscles freely to express different emotions, such as sadness, joy, and calmness without feeling discomfort or slippage of your denture.

After your trial denture is approved, it is sent to a laboratory where the teeth are affixed permanently to the plastic base and the borders are checked for proper length, fit, and thickness. During your next visit, the dentist applies a disclosing paste to all sides of the denture that are in contact with the soft tissues (to reveal whether the denture fits the soft tissues properly) and asks you to insert it. To correct areas where you feel pressure, the dentist will remount the dentures on an articulator and/or cover the chewing surfaces of the teeth with wax, paste, or paper and ask you to bite down to register the points of contact. When an error is found, the dentist grinds down the teeth before you reinsert them and wear them home.

Problems

Complete dentures are substitutes, not replacements for natural teeth. As such, they have limitations, which some but not all persons may experience:

Reduced Chewing Efficiency. Unlike natural teeth or implants, the force applied to dentures must be transferred to the tissues underneath. As a result, dentures have only about 25 percent the chewing efficiency of natural teeth.

Minor Speech Difficulties. These usually disappear within a few hours or days. Practicing reading aloud can help adapt your tongue to new dentures. If speech problems continue after you have been wearing dentures for a while, the dentist may alter the denture. If this does not correct the problem, you may want to see a speech therapist.

Resorption of Underlying Bone and Soft Tissues. Most of this occurs within the first six to eight months after teeth are removed. Many denture wearers believe their dentures are changing shape, when, in fact, it is their bone and supporting tissues that are shrinking. When this happens, the dentures may need to be relined or rebased (discussed later).

Injury and Irritation to the Oral Mucosa. Ulcerations, lesions, candida infections, and inflammation can develop. Poor nutrition and denture hygiene, alcoholism, allergic reactions, medical conditions (such as endocrine gland problems), and not removing the dentures can cause or exacerbate the difficulties. Correcting the cause helps minimize the problem.

Looseness, Especially in the Lower Denture. This can result from a retracted tongue or the inherent difficulties in keeping a lower denture in place.

Gagging and Vomiting. These reflexes may develop from dentures that are too loose or made or positioned incorrectly. They also may result from the fear of swallowing and dislodging the dentures. Saliva accumulates and triggers the gagging reflex. To remedy the problem, the cause must be identified. If the dentures are causing the problem, making the necessary adjustments may help. Sedatives, antihistamines, parasympathetic blocking drugs, and central nervous system depressants may be effective for some persons. For others, psychiatric treatment may be appropriate.

Clicking Noises During Speaking and/or Eating. These occur when the upper denture drops or the lower one becomes displaced. They may also occur if the upper and lower teeth are set too high in the base. Rebasing or remaking the dentures or replacing porcelain teeth with ones made of acrylic resin may help.

Cheilitis. Cracks or fissures at the points where the upper and lower lips meet can develop when denture teeth are not placed properly. Fabricating new dentures may correct these problems.

Additional problems associated with complete denture use, especially in the elderly and women, are discussed in Chapters 10 and 11.

Care

It is essential to keep dentures clean, to remove stains and debris, and to prevent them from developing an unpleasant odor. Debris under dentures can create pressure that encourages bone loss. See Chapter 5 for instructions on cleaning and Box 16.1 for tips on caring for your dentures.

The average life of a complete denture is about five years. A denture needs to be replaced when the biting surfaces of the artificial teeth wear or when there is significant resorption of the alveolar bone. When it no longer fits well, the denture needs to be relined. *Relining* involves resurfacing the side of the denture that is in contact with the soft tissues of the mouth to make it fit more snugly. With *rebasing,* the base of the denture is replaced and the relationship of the teeth is left the same. Rebasing and relining require impression and laboratory procedures. Both procedures are done to accommodate the denture to a change in the position of the tissues. This occurs after the soft tissues have shrunk and the alveolar

BOX 16.1

TIPS ON CARING FOR
YOUR DENTURES

• When cleaning your dentures, stand over a basin of water or soft towel to cushion their fall if they slip.

• Place dentures in warm (but not hot) water or a denture cleanser soaking solution when not wearing them.

• Remove dentures for at least eight hours every day. Constant pressure from the dentures on the supporting tissues will interfere with the blood supply to them and result in resorption of the bone and shrinkage of the soft tissues.

• Call your dentist if any part of your mouth becomes sore, irritated, or painful or your dentures become loose or uncomfortable, develop a bad odor, change color, or become stained or develop calculus deposits.

• See your dentist at least twice a year to have your dentures, the supporting tissues, and any remaining teeth examined.

• See only a dentist with a D.D.S. or D.M.D. for all your denture care.

• Have your dentist or hygienist mark your dentures with your name or Social Security number to aid in their recovery if you lose them.

• Don't make your own denture repairs.

• Don't use dental adhesives to make your dentures "fit." Short-term use of a dental adhesive while you are waiting for an appointment with your dentist is okay.

ridge on which the denture rests has resorbed. Some amount of bone resorption underneath complete dentures is inevitable. Treatment for abused soft tissues can involve one or more of the following: surgery on the tissues or bone, daily massage of the tissues to stimulate blood circulation, removal of dentures for 8 out of every 24 hours, and temporary relining of the denture.

Immediate Complete Dentures

Few persons who have lost teeth look forward to the prospect of remaining toothless for any length of time. An immediate complete denture, unlike a conventional one, is made so that it can be inserted immediately after the remaining teeth have been extracted. This confers obvious aesthetic, social, and professional benefits. It has other advantages: the denture acts as a splint to control bleeding and to keep food, saliva, and the tongue from entering the healing tissues.

An immediate denture also has disadvantages. It takes several months for the bone resorption and tissue shrinkage that normally occur after teeth are extracted. The immediate denture has to be altered to compensate for this loss of tissue. This requires relining of the immediate denture and, in some cases, a new set of dentures. This makes an immediate denture more expensive and time consuming; however, the benefit of having a denture placed immediately after the teeth are extracted versus going without teeth outweighs this disadvantage for many individuals.

Overdentures (Tooth-Supported Complete Dentures)

A variation on conventional complete dentures uses one or more natural teeth, usually in the lower jaw, to help support and stabilize the prosthesis. Teeth that are to serve as abutments may require periodontal and/or endodontic treatment before they receive a metal post and cap to provide support. Manufactured or precision attachments (e.g., ball and socket) also are sometimes used. The denture will cover the remaining tooth or teeth. In addition to the natural teeth, the denture receives support from the alveolar bone, gingiva, cheeks, tongue, and lips, as do conventional dentures.

An overdenture has benefits. The remaining roots of the teeth provide stimulation to the alveolar ridge, which encourages the repair and maintenance of bone and should result in less bone resorption. It is more stable in the mouth, especially during chewing, and there are fewer problems associated with wearing it than with conventional dentures.

It is, however, more costly and requires more visits to prepare the natural teeth to serve as abutments. Anyone considering it should use topical fluoride and must be conscientious about removing plaque from the remaining teeth to prevent caries and periodontal problems. Despite these problems, for an individual who qualifies for and can afford it, retaining even one tooth can offer a psychological lift and more support for the denture.

REMOVABLE PARTIAL PROSTHESES (PARTIAL DENTURES)

Fixed partial dentures usually are preferred by most persons. There are times, such as when the toothless span is too long or there has been too much bone loss, when a dentist may recommend a removable partial denture. For some individuals with many missing teeth, both may be used.

Partial dentures replace missing teeth by attaching acrylic or porcelain teeth to a gum-colored plastic base that is connected by a metal or acrylic frame. Metal frames provide greater support and greater stabilization.

Metal clasps, which are designed to grasp the abutment tooth or the precision attachments built into a crowned abutment tooth, help retain the partial denture in the mouth. Precision attachments are incorporated into the abutment crown and the removable partial denture frame. Although they cost more and have other disadvantages, precision attachments can be more secure and less visible.

Preplanning

To ensure successful fit, a thorough preplanning evaluation is essential. The dentist relies on the measurements derived from the diagnostic casts made from the impressions of the tissues in the mouth. If necessary, compromised teeth that would interfere with the denture may need to be extracted.

How much needs to be done to prepare the abutment teeth is determined from the study casts and the design of the denture. Crowns are necessary with precision attachments. Cast restorations for abutment teeth are not always necessary. Sometimes an abutment tooth can be altered by tooth reshaping (described in Chapter 14). How the abutment teeth are prepared varies with the individual and depends on different factors that the dentist evaluates during the examination.

A removable partial denture usually costs between $1,200 and $2,400.

Care

Partial dentures may feel clumsy the first few weeks. If the denture is difficult to insert, see your dentist. Do not try to force your partial denture into place by biting, as this can break the clasps. Be sure to remove your partial dentures at night to prevent the tissues from becoming irritated and to avoid grinding or clenching the prosthesis and damaging it. The care they require is similar to that of complete dentures, described in Box 16.1.

IMPLANT PROSTHETICS

Dental implants, which are inserted into the jaw bones, are artificial replacements for tooth roots. Artificial teeth alone or in the form of fixed or removable partial or complete dentures are affixed permanently or with clips, magnets, screws, or other attachments to the portion of the implant that sticks up through the gums. Dental implants can be used to replace one or more teeth. Implants have generated great excitement because of the many advantages they have over other dental prostheses. For example, fixed partial dentures (bridges) require tooth structure to be removed for crowns to be placed, sometimes on healthy teeth. Removable partial and complete dentures pose speaking and chewing difficulties for some individuals. Dentures may also become loose and the fear of their slipping causes embarrassment to their wearers. In contrast, a successful implant (approximately 90 to 95 percent are successful, when planned appropriately) provides close to the chewing efficiency of natural teeth, a statistic no other dental prosthesis can match. Also, because implants stimulate the alveolar bone, its resorption is either slowed or stopped completely.

Endosteal Implants

The name of the most popular and commonly used type implant is derived from the term "endosseous," meaning "within the bone." A titanium cylinder with or without threads is surgically placed in the bone of the upper or lower jaw.

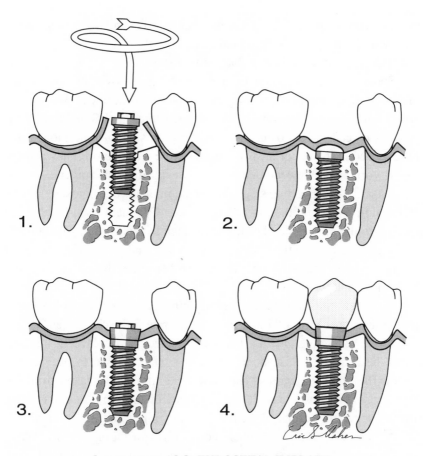

ILLUSTRATION 16.2. **ENDOSTEAL IMPLANT.**
1. The implant is surgically inserted in the bone through an incision in the gums.
2. The incision is closed, and after several months, the bone heals around the implant. **3.** An abutment cap is attached to the implant. **4.** A replacement tooth is placed over the implant abutment.

To avoid damaging the bone during implant placement, the drill speed is low and generous amounts of saline solution are used to irrigate the drill site to keep the tissues from overheating. The implants are placed carefully into the prepared sites. The implant is covered with the overlying soft tissue and allowed to heal for three to six months. The process by which bone heals around an implant has been named *osseointegration.* When osseointegration occurs, a firm contact that provides stable anchorage to the jaw is established. Implants may have other surface treatments, such as hydroxyapatite, a ceramic material that is similar in composition to bone and allows the bone to heal directly to it.

The surgical procedure is done in two stages:

Stage 1. A flap incision is made in the gums over the area to be implanted. The implants are surgically placed in the jaws. The area is closed with sutures. Healing takes between three and four months for implants placed in the lower jaw and between six and nine months for those placed in the upper jaw. If dentures were worn before, they usually can be worn again between one and two weeks after this surgery.

Stage 2. At the second stage the healed implants are exposed through an incision made in the overlying tissue. Cylinders (abutments) are attached to the implants and protrude through the soft tissue. The fabrication of replacement teeth is begun between one and two weeks later after the tissues have healed. A temporary prosthesis may be provided while the final prosthesis is being made.

Endosteal implants have a slightly higher success rate in the lower than in the upper jaw, although the success rate for each is over 90 percent. If the remaining alveolar bone is not adequate to place an implant, it may be possible to use bone grafts or synthetic bone to provide the support the implant requires. The bone for grafts can be taken from the chin area of the lower jaw, iliac crest (part of the hip), or other areas. Grafted bone can be placed on the alveolar ridges and in the maxillary sinus or nasal cavities to increase bone height in the upper jaw. When smaller amounts of bone are needed, a technique called *guided bone regeneration* can be used. In this procedure, membranes are implanted under the soft tissues and bone is encouraged to form underneath the membrane. The membranes are subsequently removed. Studies have shown that implants are successful when placed in healed grafted areas. Both bone grafting and guided bone regeneration generally involve longer healing times. Some individuals who are to receive implants need to have the inferior alveolar nerve relocated to avoid damage to it. Surgery to relocate the nerve can be done during augmentation of the alveolar ridge in the back of the mouth or placement of implants.

To assure the best outcome for implants, a patient needs:

- To be motivated to have the procedure
- To have sufficient bone support (either natural or supplemented with bone grafts)
- To have all remaining teeth and surrounding soft tissues healthy

- To be in reasonably good general and psychological health
- To practice good oral hygiene
- To have an experienced team of clinicians

Who Performs?

Implant surgery is performed by oral and maxillofacial surgeons and periodontists. The prosthodontic phase (presurgical planning and fitting the artificial teeth in the mouth) is done by prosthodontists or general dentists. Experience counts. Do not hesitate to ask dentists what training they have in the procedure, how many implants they have placed or restored, what type of implant system they use and why, and what their personal success and failure rates and those of the system they use are. In addition, you want a dentist who is committed to caring for you after the implants have been placed.

Evaluation and Treatment Planning

Careful evaluation and treatment planning before surgery is one of the keys to the success of implants. Pretreatment evaluation usually involves at least four office visits in which you see the prosthodontist or general dentist, oral and maxillofacial surgeon or periodontist, and often a radiologist. The preprocedural evaluation is the same whether implants are placed to replace one tooth or an entire arch.

To determine whether you can wear implants, the dentist conducts a thorough review of your medical and dental history, examines your existing prosthesis or prostheses and oral tissues, and evaluates your periodontal health and the relationships of your jaws. Two sets of casts (models) of the arches of the teeth and jaws are made. The first records the teeth and surrounding structures as they are before the implants are placed. On the other cast the dentist waxes in the areas of missing teeth to evaluate their effect on occlusion and the relationship of the jaws and to plan the implant prosthesis design. Radiographs are taken to determine the quantity and quality of the supporting bone and to evaluate the anatomy of the implant area. Many times it is necessary to obtain a special CT scan called a Dentascan. Sometimes during a CT scan a patient needs to wear a radiological template, an acrylic prosthesis that contains radiopaque material. This helps the prosthodontist or restorative dentist line up the implant and the artificial tooth in the correct position to each other. During treatment planning, the general dentist or prosthodontist frequently constructs the surgical templates that are used to guide the surgeon in the placement of bone grafts and/or implants during surgery.

Problems with Implants

In general, implants are well accepted and the surgery to place them involves little risk. There are, however, some risks and complications. They include:

- Injury to the mandibular nerve (which provides sensation to the lower lip and chin) during the placement of posterior implants in the lower jaw.
- Failure of the implants to heal in the bone. If the implant is loose when the artificial tooth is attached, it should be removed. The area should be allowed to fill in with bone (this takes between 9 and 12 months) before another implant is inserted.
- Bone loss if implants fail.
- Hyperplasia (overgrowth of gum tissue) around the healed implant. This usually occurs when oral hygiene is poor. Improving hygiene and using chlorhexidine mouthrinses usually reverse the problem. When discomfort or inflammation persists, gingival surgery to graft additional tissue to create an unmovable band of tissue around the implant may be needed.
- Breakage of the connection of the fixed partial denture to the implant. This may only require the replacement of a new screw to preserve the implant.

Costs and Longevity

Implants vary widely in price depending on the complexity and extent of the individual case. The cost of the implant and the surgery for each implant ranges between $750 and $1,600 (this includes the cost of the implants). The charge (additional) for fixed partial dentures or overdentures will vary with the work being done. When the cost is amortized over their expected life, implants are not as expensive as they seem, although the initial outlay is substantial. Most often, part of the expense for implants is out of pocket, as few insurance policies fully cover the costs.

BOX 16.2

CARING FOR YOUR IMPLANTS

Dental implants need to be cleaned daily to avoid bone loss.

Preparation

- Stand or sit in front of a large mirror that has good lighting.
- If you have trouble seeing close up, use reading glasses.

Cleaning Steps

1. Wrap thick floss or a sterile cotton ribbon resembling a shoelace around the abutment post and out front. A crochet hook or floss passer may help make this easier. If you like, add toothpaste.

2. Using a side-to-side motion, polish the post back and forth and up and down.

3. With toothpaste on the ribbon, clean underneath the prosthesis, using the same side-to-side or back-and-forth motion. An interproximal brush (which has a nylon-coated center wire to avoid scratching the metal posts) with toothpaste also can be used to clean the abutment posts and the undersides of the prosthesis.

4. Brush all the surfaces of the fixed prosthesis with a soft-bristled toothbrush. If you have a removable prosthesis, brush all its surfaces.

5. Brush the outer surfaces of the abutment posts and the gums with a soft-bristled toothbrush.

6. Rinse your mouth with water or an irrigator.

See your dentist

- If your prosthesis becomes loose
- For all regular appointments

CHAPTER 17

Temporomandibular Disorder (TMD)

"Temporomandibular disorder" (TMD), formerly known as TMJ, is a term for a collection of problems that affect the muscles of chewing and/or the temporomandibular joint. TMD causes a number of symptoms, but most frequently pain in the face and muscles surrounding the joint and a restricted range of movement in the jaw.

For the overwhelming majority of people with TMD, their problems are managed easily with simple care. The discomfort usually is occasional and temporary and the prognosis very favorable. For a small percentage of people, however, TMD can be a serious, debilitating, and long-lasting disorder that is difficult to treat. The chronic nature of TMD can propel some people, and sometimes the healthcare professionals who care for them, to try different treatments in a desperate attempt to eradicate the pain. Some of the treatments may be of little or no value, and some may make the condition worse. As with other persistent and painful conditions, TMD has, on occasion, attracted practitioners who promulgate unscientific remedies and procedures.

Determining who has TMD sometimes can be difficult because there is no definitive and widely accepted test to diagnose it. Because a variety of symptoms are associated with TMD, some of which are also identified with other disorders, the condition may be, at times, mis- and overdiagnosed. Despite these diagnostic hurdles, it is estimated that 6 to 10 percent of the U.S. population suffers from some form of the condition. Of this number, only about 5 percent seek treatment.

Most patients who seek treatment are women between the ages of 25 and 45. Why more women seek treatment for TMD than men is unknown, although a number of theories, none of which has been accepted or proved, have been suggested. Some experts believe that women may not necessarily suffer more from TMD but that they solicit treatment for TMD more often than men because they are more accustomed to seeking all types of medical care and seeking it earlier. Others believe women express stress differently from men. Still other experts speculate that hormone factors play a role, since the women who seek treatment for TMD are in their childbearing years. Estrogen receptors have been found in the temporomandibular joint, although the significance of this discovery, if any, is unknown.

With the recent attention TMD has been given in the media, it is tempting to think of it as a modern-day affliction, whereas it has plagued humans for centuries. Since it was first described in the medical literature in the early 1930s, TMD has been attributed to problems with muscles, occlusion, and internal derangement of the articular disc (displaced disc). Experts now recognize that the temporomandibular joint shares common characteristics with other joints, and like other joints (e.g., knees, hips) it is subject to both osteoarthritis and rheumatoid arthritis, which can be managed and treated successfully. Many problems with it will respond to the same kinds of conservative treatments, described subsequently, that are effective for injuries of other joints.

The purpose of this chapter is to help you understand the current thinking about this controversial and sometimes baffling condition, so that if you think you have TMD, you will seek appropriate diagnosis and treatment. By doing so, you may be able to avoid unnecessary, expensive, and irreversible treatments that may have lasting consequences.

THE TEMPOROMANDIBULAR JOINT AND SURROUNDING STRUCTURES

The temporomandibular joint, or jaw joint, is the hinge that connects the mandible, or lower jaw, to the temporal bone at the sides of the head, or skull. It allows us to perform different movements with the mandible (opening and closing, side to side, and forward and back), so we can chew, swallow, and talk. You can feel the joint move if you place your fingers in front of your ears when you open your mouth.

To accomplish these jaw movements, the temporomandibular joint is fitted into the glenoid (articular) fossa, a cavity in the cranium, the part of the skull that houses the brain at the base of the skull, behind the upper and lower dental arches (see Illustration 17.1.) When the mouth is opened and closed, the end of the mandible, the condyle, moves forward and back along the articular fossa and eminence. An articular disc of fibrous tissue fits over the condyle to cushion this movement. Special fibrous tissue permits the disc to slide over the condyle as the mandible moves.

Ligaments, strong semielastic bands of connective tissue, attach the disc and mandible to the skull. These ligaments prevent the jaw from opening too widely and the disc and condyle from slipping. A specialized part of the joint produces synovial fluid, a slippery film that coats the inside of the joint and lubricates its movement.

Muscles stretch from the mandible to the skull and help control the jaw as it moves. The strong jaw-closing muscles usually are the ones that

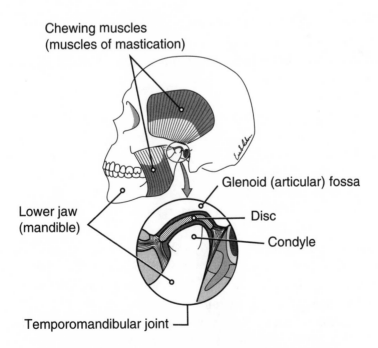

Chewing muscles
(muscles of mastication)

Glenoid (articular) fossa

Lower jaw
(mandible)

Disc

Condyle

Temporomandibular joint

ILLUSTRATION 17.1. **TEMPOROMANDIBULAR JOINT.**

become painful in TMD. The muscles responsible for opening the jaw are situated in the front of the neck above the Adams apple (the bulge of thyroid cartilage on the voice box).

S Y M P T O M S　O F　T M D

TMD can produce a wide variety of symptoms, many of which are similar to those of other, unrelated disorders. For its ability to mimic sinus, neurological, ear, dental, and other problems, TMD has been dubbed the "great imposter." This facility to masquerade as another disorder can result in misdiagnosis. It also may mean that a more serious medical disorder erroneously may be attributed to TMD and treatment for it delayed. For these reasons, diagnosing TMD may be difficult and require patience and sometimes perseverance by both dentist and patient.

Most individuals with the condition experience one or more of the symptoms listed below in the approximate order of their prevalence:

- Pain in the face or head region. This can be in or around the ear or jaw joint.
- Noises. These include clicking, grating, or popping sounds when the jaw is opened or closed.
- A decrease in the range of jaw movement.
- Sore jaw muscles.
- Headache.
- A temporary or permanent locking of the jaw.
- Pain when yawning, chewing, or opening the mouth, especially widely.
- Inability to chew properly.
- Bruxism (tooth grinding).
- Tooth pain for other than dental reasons.

At one time or another nearly everyone has one or more of these symptoms. Just because you have one of them does not mean necessarily that you have TMD. The following descriptions of some of the symptoms may clarify the confusion regarding them.

TMD can produce a variety of different sounds emanating from the jaw. Clicking or popping noises result when the disc slips in and out of its position. A grating sound results when the bones rub against each other and produce friction. This usually is caused when the disc moves out of proper position or perforates (develops a hole allowing the bones to rub against each other without cushioning). Arthritis of the temporomandibular joint may produce a grating sound. Temporomandibular joints that produce sounds but do not cause pain or other problems do not need to be treated.

Headaches related to TMD cause a generalized ache or a pain in the temple and may result from the repeated contraction of muscles of the head and neck from clenching the jaw. Headaches unrelated to jaw movement, jaw clenching, or chewing may not be related to TMD. Numerous other medical conditions produce headache and may require further evaluation by other specialists.

WHAT CAUSES TMD?

There are many causes of and factors that contribute to TMD. Sometimes the cause is obvious, such as an injury; other times the cause cannot be identified. TMD is seen in persons who experience the following:

Injuries to the Jaw

Direct or indirect injuries to the jaw from motor vehicle accidents, falls, fights, intubation during an operation, and exaggerated jaw movements can damage the temporomandibular joint. The damage can result from:

Trauma to the Chin. The impact is transmitted to the jaw joint.

Stretching the Jaw Open Too Wide, beyond the range of elasticity of the ligaments. This can happen during yawning or opening the mouth wide for a large quantity of food, for example, a hero sandwich. The joint can also sustain damage from dental and medical treatments that require the mouth to remain open wide for an extended period of time, as well as from surgeries performed under general anesthesia (especially in patients with small mouths), which involve spreading the jaws wide to accommodate the breathing (endotracheal) tube.

Grinding and Jaw Clenching

Oral habits, such as grinding the teeth, clenching the jaw, or biting the fingernails, increase the use of the jaw muscles and the force on the temporomandibular joints. This can cause the muscles to go into spasm and become sore. Individuals who clench their jaws while sleeping frequently complain of a sore jaw when they wake in the morning. A dentist usually can detect habitual jaw grinding by the flattening of the tooth cusps it can cause.

Stress

Although experts have been unable to point to a specific characteristic that distinguishes the person who suffers from TMD from one who does not, some dentists claim that some sufferers seem tense and under stress. When under pressure, some people unknowingly clench their jaws. This may be an instinctual response, a vestige of our evolutionary heritage. When confronted with an enemy, primitive humans had two choices: to fight or flee. Although neither of these is entirely acceptable in our culture today, we are still programmed to react with the same physiological responses as our ancestors did. Our bodies release adrenaline, our hearts pump faster, our muscles tense and contract, and our blood pressure spikes. For some people, some of the muscles that tighten are those surrounding the jaws and temporomandibular joint. Persistent jaw clenching will overtax the muscles and make them sore and painful. A constant level of stress can also lead to depression and a lowering of the pain threshold.

Malocclusion

When TMD was first identified, it was attributed to a problem with occlusion, or how the teeth of one dental arch contact those of the other. How much, if at all, occlusal problems contribute to TMD remains controversial, but recent scientific research does not give strong support to the role of malocclusion in the genesis of TMD.

A reason for this is that the position of the jaws and how the jaw moves does not rely on occlusion alone. Instead, they depend on the interrelationship of three things. The first is the way the bones, cartilage, ligaments, and disc in the temporomandibular joint are arranged. Second, the muscles attached to the jaw determine how it opens and closes. And finally, the position of the teeth contribute to the final position of the closed jaw. The joint, muscles, and teeth together (and not the position of the teeth alone) determine the movement and position of the jaw. They must all function properly for the jaw to feel comfortable. Fortunately, all these structures can accommodate to changes from minor injuries and aging. Many people with malocclusion do not have TMD. Many times malocclusion may be the result of TMD, not the cause.

If there is strong evidence for malocclusion as a factor in TMD, the traditional method for handling this has been to adjust the bite (change the occlusion). There are several ways to do this. The first, called occlusal adjustment, is to grind away small amounts of the tooth structure. Doing this alters the way in which the teeth come together when they are closed. Other methods include changing the shape of the teeth by crowning them or moving them with orthodontic treatment. These procedures have been used to treat TMD with mixed results. Neither method should be contemplated until after conservative treatments are tried and there is documentable evidence that malocclusion is a contributing factor.

DIAGNOSIS OF TMD

TMD involves problems with either the muscles or the temporomandibular joint itself or, more commonly, both. The following are four of the most common diagnoses of TMD:

Myalgia (Muscle Pain)

Other terms for pain that arises from numerous muscles include myofascial pain and dysfunction, myositis, and myofascitis.

Internal Derangement

Also called anterior disc displacement, this is used when the disc in the temporomandibular joint is displaced, or slipped, usually in front of the condyle. When this occurs, the bones move on the ligament, not on the cushioning the disc provides. As a consequence, the jaw cannot open fully. Recent research suggests that disc displacement is the result and not the cause of TMD. Some current studies indicate that biochemical changes in the synovial fluid may cause inflammatory changes and cartilage breakdown. The subsequent failure of the synovial fluid to lubricate the joint as it moves leads ultimately to disc displacement. Doctors now understand that many joints with disc displacement are fully capable of healing, even with the disc out of proper position.

Arthritis

Different types of arthritis can afflict the temporomandibular joint. Osteoarthritis, frequently called wear-and-tear arthritis, is the most common.

Synovitis

The synovial membrane of the joint becomes inflamed; this causes swelling, tenderness, pain, and restricted range of motion.

WHO SHOULD TREAT TMD?

Because of its ability to mimic other disorders, many patients with TMD visit a number of different doctors before coming to a dentist who is experienced in diagnosing and treating the condition. If you think you have TMD, your general dentist is a good place to start. Although the diagnosis and treatment of TMD does not constitute a separate dental speciality, many dentists are becoming more informed so that they can render appropriate treatment or make referrals to dentists who can. Before being treated, ask the dentist what his or her qualifications in the field are. (See Box 17.1 for advice on seeking care.) If your general dentist or the dentist to whom he or she refers you prescribes a treatment that you believe will be irreversible or expensive, you should seek a second opinion at, for instance, a dental school or hospital TMD pain clinic.

THE EVALUATION

A thorough evaluation of TMD involves some or all of the following.

BOX 17.1

TREATMENT TIPS FOR YOUR TMD

• Avoid being treated by a dentist or physician who adheres to only one approach.

• If possible, seek treatment from doctors affiliated with a recognized pain clinic.

• Seek a multidisciplinary team of healthcare professionals, such as a dentist, neurologist, physical therapist, and psychologist (if needed). It is best if they all share the same philosophy for treating TMD.

• Get an accurate and specific diagnosis.

• If you have doubts about your diagnosis and/or treatment, seek a second or even a third opinion.

• Ask your dentist or physician why each treatment is being prescribed and what it is to accomplish.

• Always try conservative and reversible treatments first. These include heat, massage, physical therapy, a soft diet, reducing stress, overcoming oral habits (e.g., chewing ice or grinding your teeth), or the use of a mouthguard at night.

• If a mouthguard has been prescribed, be sure to have your progress reevaluated after three or four months of use.

Interview

The time a dentist takes talking with you and taking a detailed history is potentially the most valuable aspect of diagnosing your TMD. Some dentists elicit the information via a questionnaire, whereas others ask you directly. The relevant information includes:

• What is your chief complaint? Which symptom (e.g., pain, clicking) do you feel needs the most urgent attention?
• Where does it hurt?

- How does it hurt? Is it a dull ache or a sharp pain?
- Is there a pattern to the pain? Does it appear in the morning, every morning?
- How long has it hurt or bothered you?
- What makes it better? What makes it worse?
- When did you first notice it? This is especially important for identifying a specific event that might have precipitated the problem.
- Has it become worse since you first noticed it?
- Do you have any oral habits, such as nail biting, jaw clenching, or teeth grinding?
- What treatments have you already tried?
- Does it affect your social and personal relations and your professional and recreational activities? If so, how and to what extent? Because many factors can exacerbate TMD, including stress, if chronic pain is suspected, some dentists will refer a patient to a psychologist for a psychological evaluation.
- How is your general health? Do you have any other health problems or complaints? Some medical conditions, such as rheumatoid arthritis or lupus erythematosus, can affect the temporomandibular joint in the same way they affect other joints. Muscle disorders, such as dystonia (characterized by irregular muscle spasms), can affect the jaw muscles. Neurological disorders, such as multiple sclerosis, can produce TMD symptoms.

Examination

The physical examination by an appropriately trained dentist remains the gold standard to evaluate TMD. The exam can be conducted simply; the dentist uses hands, a stethoscope, and a ruler. In a TMD exam, the dentist:

- Palpates the muscles of the jaw to determine whether there is soreness.
- Evaluates and measures the range of motion of the jaw, that is, how wide it can open and how much lateral (side-to-side) motion it has. Individuals who have TMD usually cannot open their mouths as widely as normal, although some are able to open them more widely.

- Listens to the sounds the jaw joint makes. Although this is usually done through a stethoscope, some dentists use their fingers to feel vibrations.
- Examines all soft and hard dental tissues to rule out dental diseases, such as caries, periodontal disease, and dental infections, and notes extreme malocclusions.
- Examines the head and neck. This can include a cranial nerve evaluation for individuals with suspected neurological problems. Consultation with other specialists, such as neurologists or otolaryngologists, may be required.

Imaging Studies

For many patients imaging studies may not be needed. Sometimes, however, they are necessary to visualize the structures of the jaw, head, or neck. Although various imaging studies can detect and verify joint problems, muscle problems usually cannot be seen. (See Chapter 21 for an explanation of the ones not described here.)

Transcranial Radiographs. These are radiographs taken across the skull with the jaw open and closed. They are useful in revealing severe problems with the condyle and glenoid fossa.

Panoramic Radiographs. These are valuable for viewing the entire upper and lower jaws on one film. They can reveal severe abnormalities of the bone, tumors, elongations of bones, infections, or old injuries.

Tomograms. These are sophisticated radiographs, in which a cross section of an anatomic structure is revealed. Tomograms can show detailed views of the condyle and the glenoid fossa.

Arthrograms. With this imaging study, radiopaque dye is injected into the temporomandibular joint and a radiograph is made. The dye surrounds and outlines the disc to reveal displacement or perforation.

Computed Tomography (CT). The computerized radiographs that are produced by this procedure can detect problems with the bones of the joint and disc.

Magnetic Resonance Imaging (MRI). This technique uses powerful magnetic fields to produce images of body tissues. It can detect problems involving the articular disc, bones, and inflammation, as well as soft and hard tumors in the joint. Because it does not expose the patient to radiation or dyes, MRI is surpassing CT and arthrography in many instances. MRI is seldom the first test given as it is expensive, not available in all communities, and not always covered by insurance.

Laboratory Tests

Laboratory blood studies and other tests may be ordered to help confirm the diagnosis when the physical examination and interview indicate that a patient's TMD may be related to a systemic disorder. Some examples include rheumatoid and psoriatic arthritis, lupus erythematosus, and temporal arteritis.

Other Methods

Although medications, local anesthesia blocks, mouthguards, and arthroscopy are used to treat TMD, they can, on occasion, be instrumental in diagnosing them. For example, a trial of carbamazepine, a medication used to treat the symptoms of trigeminal neuralgia, can help diagnose it and rule out TMD. Although arthroscopy (described subsequently) usually is used as a treatment, it can also be used with imaging studies to detect adhesions and perforations of the disc, as well as other abnormal conditions, some of which may require open joint surgery.

TREATMENTS

Research has shown that 80 percent of TMD patients will be relieved of their symptoms by one or a combination of the conservative and reversible treatments, described here. At the Temporomandibular Disorders and Facial Pain Clinic at Columbia University, the least invasive, reversible, and most conservative medical management is the first treatment provided. Conservative treatments include such therapies as soft diet, heat and/or cold therapy, muscle exercise and massage, mouthguards, and medications. Reconstructive open joint surgery and crowning the teeth are considered aggressive forms of treatment. No one should start treatment without first having a thorough diagnosis and evaluation by a qualified dentist or physician.

Any treatment you receive for TMD should be related to the diagnosis of what is causing your pain. Therefore, if you are given a diagnosis of TMD, you should ask the dentist or physician, "What specifically is causing this problem? Is it a disc? Is it stress? Is it muscle? What do you think happened?"

Soft Diet

To give the muscles and joints relief from activity, patients with TMD are instructed not to bite into foods that require that they open their mouths wide (e.g., a thick sandwich), to avoid crunchy or hard foods (e.g., bagels and carrots), and to cut food into small pieces. Most patients benefit by following a soft, or no-chew, diet, which includes foods like yogurt, scrambled eggs, cottage cheese, and mashed potatoes. Individuals who are in extreme pain may be put on a semiliquid diet. If the pain is from inflammation caused by a minor injury, adhering to this soft-diet regimen for two weeks usually is sufficient. Patients with chronic TMD, however, may need to follow a soft diet for an extended period of time.

Heat and Cold

Moist heat or cold, in the form of ice packs or a fluorimethane spray (a liquid spray that is very cold when it touches the skin), applied to the muscles of the jaw, helps inhibit pain. After using hot or cold packs (both are equally effective), mild stretching exercises should be performed to relax the muscles.

Muscle Exercise and Massage

Movement is vital to nourish and lubricate the temporomandibular joint and to keep the jaw muscles healthy. A daily exercise regimen, including massage and stretching sore muscles, may be suggested by the dentist, physician, or physical therapist. Before starting any jaw exercise program, an evaluation by a dentist or physician is required. (A referral to a physical therapist also may be needed.)

A simple exercise device, E-Z Flex, has been developed by doctors at Columbia University to improve the range of jaw movement, promote healing of the temporomandibular joint, and gently stretch sore jaw muscles. E-Z Flex consists of a mouth piece inserted between the teeth with a fluid-filled tube connected to a hand pump. When the hand pump is squeezed, hydraulic motion is transferred to the mouthpiece. This gently stretches the temporomandibular joint and attached muscles. (See Box 17.2 for simple jaw exercises.)

Ultrasound

Deeply penetrating heat from an ultrasound unit is effective for a joint that lacks mobility from scar tissue, fibrosis, or muscle spasm. Ultrasound is applied by a physical therapist or doctor.

Transcutaneous Electrical Nerve Stimulation (TENS)

TENS (described in Chapter 19) can be effective in relieving facial pain. It can be administered in the office by the dentist or at home by the patient.

Mouthguards

Although there are many variations, there are two basic types: those that reposition the jaw and those that do not. Because the repositioning types change the occlusion irreversibly, they should be used infrequently, if at all, and only after the nonrepositioning mouthguards have been tried.

The nonrepositioning types are flat and cover an entire upper or lower dental arch. They snap on over the teeth to prevent the jaws from closing and the teeth from contacting each other and can be removed easily for cleaning. They are made of either hard (acrylic) or soft thermoplastic material. The soft guards are not as durable as the hard guards, nor can they be adjusted to an individual's bite as well.

Mouthguards are not without some degree of risk. If made improperly, they can cause caries, inflame gingival tissues, or unintentionally

B O X 17.2

EXERCISES FOR TMD

As part of conservative treatment for TMD or following surgery for it, dentists or oral and maxillofacial surgeons may recommend a regimen of simple jaw exercises, the same or similar to the ones listed here, to stretch the muscles involved in moving the jaw.

The exercises, which can be done at home or work, are best done in a number of short sessions lasting no more than three minutes each. If you do them in front of a mirror, you can check whether you are doing them correctly and monitor your progress. Before performing these or other exercises, be sure to obtain your dentist's approval. After completing the exercises at home, apply either moist heat or cold to the sore muscles for five minutes.

Exercise 1—Stretch Open

1. Open your mouth as wide as you can *without* causing discomfort.
2. Hold open for five seconds.
3. Close your mouth, relaxing without the teeth touching.
4. Massage the muscles with your fingers while you rest for five seconds.
5. Repeat five times at one session, five times each day.

Exercise 2—Isometric Open

1. Place two fingers under your chin.
2. While trying to open your mouth, push up with your fingers to resist opening.
3. The resistance from the fingers is applied as gentle force to the chin for five seconds. (There is no real movement of the jaw, just resistance to opening.)
4. Rest five seconds and massage the muscles with your fingers.
5. Repeat five times, five times each day.

If done properly, the large jaw closing muscles should relax.

change the relationship of the dental arches and move teeth. When made correctly, mouth guards can:

- Take pressure off the jaw joint by separating the teeth. A mouth-guard reduces irritation to an inflamed joint by preventing the condyle from fully seating in the glenoid fossa, which occurs every time the teeth come into contact with each other, such as during swallowing or clenching.
- Decrease muscle activity.
- Make the wearer aware of oral habits, such as grinding.
- Provide a placebo effect for some individuals.
- Compensate for an uneven or uncomfortable bite.

Initially most mouthguards require the dentist to make minor adjustments, which can involve several follow-up visits. The mouthguard may need to be ground down to establish an even and comfortable bite or have a liner applied to it to make it more comfortable.

How long someone wears a mouthguard depends on the nature of his or her TMD. People who grind their teeth usually benefit most from wearing the appliance at night, whereas those who clench their jaw at specific times during the day, such as while at the gym lifting weights, usually will want to wear the device at these times. Wearing a bite plate 24 hours a day is not recommended since this may alter the position of the jaw. When symptoms resolve, many people can stop wearing them, although some people need to wear their bite plate at night indefinitely.

Relaxation Techniques

Different stress-reduction techniques, which include biofeedback, relaxation training (e.g., contracting and relaxing muscles), and breathing exercises, can help reduce the pain and restricted movement of the temporomandibular joint that are aggravated or caused by muscle contraction.

Medications

The following types of medications are prescribed for TMD:

Nonsteroidal Anti-inflammatory Drugs (NSAIDs) and Steroids. Reduce swelling in the joint and muscles. There are approximately 25 prescription NSAIDs and numerous over-the-counter products available. The most common are aspirin and ibuprofen. When NSAIDs are not successful, a short-term regimen of oral steroids or an injection of steroids into the temporomandibular joint may be tried. Although steroids are much more effective at reducing inflammation than NSAIDs, long-term use of steroids is not advised, as they can cause osteoporosis and many other serious side effects.

Muscle Relaxants. Help relax contracted muscles and may be beneficial for individuals who grind their teeth and clench their jaw at night.

Antianxiety Medications. Reduce anxiety and relax tight muscles. An example is Valium and there are others.

Narcotic Analgesics. Are sometimes used, but not for more than two to three weeks, to manage the flare-up of pain in patients with chronic TMD or the acute pain after surgery.

Antidepressants. Can be powerful tools to alleviate chronic pain (that which persists for more than six months). After experiencing chronic pain, many persons also develop symptoms of depression, including fatigue, difficulty sleeping, loss of appetite, decreased energy, and decreased ability to concentrate and enjoy life. Since the chemicals involved in both depression and pain are often the same, antidepressant medications that reduce depression also influence one's perception of pain. The most commonly used are the tricyclic antidepressants, such as amitriptyline (Elavil) and nortriptyline (Pamelor). They are effective for pain relief in doses much smaller than those used for depression.

Trigger Point Injections

Injecting local anesthetic through a needle into areas of muscle tenderness can alleviate muscular and neurological pain. Following the injection, the muscle should be stretched. This therapy usually is reserved for individuals whose pain has not responded to simpler therapy. Injections of anesthetic can also be used to diagnose and locate the source of pain.

REEVALUATION

A patient who is being treated for TMD needs continual monitoring and reevaluation and, at times, reexamination. If after three or four weeks of conservative treatment you are still experiencing symptoms, your dentist should reevaluate your diagnosis to be certain that a more serious disorder is not being overlooked. If the diagnosis remains TMD and you are not responding to conservative treatments, your dentist may modify the original treatment. As examples, if one medication disturbs your stomach, you may be given another, or if you are still eating chewy foods, you may be put on a softer diet.

If these things have been done and you still are not better with conservative treatments after three to six months *and* your problem is associated with the jaw joint (and not confined to the muscles), it is appropriate for your dentist to refer you to an oral and maxillofacial surgeon for further evaluation.

SURGICAL ALTERNATIVES

Many surgical procedures exist for the treatment of temporomandibular disorders. Which procedure is used depends on the specific needs of the problem and patient. Surgery can be performed either arthroscopically or through an incision that exposes the joint (open joint procedure). Brief descriptions of some of the surgical procedures are given here.

Individuals with TMD may be candidates for surgery if documented pathology or structural abnormalities exist that are surgically treatable (e.g., disc derangement and hypermobility) and some of the following criteria exist:

- There is pain or dysfunction, such as locking or limited jaw movement, which is intolerable.
- Jaw function is restricted.
- Nonsurgical therapy has failed to provide relief.
- The symptoms are getting progressively worse or are staying at an intolerable level.

When surgery is indicated and used as part of a comprehensive management plan, successful outcomes can be expected. The experience of the surgeon and diligent postsurgical physical therapy are critical factors involved in the outcome.

Arthroscopy

In this surgical approach, an arthroscope, which consists of a tiny (1.9 millimeters in diameter) lens and light, is inserted through a narrow hollow tube called a cannula, into the joint. The images of the joint and surrounding structures can be viewed either through the arthroscope itself or on a video camera, which magnifies them. Reconstructive surgical procedures can be performed by working through a second small cannula placed into the joint.

Arthroscopic surgery is less invasive and produces less scar tissue, and is usually followed by a quicker restoration of jaw function than open joint surgery. It results in small puncture wounds that usually require no sutures and leave only small marks. In selected cases, arthroscopic surgery can be performed under local anesthesia and sedation in an oral and maxillofacial surgeon's office, rather than in a hospital.

It is important to remember that, due to the small size of the joint,

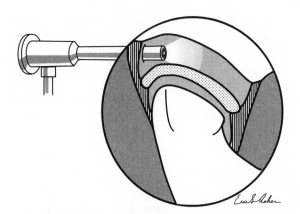

ILLUSTRATION 17.2. **ARTHROSCOPIC SURGERY.**
An oral surgeon can inspect the condition of and damage to the inside of the temporomandibular joint with an arthroscope, inserted directly into the joint.

the arthroscope, and the cannula, this is a minimally invasive surgical technique. Joint lavage (irrigation) and lysis (cutting) of adhesions (scarbands) are the most commonly performed arthroscopic procedures. As with any surgical procedure it carries potential risks. However, the incidence of complications is exceedingly small. These include the risk of damage to the middle ear, which can result in hearing loss; injury to the facial and/or trigeminal nerves, which is less likely to occur than with open joint surgery and may result in paralysis of some facial muscles; and the possibility that the small instruments will break and open joint surgery will be needed to retrieve them. Probably the greatest risk of any surgical procedure is failure to resolve the patient's pain or dysfunction. Arthroscopy demands a high level of experience and precision by the surgeon.

As a diagnostic tool, arthroscopy affords a good view of the following problems with the temporomandibular joint: displacements and perforations of the disc, synovitis, osteoarthritic destruction, and adhesions. Following this diagnostic look, the surgeon can treat based on the pathology that is seen. Adhesions and arthritic tissue can be removed, perforations of the disc can be debrided, and inflamed tissue can be trated with injection of medications under direct visualization.

Reconstructive Open Joint Surgery

Open Temporomandibular Joint Surgery. Another surgical option is open joint surgery, also called *TMJ arthrotomy.* It involves an incision in front of the ear, with the surgeon directly manipulating the structures inside the joint. Since there is an incision, sutures are required and overnight hospitalization is often necessary. The recuperation for this surgery takes longer and the potential for forming scar tissue is greater than with arthroscopic surgery. TMJ arthrotomy should be reserved as treatment for patients who have the formation of severe scar or bony tissue in the joint, tumors in the joint, or severe destruction of the bony structures of the joint. Passive motion exercises are an essential part of the rehabilitation following both arthroscopy and arthrotomy. Some of the potential complications following TMJ surgery include failure to relieve symptoms, decreased jaw opening, nerve injury, ear complications, and changes in the bite. Therefore, it is extremely important that your surgeon be highly skilled and experienced in this field.

Temporomandibular Joint Reconstruction. Although rare, there are some patients who develop an extremely rapid destructive process within the temporomandibular joint. This can be due to systemic rheumatologic conditions, tumors, or for unknown reasons (called idiopathic condylar resorption). These conditions cause such significant destruction in the joint that there is often a change in the occlusion. Surgical treatment may involve removal of the condyle and reconstruction of the joint, usually with the patient's own tissues, such as a rib graft or other bone graft sites. However, in some instances where the degenerative process is slow, the surgeon may opt to wait for the destructive process to cease, and then correct the occlusion with a combination of orthodontics (braces) and orthognathic surgery (see Chapter 18).

Temporomandibular Joint Implants. Total joint replacement with implants remains a controversial area. Although there have been several joint replacement systems available, most of these have not withstood the test of time. Research is currently being undertaken to find the most ideal temporomandibular joint replacement material. In the late 1970s and early 1980s an artificial material composed of teflon and Proplast (called a Vitek implant) was used in the repair of temporomandibular joints. This material is prone to premature wear, which can result in an inflammatory arthritis that produces pain and joint dysfunction. Current recommendations include the removal of this material from all joints, even if symptoms are not present. If you have had surgery for the temporomandibular joint in which an artificial material was used, contact your surgeon to determine if it was a Vitek implant and, if so, what steps to follow.

Disc Repositioning. In this procedure a disc that is displaced but whose structure is otherwise near normal is repositioned.

Discectomy (Disc Removal). Part or all of the disc may be removed when it cannot be repositioned because it is too severely damaged. Following discectomy, the disc may be replaced. The ideal replacement material has not as yet been determined. Examples of materials currently being used include: cartilage taken from the patient's ear, a graft of dermis (skin) harvested from the patient or a muscle/tendon flap from the temporalis muscle (muscles used for chewing). Replacing the disc may prevent bone changes, pain, joint noises, and adhesions, which can develop following the surgery.

Surgeries on the Condyle and Joint Fossa. These are performed on individuals whose temporomandibular joint has been damaged by degenerative arthritis, trauma, or other causes. Different procedures are performed, depending on the type and extent of the damage and its location. When the destruction is extensive, the damaged surface of the condyle may be shaved surgically or removed. Irregularities on the surface of the condyle are reshaped when the damage is less extensive. A number of procedures have been suggested to replace bone that has been removed, including a bone graft harvested from the patient's fifth, sixth, or seventh rib and secured with wire screws or plates.

Total Temporomandibular Joint Reconstruction. In patients who have lost their condyle as a result of severe degenerative arthritis, trauma, or surgery, total joint reconstructions can be performed. A prosthesis constructed of human-made material, usually a combination of plastic and metal, can be used. Prosthetic joints should not be used in children because they are still growing or in persons with systemic diseases, infections, or allergies that would interfere with healing. Reconstructing the joint with bone and cartilage grafts from the patient is also done. Joint replacement, similar to other types of joint surgery, requires aggressive postsurgical physical therapy to be successful.

Other Types of Surgery

If, during treatment for TMD, it is determined that correcting an existing malocclusion can improve the short- or long-term prognosis, a combination of orthodontic therapy and orthognathic surgery (see Chapter 18) may be required. This combined therapy may be appropriate for an open-bite malocclusion, which, if corrected, will provide a stable occlusion for someone who responded to splint therapy. Orthognathic surgery is performed as part of the overall treatment plan for the TMD. It is not joint surgery but is done to improve the relationship of the jaws.

The following organization will send a packet of information on TMD to anyone who calls or writes requesting it.

National Oral Health Information Clearing House
1 NOHIC Way
Bethesda, MD 20892-3500
301-402-7364
Call between 9:00 A.M. and 5:30 P.M. Monday through Friday EST.

CHAPTER 18

Oral and Maxillofacial Surgery— More than Removing Wisdom Teeth

Surgery on the Maxilla (Upper Jaw)
Surgery on the Mandible (Lower Jaw)
CLEFT LIP AND PALATE
OBSTRUCTIVE SLEEP APNEA

ITS SCOPE

In recent years, oral and maxillofacial surgeons have expanded their practices to encompass a wide range of dental, skeletal, and facial problems. This chapter will familiarize you with many of the procedures they perform and the reasons for them. Space does not allow detailed descriptions for each of them. The surgical placement of implants and surgeries for temporomandibular joint disorders, procedures oral and maxillofacial surgeons also perform, are covered in Chapters 16 and 17, respectively.

If you require oral surgery that is outside the realm of what your general dentist is qualified for or feels comfortable performing, he or she will refer you to an oral and maxillofacial surgeon. If you want more information or a referral to an oral and maxillofacial surgeon in your area who specializes in a certain procedure, call the American Association of Oral and Maxillofacial Surgeons, listed in Appendix 1.

EVALUATION

To diagnose your problem, the oral and maxillofacial surgeon takes a detailed history of your past and present oral and medical conditions and performs a physical evaluation. Laboratory tests (e.g., complete blood count and urinalysis) may be required for diagnosis and are usually required for preoperative evaluation, as are imaging tests, such as panoramic and other radiography, computed tomography (CT scans), and magnetic resonance imaging (MRI). Complete evaluation of a dentofacial deformity (see the section "Orthognathic Surgery") includes a cephalometric analysis and a model of the teeth and supporting structures.

Before surgery, depending on your medical condition, some of the precautions described in Chapter 12 may be taken. Donating your own blood is recommended if you are undergoing an operation that normally requires blood transfusions 10 percent of the time. Before undergoing anesthesia, it is very important to tell the surgeon and anesthesiologist about any medications you have been prescribed or are taking on your own. The surgeon should also give you specific postoperative instructions to follow to minimize complications and to hasten and make your recovery easier. It is best if you review these instructions with the surgeon before the operation to be certain that you fully understand them and can make any special preparations if required.

COMPLICATIONS

All surgeries carry potential risks. In addition to the risks of anesthesia, the risks of oral surgery can include scarring, infections, nerve damage, changes to the occlusion, and damage to teeth. Before consenting to oral surgery, you should thoroughly discuss with the surgeon the potential risks and anticipated benefits of the proposed procedure, as well as alternatives if there are any.

REMOVAL OF TEETH (EXTRACTION)

The surgical procedure oral and maxillofacial surgeons most commonly perform is the removal of teeth (extraction), including the third molars (known as wisdom teeth). Although most third molars are removed because they are impacted (cannot fully erupt because of an obstruction), nonsymptomatic third molars should not be removed routinely without a complete and thorough evaluation and a discussion of the potential problems that may arise.

Reasons for Extraction

By the time a child reaches 17 or 18 years of age, most dentists are able to determine whether there is sufficient room for the third molars to erupt fully. Most dentists will recommend that impacted third molars be removed for the following reasons:

Gingival Inflammation. This occurs most often when the impacted third molar(s) erupts partially and the gingiva overlies part of the tooth. This overlying tissue can easily become inflamed or infected either from bacteria and debris trapped between it and the crown of the tooth or from the trauma of an erupted opposing third molar biting down on it.

Dental Caries Involving the Second Molar.

Periodontal Bone Loss Involving the Second Molar.

Cysts and Tumors of the Jaw. Recent research has shown that left alone, only a small percentage of impacted third molars develop cysts or tumors. The lesions, however, may not cause symptoms and can grow quite large before detection.

Interference with Orthodontic Treatment or Its Results.

Pain. Occasionally an impacted third molar will produce jaw pain without signs of infection or caries. Other causes of the pain should be ruled out first.

Root Resorption. Erupting third molars occasionally cause the teeth next to them to resorb.

Dental Prostheses. Before fabricating a removable or fixed prosthesis, any impacted teeth underlying areas the prosthesis rests on should be removed to prevent bone resorption, perforation of the oral mucosa, pain, and possible infection.

Prevention of Jaw Fracture. An impacted third molar makes a thin lower jaw more susceptible to fracture.

Considerations for Extraction

Before third molars are removed a number of factors need to be considered, including:

Age. Older persons do not tolerate surgery as well, nor do they heal as quickly as younger persons do. Impacted third molars that are covered with bone and are not troublesome in older patients usually are not removed. The dentist will continue to monitor them and make panoramic radiographs every several years to be certain no problems develop.

Tooth Position. Surgery may not be performed if removal of the impacted tooth risks damage to the adjacent structures that would be more significant than the potential benefits of removing the impacted molar. The surgery may be less risky if impacted teeth are extracted before age 20. One reason for this is that the tooth roots are not formed completely and less of the surrounding bone needs to be removed. Also, incompletely formed roots mean there is more space between the roots and the inferior alveolar nerve. As a result, more bone must be removed, and the risk of damaging the nerve increases.

Surgery

In most cases, teeth are removed as an office procedure under local anesthesia (with or without sedation) or general anesthesia. To remove a tooth that is impacted in the bone, an incision is made in the soft tissue over the impacted tooth. The surgeon removes as little bone as possible to gain access to the tooth and the underlying bone. The tooth is either removed with forceps or an instrument called an elevator or cut into pieces with a drill and removed. The socket is irrigated with sterile saline and any rough edges of the bone are filed down and smoothed. The incision is then closed with sutures (often ones that dissolve).

Recovery

Although the amount of pain patients feel afterward varies, a tooth that is deeply impacted usually requires more surgery and is accompanied by more bleeding, swelling, and pain than one that is not as deeply impacted. Analgesics, most commonly aspirin or acetaminophen with codeine, and nonsteroidal anti-inflammatories (e.g., ibuprofen) are given routinely. Antibiotics (most often penicillin) are frequently prescribed.

Surgeons recommend slightly differing postoperative regimens. Patients who will be sedated should be sure they understand the instructions before the extraction. Ice applied to the cheeks and jaw (20 minutes on and 20 minutes off) for 24 to 36 hours after surgery can minimize swelling and pain. Placing a folded gauze sponge over the extraction site and biting with firm but gentle pressure can control postoperative bleeding. If bleeding (not a small amount of oozing) persists after a few hours of pressure, contact the surgeon. An effective way to keep the surgical site clean to promote healing is to rinse with warm salt water (one-half teaspoon salt in a glass of warm water) three times each day for five days starting 24 hours after the extraction. If pain or swelling begins to increase three days after surgery, call the surgeon.

Complications

Complications occur in up to 10 percent of surgeries to remove third molars. The incidence of complications increases with the difficulty of the surgery, the patient's age, and the experience and training of the surgeon.

The most common complication is dry socket (alveolar osteitis). Dry socket is reported to occur approximately 5 to 8 percent of the time after the removal of impacted lower third molars. Although some controversy exists regarding the cause(s) of dry socket, it is easiest to think of it as the delayed healing of a tooth socket following extraction. The condition can be very painful for the three to five days it lasts before it resolves. It seems to occur more frequently in persons who smoke cigarettes and in women who are taking oral contraceptives. Using a mouthrinse containing chlorhexidine before and after surgery may reduce the risk of dry socket. Treatment usually includes some cleaning (debridement) of the socket and placement of a medicated dressing in the socket. This produces almost immediate relief of pain. The dressing should be changed daily until the pain substantially diminishes. Other complications that occur occasionally include damage to the inferior alveolar nerve (located in the lower jaw).

INFECTIONS

Infection caused by teeth usually results from deep decay (caries) that involves the pulp or bone surrounding the tooth. The infection usually involves only nearby structures but can spread to the head and neck. Symptoms of dental infection can vary. Even with treatment, symptoms can include swelling of the face or below the jaw, pain, difficulty opening the mouth, fever, and tenderness. If any of these occur, it is critical to seek treatment immediately. Failure to do so can result in the spread of the infection to areas such as the orbit (around the eye, which can result in blindness), the brain, and the chest. Infections in these areas can be fatal. If the surgeon is concerned about the spread of infection, the patient will be hospitalized and placed on intravenous antibiotics.

Panoramic, periapical, and other radiographs may be made to diagnose dental infections. CT scans and MRIs also are used to diagnose and determine the location, extent, and spread of the infection.

Treatment usually involves four steps: removing the cause, surgical drainage, antibiotics, and supportive care. Until the cause of the infection can be treated, antibiotic therapy is vital. An incision and drainage procedure is often required. It can be performed in the office if the infection is localized and pointing into the mouth. If the infection has spread to areas beyond the mouth, the procedure may need to be done under general anesthesia in a hospital. Antibiotics may be administered intravenously rather than by mouth. When the immediate problem is resolved, the dental cause of the infection (if not treated as part of the incision and drainage procedure) must be treated as soon as possible with root canal therapy, extractions, or other procedures or the infection may return.

SINUS DISORDERS

The sinuses are openings or cavities in parts of the facial bones. They are lined with mucous membranes that, when irritated or infected, may thicken and block the sinuses, and so cause acute or chronic infection or sinusitis. Occasionally untreated acute sinusitis can spread to infect the eyes and brain and can result in meningitis, blindness, and possibly death. Radiographs and CT scans are used to detect the condition and confirm the diagnosis.

Acute sinusitis of the maxillary sinuses (under the eyes and on either side of the nose) most commonly is precipitated by the rhinoviruses responsible for the common cold. It also can occur when maxillary teeth become infected by tumors in the upper jaw, or injuries to the face. Symptoms of acute maxillary sinusitis include severe pain in the cheeks, headaches, fever, and lethargy.

Chronic sinusitis (lasting over three months) can result in a foulsmelling discharge from and stuffiness of the nose, bad breath, headaches, cough, lethargy, and depression.

Treatments include the use of antibiotics (usually ampicillin or amoxicillin), decongestants to shrink the inflamed sinus membranes, analgesics to relieve pain, inhalation of warm steam, and irrigation of the sinus with saline as prescribed by the doctor. If the condition is not controlled medically or the infection begins to spread, surgery usually is required.

Different surgical approaches are taken depending on the sinus involved and the extent of the infection. For some conditions, endoscopic surgery is the surgical approach of choice. An endoscope (telescope) is used to drain sinuses and to remove inflamed and infected sinus tissue. To remove benign cysts, tumors, and polyps and retrieve teeth from the sinuses, a more conventional surgery, called a Caldwel-Luc procedure, is performed under general anesthesia. In this procedure, an incision is made around the necks of or above the upper teeth. A hole is made through the bone into the maxillary sinus. Both types of sinus surgery are most often performed on an outpatient basis.

TRAUMA

Injuries to the teeth and face can run the gamut from chipped, loose, displaced, or avulsed teeth to potentially disfiguring and sometimes lifethreatening fractures involving the upper and lower jaws, nose, cheeks, and orbits (bones around the eyes). Listed here are some of the more common facial injuries oral and maxillofacial surgeons treat.

Dental Injuries

Teeth can be fractured from a variety of causes, including automobile accidents, domestic violence, child abuse, sport activities, and accidental falls. Radiographs usually are taken to reveal the extent of damage to the teeth and alveolar bone.

Injuries confined to the enamel can be repaired cosmetically by bonding (see Chapter 14). Fractures of the crown that expose the dentin should be covered, preferably with calcium hydroxide (pulp capping) as soon as possible. Fractures of the crown that expose the pulp usually require root canal therapy or extraction. Pulp capping can be used if the patient is young or the pulp exposure is minimal. Teeth that have become loose from the trauma are often stabilized by bonding or wiring for two to four weeks.

Permanent teeth in children that are pushed into the socket (intruded) are usually left alone for two to three months to see whether they will reerupt. An intruded primary tooth is usually extracted to prevent damage to its permanent successor. Permanent teeth that have been displaced (moved in a direction other than intruded) are repositioned and stabilized from two to four weeks. Radiographs should be taken to determine whether the roots have been fractured. If the pulp dies (this can occur soon after the trauma or later), root canal therapy must be performed.

Which course of treatment is taken for a tooth that has been knocked out (avulsed) depends on how long it has remained out of its socket. Overall, permanent teeth that are replaced in children have a better success rate than those in adults. For children there is 90 percent success if the tooth is replanted within 90 minutes. After 90 minutes the success rate drops to below 50 percent. Avulsed teeth should be transported, with the patient to the dentist, in a clean container. Milk is a good solution to keep the tooth moist, or it can be placed in the mouth under the tongue. After it is replanted, a tooth usually is stabilized for two or three weeks. Although the rate of infection following replantation is low, some dentists give their patients antibiotics and, if it is not up to date, a tetanus immunization. Even if the tooth stabilizes it may be lost through the process of resorption, in which the root is slowly dissolved away. Root canal therapy is usually necessary for teeth that have been more than moderately displaced. The teeth need to be radiographed yearly to monitor for root resorption.

Trauma over a larger area can result in a *fracture of the alveolar bone* or tooth socket and displacement of the tooth and its bony socket. Treatment for this injury is similar to the repair of any other fracture. Under local anesthesia, the fracture is reduced (moved back into position with finger pressure) and the fractured segment is stabilized with wires or appliances.

Facial Fractures

To restore the form and function of a displaced fractured facial bone, it must be reduced, fixed or immobilized, and stabilized for four to six weeks. (*Reduction* refers to moving a fractured bone to its normal position. *Fixation* refers to reconnecting a fractured bone with screws, plates, and/or wires to hold it in position after it has been reduced. *Stabilization* is done with various devices to immobilize the fractured bone to allow it to heal.) For obvious reasons, a cast, which is commonly used to stabilize a broken arm, cannot be put on the head to stabilize a broken lower jaw. Occasionally a traction device that resembles an erector set is used. More commonly the jaws are stabilized by wiring them closed.

Fractures of the Jaw. Fractures of the mandible (lower jaw) are treated by an open or closed reduction. During an *open reduction* the fractured bone is exposed, usually by an incision. It is then directly reduced (the surgeon can see it) and fixed with plates, screws, or wires. During a *closed reduction* the fractured bone is aligned from outside, without being directly exposed by an incision. To permit healing, the fractured bone ends must be stabilized by wiring the jaws together for four to six weeks. If an open reduction is done and the fracture is fixed with plates and/or screws, the jaws may not need to be wired closed to heal. Even when treated, fractures of the condyle (the end of the mandible), can result in temporomandibular dysfunction, such as internal derangement and ankylosis, and cause pain, noise, and difficulty opening the mouth.

Fractures of the maxilla (upper jaw) are not as common as fractures of the lower jaw. They most often result from a substantial injury to the face. Upper jaw fractures are usually repaired by open reduction and fixation with plates and screws.

Fractures of the cheek bone (zygoma or malar bone) most commonly occur as a result of sports injuries or fights. They are usually repaired similarly to upper jaw fractures. Symptoms may include double vision, numbness of the cheek, and difficulty opening the mouth. The fractured cheek may appear flattened. Treatment may be delayed until the swelling subsides. Occasionally a "blow out fracture," in which only the floor of the orbit (the bone around the eye) is fractured, occurs. Symptoms often include double vision. Multiple fractures of the orbital floor can cause the eye to look sunken. When double vision lasts longer than two weeks or is the result of a trapped eye muscle, surgery is usually required. During this procedure a human-made material or a bone or cartilage graft from the patient may be used to reconstitute the orbital floor.

Fractures of the Nose. Not every fracture of the nose requires repair. Fractures that produce an unacceptable deformity of the nose or that result in the obstruction of an airway are usually repaired by repositioning the nasal bone and cartilage. Repair may be done immediately following injury or be delayed until the swelling has subsided. To maintain the repair of the fractured nasal bones, either a premade splint is secured in place or a combination of tape and plaster is used. Fractures of the nose may also require packing of the nose to control bleeding or hold it in place.

Fractures of the Frontal Bone. When the bone of the skull that forms the forehead and frontal sinus is injured, damage can also be sustained by the orbits, nose, and cranium (skull). For extensive injuries of these areas, consultation with a neurosurgeon is usually requested.

As with all injuries involving the face, between 6 and 12 months after the initial surgery, additional surgery may be required to correct residual deformities. This may involve the use of human-made material and/or grafting bone from the patient's rib, hip, or skull, and correcting scars from lacerations or surgery.

SALIVARY GLAND DISORDERS

Disorders of the salivary glands include infections, obstructions, and chronic conditions, such as Sjögren's syndrome and benign or malignant tumors. Symptoms of benign disease include enlargement of the affected gland (as with the viral disease parotitis or mumps), pain, and a decrease or increase in the amount of saliva secreted. Tumors of the salivary glands cause enlargement but rarely pain.

Tests

Various tests aid in detection. Radiography commonly is used to reveal the presence of calculi (abnormal stones of mineral salts); CT scans and MRIs are useful to show masses in and adjacent to the glands; ultrasonography helps differentiate solid masses from cysts; and sialiography can detect calculi and other obstructions, as well as cysts and tumors.

With sialiography a catheter is inserted into the duct of the salivary gland, through which contrast medium is injected. Radiographs are then taken. A biopsy of a minor salivary gland in the lower lip may confirm the diagnosis of Sjögren's syndrome and sarcoidosis (a condition of unknown cause in which lesions develop around many organs, including the liver, lungs, spleen, and skin).

Treatment

Treatment depends on the condition that is causing the salivary gland disorder.

Sialadenitis. In this infectious condition, usually a parotid salivary gland (in front of and below the ears) swells; becomes tender, firm, and painful; and exudes pus but little saliva. The acute form most often occurs after surgery or in elderly, malnourished, dehydrated, and/or chronically ill persons. Treatment involves giving fluids and appropriate antibiotic therapy. The chronic form, most often associated with Sjögren's syndrome, is treated with systemic antibiotics and irrigation of the parotid duct with antibiotics.

Sialadenosis. This is a noninflammatory enlargement of a salivary gland, most often the parotid. It can result from malnutrition or other nutritional disorder (e.g., pellagra, beriberi), alcoholism, allergy, or the injection of an iodine-containing compound. Treatment aims at removing the underlying cause.

Obstructions. Trauma from a bite to the lip or cheeks or from other injuries can create *mucoceles,* lesions that result from damage to the ducts of the minor salivary glands. Some of these lesions disappear on their own, but most recur, particularly on the lower lip. When they persist or recur, the mucoceles, along with the involved minor salivary gland, need to be removed.

Ranulas are cysts, which can become quite large, that occur under the tongue in the floor of the mouth. Generally they do not disappear but instead reform, increasing and decreasing in size, as saliva leaks out into the surrounding tissue. Ranulas must be treated surgically.

Saliololithiasis, the formation of calculi within the ducts of major or minor salivary glands, occurs most often in men between the ages of 30 and 50. The stones within the glands usually cause less pain than those within the ducts. The partial obstruction of the duct by a stone will cause temporary swelling of the gland after eating from the increase in saliva. At other times it may cause no symptoms. If not treated, the salivary glands can become inflamed or infected. Antibiotics, analgesics, and surgical drainage of pus are used to treat an acute condition, after which the sialolith is removed surgically.

Tumors. Salivary gland tumors are uncommon. The most common tumor of the parotid gland is benign and called a mixed tumor or pleomorphic adenoma. A tumor that occurs in the sublingual gland has the greatest likelihood of being malignant. Benign tumors usually cause no symptoms and are slow growing. Malignant tumors grow more rapidly. Neither usually causes pain. When the facial nerve (which moves the muscles of the face) is affected, it usually indicates a malignancy. Both benign and malignant salivary gland tumors must be removed surgically.

CYSTS AND TUMORS

Nonmalignant Masses

Cysts and benign tumors are abnormal lesions that can develop in many areas in and around the mouth. They are almost always caused by problems with teeth (e.g., teeth that are unerupted, missing, or impacted). Depending on their size, location, and nature, the surgeon may remove the whole lesion or a part of it for biopsy. Cysts and benign tumors, such as the fibroma, require complete surgical removal. A few require complex surgery. For example, with the ameloblastoma, a tumor that occurs in the jaw bones, it is necessary to also remove some of the normal surrounding bone. This lesion has a high recurrence rate because it can extend minute fingers of cells into the surrounding tissue, and these cells can be left behind during removal. If a benign cyst or tumor has grown very large, the jaw bone can fracture spontaneously or during surgery. If this happens, it requires repair and reconstruction.

Malignant Tumors

Squamous cell carcinoma is the most common malignant (cancerous) tumor of the oral cavity. It can enlarge and spread both locally and to adjacent lymph nodes of the neck. Other types of oral cancers can spread to distant parts of the body (metastasize) through the bloodstream.

Treatment of oral cancer depends on the type of tumor. Early squamous cell cancer can be treated with surgery and/or radiation. Late disease usually requires surgery and radiation therapy. Chemotherapy is usually used as auxiliary therapy. Surgery often involves a radical neck dissection, the removal of the lymph nodes in the neck. If a large area of tissue needs to be removed, reconstruction is usually necessary to restore a patient's function and aesthetics. Reconstruction may be performed at the time the tumor is removed or may be delayed. Reconstruction techniques can include metal plates, bone grafts and soft tissue flaps, and complex grafts of bone, muscle, and skin, called free flaps. With free flaps, blood vessels in the neck are connected to blood vessels in the graft.

ORTHOGNATHIC SURGERY

The word "orthognathic" is derived from the Greek, *orthos,* meaning "straight," and *gnathos,* meaning "jaws." Orthognathic surgery is performed to correct a variety of skeletal (dentofacial) deformities of the upper and lower jaws. These deformities are usually accompanied by a malocclusion. Dentofacial deformities most often become apparent during development. They can be caused by genetic or acquired factors, such as trauma.

Surgery for Facial Imbalances

Orthognathic surgery is performed to correct facial imbalances, including the following:

Lower Jaw. With *retrognathia,* the lower jaw is small or underdeveloped and the chin appears receded. With *prognathism,* the lower jaw is overdeveloped, the chin juts forward, and the lower teeth may be in front of or overlap the upper teeth.

Upper Jaw. When there is *vertical maxillary excess,* the upper jaw is long or overdeveloped, the smile may appear "gummy" and the teeth may not meet. When the upper jaw is underdeveloped, a condition called *vertical maxillary deficiency,* the upper lip may appear sunken, the upper teeth may look receded. The upper jaw may also be receded or protruding.

Asymmetric Jaws. Sometimes one side of a jaw may develop more or less than the other; this makes the face look off center.

Open Bite Malocclusion. When the teeth do not meet, an open bite exists.

These facial imbalances not only make the face and jaws appear out of proportion but can cause problems with speech, occlusion, oral health, and chewing. The decision to undergo orthognathic surgery usually is made to improve the functioning of the jaws and teeth (e.g., to correct a problem with occlusion or make eating less difficult) and/or to improve the appearance of the face.

Orthognathic surgery is most often performed in conjunction with orthodontic therapy. It involves a team effort between the orthodontist and the oral and maxillofacial surgeon. Before surgery an orthodontist uses braces to move the teeth into the position they will be in after surgery. Third molars or other teeth may need to be extracted before orthodontic treatment to make space for the movement of the teeth. This phase of treatment can take between 6 and 18 months. Following surgery, orthodontic treatment is continued until the teeth are finally aligned. Following the removal of the orthodontic appliances, a positioner (a flexible plastic mouthpiece) or retainer is usually required to secure the teeth into their new positions.

Pretreatment evaluation is done by both the orthodontist and surgeon. The orthodontist will evaluate the teeth and bite using the casts, cephalometric analysis, panoramic radiographs, and other aids described in Chapter 15. The oral and maxillofacial surgeon also analyzes the records and models to determine how to reposition the bones surgically.

The entire process can take between 24 and 30 months. During this time patients visit the orthodontist and the oral and maxillofacial surgeon, as well as their general dentist for checkups and cleanings.

Orthognathic surgery is performed under general anesthesia in a hospital or outpatient surgical center. The surgery lasts between one and six hours. The newly positioned bones are prevented from moving by fixation appliances (screws, plates, and/or wires) until the bone has healed. Plates and screws usually are not removed, whereas wires, which keep the mouth closed to prevent the jaws from moving, are taken off in four to six weeks.

Surgery on the Maxilla (Upper Jaw)

Surgery on the upper jaw moves it forward, backward, up, or down. The operation leaves no facial scars, since the surgeon gains access to the jaw from within the mouth, most often under the upper lip. The upper jaw is cut horizontally and the lower portion of it is moved. To raise or lower it, a wedge of bone may be inserted or removed. The jaw is then immobilized with plates, pins, and screws. New bone will grow to fill in any spaces created.

The traditional method of expanding the width of the hard palate is with rapid palatal expansion (RPE) orthodontic appliances. In some instances, surgery is performed to assist the expansion.

Surgery on the Mandible (Lower Jaw)

Surgery on the lower jaw is done to make the lower jaw appear less or more prominent. As with the surgery on the upper jaw, a number of different techniques are used, most of which create no facial scars. After the cuts in the bone are made, the jaw is moved and fixed into position with plates, screws, and/or by wiring the jaws together.

Oral and maxillofacial surgeons can also operate on the chin alone, to make it more or less pronounced. To accomplish this, the bone on the end of the mandible is cut and pulled forward, backward, or downward to change the length of the chin. The new position is stabilized with wires,

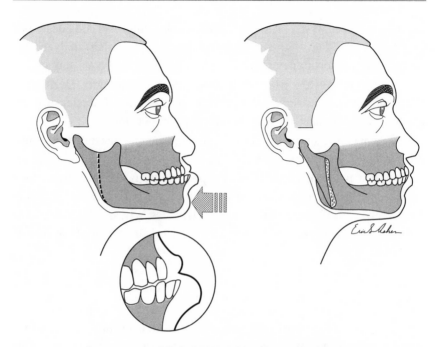

ILLUSTRATION 18.1. **ORTHOGNATHIC SURGERY.**
This surgery is performed to make the lower jaw less prominent and to correct the malocclusion (the bite between the lower and upper teeth). To accomplish this, the surgeon cuts the jaw, repositions it, and secures it in place with plates, screws, and/or wires.

plates, or screws. Since the incision is made through the mouth, this procedure, too, leaves no facial scars.

CLEFT LIP AND PALATE

Surgical intervention to repair the cleft lip or palate begins at three months and continues throughout childhood and sometimes into adulthood.

Surgery for a cleft palate, done at 12 to 18 months, brings the edges of the cleft or separation together and creates a seal between the nasal and oral cavities in the region of the hard and soft palate. Its primary goal is to encourage normal speech development.

Some children with cleft palates also have clefts that extend through the alveolar bone. This disturbs the alveolar ridge that supports the teeth. Bone grafts, usually from the hip, done at age 7 to 9 years, provide periodontal support for existing teeth and a path for the eruption of the canine tooth. Before the additional bone grafting, orthodontic treatment usually is done to correct cross bites and align the front teeth. Before, during, and after grafting, orthodontic appliances are worn to prevent the teeth from returning to their original positions. Both the bone grafting and expansion surgery are usually performed under general anesthesia in an operating room.

The normal growth and development of the face and jaws is affected by the cleft and the surgery done to repair the cleft. Subsequent surgery can repair these deformities. Following the correction of the skeletal and dental problems, deformities in the soft tissues, such as those that occur in the lip and nose, can be repaired.

Children with clefts are best managed by teams of professionals, which, in addition to surgeons, include pediatricians, neurosurgeons, ophthalmologists, audiologists, speech therapists, geneticists, psychiatrists, psychologists, orthodontists, pediatric dentists, prosthodontists, and social workers. Although the therapeutic interventions are time consuming, the benefits are great. Children born with disfiguring clefts who have received comprehensive therapy can expect to achieve very acceptable appearance and function.

OBSTRUCTIVE SLEEP APNEA

Sleep apnea is the cessation of breathing for at least ten seconds while sleeping. Someone with the disorder may be awakened during the night as many as 600 times, with each apneic episode lasting between 15 and 60 seconds. The total amount of time devoted to the apneic episodes can equal as much as one-half the night's sleep. Individuals with sleep apnea frequently feel fatigued during the day; this can interfere with their work and personal relations. Sleep apnea can also result in automobile and work-related accidents. In rare instances, the condition can cause sudden death. Bed partners often complain about the loud snoring, which is interrupted with the apneic episode when the person stops breathing for a short time.

The airway in someone who experiences sleep apnea may be

obstructed by tonsils, adenoids, a deviated nasal septum, or very occasionally a tumor in the nasal pharynx. Although dentofacial deformities are found in some but not all persons with sleep apnea, their correction sometimes relieves the problem.

Evaluation includes a physical examination with fiberoptic endoscopy, radiography, cephalometric analysis, CT scans, and polysonography. This last test is done in a sleep laboratory where the patient's sleep is monitored for the night. It includes an electroencephalogram (EEG) to measure the electric impulses made by brain cells, electrooculogram (EOG) to measure electrical impulses in the eye, electromyelogram (EMG) to measure electric activity in muscles, and electrocardiogram (ECG) to record the heart's electric activity.

Management of sleep apnea includes both surgical and nonsurgical therapies. Nonsurgical therapy includes splints to reposition the lower jaw, decongestants, snore alarms, and a mask device called CPAP. Surgical treatments include nasal septal surgery, tonsil and adenoidectomies, uvulopalatopharyngoplasty, laser-assisted uvuloplasty (LAUP), orthognathic surgery, and tracheostomy. Although a *tracheostomy* almost always results in a cure, this radical surgery, in which a tube is inserted through the neck into the trachea, leaves the patient disfigured and vulnerable to pain, infections, and bleeding. As such, it should be restricted to persons whose sleep apnea results in life-threatening cardiac dysrhythmias (irregularities or other abnormalities in the rhythm of the heart). With *uvulopalatopharyngoplasty,* the tonsils, adenoids, and uvula (the small, cone-shaped tissue that hangs down from the middle of the soft palate) are removed, along with some of the back margin of the soft palate. This surgery is highly successful for persons whose apnea is caused by an obstruction of the soft palate and tonsils. The *LAUP* procedure, effective in some patients, uses a laser to remove a small portion of the soft palate and uvula. The procedure is repeated a number of times until the patient experiences relief.

Orthognathic surgery, which involves advancing only the lower jaw or, in a more recently developed technique, advancing both the upper and lower jaws, is most effective for individuals whose sleep apnea is caused by airway obstruction at the level of the soft palate and the base of the tongue. The surgery on both jaws usually is performed only on persons whose obstructive sleep apnea is severe, who are obese, for whom other therapies have failed, and who have a lower jaw that is retruded severely but otherwise have normal skeletal development. Orthodontic treatment usually is done before or after both types of surgeries to prevent malocclusions and limitations on the amount of jaw advancement that can be accomplished.

PART VI

DENTAL FEARS,
EMERGENCIES,
AND
CONTROVERSIES

CHAPTER 19

Pain: Controlling It and Conquering Your Fear of It

T eeth are extremely sensitive, as anyone who has had a toothache can attest. The pain from an aching tooth has been described in various literary works. In Shakespeare's play *Much Ado About Nothing,* Leonato says, "There was never yet philosopher that could endure the toothache patiently." Throughout the ages, different cultures have devised prayers, chants, and cures to deal with their dental sufferings (including sticking the gums with a splinter or nail and driving it into a tree to "transfer" the pain). During medieval times, Christians felt victims brought the pain on themselves by committing egregious sins.

Fortunately, we no longer have to resort to lucky charms or bite bullets to endure our dental woes. The armamentarium of medications and techniques dentists now use routinely can render dental diseases and treatments painless. Even so, too many people remain fearful of dental care.

WHAT IS PAIN?

We all know pain when we experience it, yet it is a difficult concept to describe. Although there is no simple definition, it is generally accepted that pain is an unpleasant sensory experience usually initiated by some type of noxious stimulus. This is conducted via nerves to the central nervous system where it is perceived as pain.

Pain has a dual nature. *Pain perception,* how the painful impulse is produced and transmitted to the central nervous system and then perceived, is similar in all healthy persons. *Pain reaction,* how someone responds to the pain, varies between individuals and can change from day to day in the same person. How much pain we can tolerate (our pain thresholds) is influenced by our emotional states, fatigue (we feel more pain when we are tired), ages (in general, older persons tolerate pain better than younger persons, including children), and fears and anxieties (which decrease our pain thresholds).

Dentists today can alleviate both aspects of pain. By employing the different modalities and medications explained in this chapter, the physiological perception of pain can be eliminated and our negative reactions (anxieties) to it can be reduced greatly, if not banished completely.

REDUCING ANXIETY

In a survey asking people to list what they feared, visiting the dentist ranked second, behind public speaking. Between 6 and 14 percent of the population is so anxious about dentistry that it puts off visiting the dentist until the pain becomes so severe that it can no longer be endured. As a consequence, the treatments these people need may be more involved and more anxiety provoking than they would have been had the problems been detected and remedied earlier.

Many dental patients are mildly to moderately fearful of dental care. Even though these individuals visit the dentist routinely, they do not find it pleasant. While sitting in the dental chair, they experience low levels of stress, with an elevated heartbeat and sweaty palms.

Most people who are apprehensive about receiving dental care either have had a negative prior experience at the dental office or have heard stories from others and formed a preconceived negative notion about dental treatment. People who are 30 and older may remember their childhood trips to the dentist, when they had numerous carious lesions filled using lower-speed drills and no local anesthesia. Today, with the advent of high-speed drills and topical and local anesthetics being commonly used for restorative procedures, everyone's visit with the dentist can be painless or nearly so.

You and your dentist can make your dental visit more pleasant using the following methods.

Nondrug Methods

Rapport with Your Dentist. One of the most effective methods to reduce anxiety about dental treatment is to establish a good relationship with your dentist and dental hygienist. A sympathetic dentist with whom you can share your feelings will tailor treatments to accommodate both your dental needs and fears. Your dentist should discuss the different options for pain and anxiety relief with you and let you know realistically what to expect.

If you are very apprehensive, you may need to shop around before choosing a dentist who is committed to helping you and who will take the time to reassure you and provide the techniques and support you may need. Be sure to select a dentist who is available 24 hours a day if you have an emergency following treatment. In addition, choose a dentist who will provide you with posttreatment pain and antianxiety medication if you need it. (See also Box 19.1.)

Guided Imagery. There are many ways of harnessing the power of your imagination so that you can feel more relaxed while in the dental chair. One is to imagine that with every breath you take in you are breathing in calmness and with every breath you expel you are releasing tension and worry. As you breathe slowly and rhythmically, imagine this feeling

---

BOX 19.1

TIPS FOR MAKING YOUR VISIT TO THE DENTIST LESS STRESSFUL

• Choose a dentist with whom you have a good rapport and can comfortably discuss your anxiety over dental care.

• Schedule your visit early in the day so you don't spend the day worrying about it.

• Get a good night's sleep. (Rest lowers your reaction to pain.)

• If your dentist recommends it, arrive at the office 30 to 60 minutes early to take an antianxiety medication (e.g., Valium or Ambien). Make sure you have arranged to have a responsible adult take you home.

• Be sure your dentist explains why you need treatment and what is involved in each step. Being knowledgeable will give you a sense of control over the situation and take away your fear of the unknown.

• Accept that a certain amount of anxiety is normal.

• Bring a tape recorder with earphones along with your favorite music to listen to during treatment.

• Schedule short visits. If possible, have different procedures performed at separate appointments.

• Visit regularly. Postponing visits increases the likelihood that small dental problems will become bigger problems that will require more extensive and expensive treatments.

• If it makes you feel more comfortable, ask a trusted friend or family member to come with you to the dentist.

• Decide with your dentist before treatment what signal (a raised hand or a nod) you can use to indicate if you are becoming uncomfortable or apprehensive.

• Tell your dentist what your specific fears are. Some people fear the injection, some fear the noise of the instruments, some feel claustrophobic (from the dentist working close to them or from the nose cone for nitrous oxide), and some do not like the loss of control.

• Use your imagination before and during the procedure to feel calmer. (See the section "Guided Imagery.")

• Use distraction techniques during the procedure. Focus on a picture on the wall or music, or breathe slowly and rhythmically, counting each breath.

• Reward yourself with a treat (e.g., a movie or a book) afterward.

• Be kind to your family and friends. Fear is contagious. Don't tell dental care tall tales. If you are anxious about visiting the dentist, you may easily pass your fears to your children or to others.

• Parents should avoid the use of dental treatment as a threat and should not instill fear in their child before a visit.

• See the dentist for routine evaluation and cleaning prior to any invasive procedures.

going into every part of your body. Or, if you prefer, imagine that you are in your favorite place. This might be on a beach, in a garden, on a boat, or by a meadow or lake. Practice these exercises before visiting the dentist so that they are effortless for you to do once there. You can develop these visualization skills on your own or have a session or two with someone trained to guide you through these and other exercises. To find a practitioner, consult the Academy for Guided Imagery, P.O. Box 2070, Mill Valley, CA 94942, telephone 800-726-2070, or the American Holistic Medical Association and the American Holistic Nurses Association, 4101 Lake Boone Trail, Suite 201, Raleigh, NC 27607.

Hypnosis. Hypnosis produces an altered state of consciousness by focusing the attention so that concentration on other stimuli (e.g., needles, anxiety) is reduced. Hypnosis was first used in dentistry in 1837 to provide sole pain relief for an extraction. Ten years later it supplied the only analgesia for the removal of a tumor from a patient's jaw. With the discovery of anesthesia, hypnosis fell out of favor as a way of blocking pain during dental treatments. Recently, however, there has been a resurgence of interest in it.

Some studies have shown that over 90 percent of patients who use hypnosis can undergo many dental procedures without the use of anesthesia. Hypnosis can be especially valuable for patients who are unable to use local or general anesthesia, such as those with allergies or idiosyncratic reactions to drugs, or who are extremely anxious about injections. It can also be used successfully to treat some chronic (benign) facial pain, to encourage oral hygiene, and to help denture wearers adapt to their prostheses.

To learn more or to find a hypnotherapist and/or a dentist who uses hypnosis in practice, ask the International Medical and Dental Hypnotherapy Association, 4110 Edgeland, Suite 800, Royal Oak, MI 48073, telephone 800-257-5467 or 810-549-5594, or the National Society of Hypnotherapy, 2175 NW 86 Street, Suite 6A, Des Moines, IA 50325, telephone 515-270-2280.

Electronic Anesthesia (EDA). A newer alternative to local or topical anesthesia is electronic anesthesia (EDA). This works on the same principle as transcutaneous electrical nerve stimulation (TENS), used in physical therapy to relieve pain. A small current of electricity is sent via surface electrodes through disposable pads that are placed on the mucosa, usually beneath the teeth that are undergoing treatment. EDA can anesthetize an area to receive an injection or provide enough pain relief so that anesthesia is not required for simple restorative processes, such as placing amalgam and composite fillings, cementing crowns, and periodontal scaling.

EDA has advantages: it is noninvasive, uses no needles, and incurs no posttreatment numbness, speech problems, or adverse reactions to anesthesia. It has the added benefit that it is controlled by the patient. After the dentist places the pads in your mouth and establishes your baseline tolerance, you can maintain or increase (but not decrease) that level.

It cannot be used on persons who have pacemakers or epilepsy, are pregnant, or have histories of heart problems, cerebrovascular accidents, or transient cerebral ischemia.

Pharmacologic Methods

Medications. Valium or another antianxiety medication, which your dentist can prescribe, can be taken 30 to 60 minutes before an appointment to help you relax. Since you should not drive while on the medication, be sure to have someone else take you to and from the dental office.

Sedation. Although the local anesthesia dentists use should eradicate pain, many anxious patients prefer the additional use of nitrous oxide with oxygen or intravenous sedation to decrease anxiety and produce conscious sedation. Some individuals who are extremely apprehensive even request the deeper state of sedation produced by general anesthesia. See the following sections for descriptions of these techniques.

PAIN CONTROL

The following are different ways dentists can manage pain before, during, and after dental treatment.

Pretreatment Medication

Taking a nonnarcotic analgesic medication, such as ibuprofen, aspirin, or acetaminophen, before potentially painful dental treatments, among them periodontal procedures and extractions, has been shown to reduce the need for narcotic medication afterward. This is especially beneficial for patients who are unable to take narcotics, such as those who have substance addictions. (Nonnarcotic or nonopioid analgesic medications are not related to or derived from morphine or its related substances.)

Local Anesthetics

Local anesthetics are commonly used before many routine dental procedures to relieve pain during treatment. They are injected slowly into the oral mucosa and connective tissues in the mouth to anesthetize the area where the treatment will occur. The agents used most frequently are lidocaine (Xylocaine), usually with a small amount of epinephrine; mepivacaine (Carbocaine), used with the vasoconstrictor levonordefrin or alone, and, less frequently, prilocaine and marcaine, with and without epinephrine. The local anesthetics without epinephrine are well suited for use in persons with untreated hyperthyroidism and certain adrenal medullary tumors, in persons taking some antihypertensive and antidepressant medications, and in persons at risk for cardiac arrhythmias.

A topical anesthetic can be applied at the site of the injection to take the sting out of the injection. To numb the area effectively, it needs to be left on for at least two minutes before the local anesthetic is injected. If you are not offered a topical anesthetic and would like one, request it.

Conscious Sedation

Conscious sedation is a state in which you are less aware than usual of what is going on around you. If you are consciously sedated, you do not require assistance to breathe and swallow as these reflexes remain intact. Although the different types of conscious sedation and even general anesthesia are used most often because patients are uneasy about a dental procedure, medications with analgesic (pain-reducing) effects can also be added. Sedative drugs may be delivered orally, by inhalation, intravenously, or intramuscularly.

Nitrous Oxide with Oxygen. Nitrous oxide, commonly called laughing gas or sweet air, has become increasingly popular in recent years. It produces a light level of conscious sedation to decrease anxiety and, to a slight degree, the perception of discomfort.

To administer it, nitrous oxide is mixed with varying amounts of oxygen and inhaled through a hood placed over the nose. It produces a tingling in the toes and fingers (some patients hear white noise) and a sense of relaxation.

Nitrous oxide has many advantages. It can be titrated, so that the dentist can administer more or less of it a the patient requires (compared to oxygen). It is reversible almost immediately, so the effect lasts only as long as it is being inhaled, and it can be turned off midprocedure if you do not like it.

It produces few side effects, but may produce nausea, so a full stomach should be avoided, though light meals are acceptable. You must have someone accompany you to the dental appointment. Nitrous oxide can be used on most people, including those with cardiac problems or asthma; it is not appropriate for individuals who have difficulty breathing through the nose, are claustrophobic, pregnant, or have emphysema.

Many general dentists are prepared to use nitrous oxide. Some states require dentists to obtain a certificate to administer it.

Intravenous Sedation. In some cases nitrous oxide may not provide sufficient anxiety control, especially in long procedures, so intravenous sedation may be a preferable technique. With this method of conscious sedation, the medications are introduced intravenously (through the bloodstream), usually in a vein in the arm, to achieve varying levels of sedation. In the shallower level of sedation, the patient is awake and breathing and swallowing on his or her own. In the deeper levels of sedation, the patient is much less apt to remember what is going on but can be aroused. All persons who are sedated intravenously must have another person take them home and should refrain from oral intake six to eight hours prior to the procedure.

To produce these effects, a mixture of medications is used. This can include varying amounts of a sedative or antianxiety drug, such as the benzodiazepenes (e.g., Versed or Valium); a narcotic, such as meperidine (Demerol) or fentanyl (Sublimaze) for pain relief and euphoria; and sometimes a barbiturate, such as methohexital sodium (Brevital), for the patient to reach a deeper level of sedation. The topical anesthetics, ethyl chloride in spray form or EMLA, which stands for eutectic mixture of local anesthetic, can be applied to the skin, so that the intravenous line can be started without discomfort. Most of the medications used for intravenous sedation have amnesic qualities, so you will have difficulty remembering what happened. They can be given comfortably in a dental office by an appropriately trained dentist.

Because levels of consciousness or sedation are a continuum, patients can easily slip from a lighter stage, in which they can maintain their breathing and swallowing reflexes, to a deeper stage (induced with general anesthesia), in which they cannot breathe on their own. In case a deep stage of sedation is reached inadvertently, it is imperative that all dental personnel be highly trained in airway management and emergency techniques. For this and other reasons, almost every state requires that a dentist receive a certificate and training in anesthesia and be certified in advanced cardiac life support before administering sedation intravenously or intramuscularly. As a consequence of these restrictions, not every dentist offers it.

If you are considering having intravenous or intramuscular sedation, it is important to find out what anesthesia training the dentist who will be treating you has had. Since all oral and maxillofacial surgeons receive at least four to six months of operating room anesthesia training and three years of ambulatory anesthesia training as a requirement for their specialty, you can be assured they have the appropriate training. If, however, a general dentist is going to perform intravenous sedation, you should ask whether he or she has completed an accredited dental anesthesia residency program or has met the state requirements to perform intravenous sedation. You also should find out how often the dentist administers it.

There should be a minimum of two dental personnel present, one appropriately trained person to administer the anesthesia and monitor the patient and the other to perform the procedure. Ideally, every member of the office staff (from secretary to dentist) at an office where anesthesia is given should be trained in performing basic life support.

Other Methods. Medications to induce sedation can also be delivered intramuscularly (through an injection), orally (by liquid or tablet that is swallowed), and rectally (usually in suppository form). Medications in liquid form frequently are given to sedate children. The intramuscular route is sometimes best for patients who are mentally retarded. Rectal suppositories are used most often for children or physically or mentally challenged persons to begin general anesthesia or to proceed with a treatment.

General Anesthesia

General anesthesia is seldom used for routine dental procedures. Exceptions are many surgical procedures, such as surgery on the jaw to correct congenital or acquired deformities and for cleft lip and palate correction. It may be the only technique that will be tolerated by some persons, among them individuals who are *extremely* anxious, or have mental or physical conditions, such as Down syndrome, mental retardation, autism, cerebral palsy, or multiple sclerosis, and young children unable to cooperate. In addition, many dental patients who may be able to endure procedures that require one to two hours to complete with intravenous sedation, may not be able to cope with longer procedures, unless they are "put under."

General anesthesia produces losses of pain and memory and a partial or total inability to breathe, cough, and swallow on one's own. These functions must be monitored and maintained artificially by the anesthesiologist with endotracheal tubes (breathing tubes) and other equipment. As with other types of sedation, with the exception of nitrous oxide, individuals who have undergone general anesthesia must have an adult escort them home.

Many of the same medications used in intravenous sedation are also used in general anesthesia. They are delivered intravenously and by inhalation through face masks and endotracheal tubes, with oxygen and sometimes nitrous oxide and oxygen to increase the effect of the barbiturate. Equipment, including pulse oximeters, EKG, sphygmomanometers, end tidal CO_2 and temperature monitors, and esophageal stethoscopes to monitor vital functions, is also required.

General anesthesia during dental procedures can be performed in a dental office or dental surgical facility or in a hospital operating room on an ambulatory basis. For short (less than 30 minutes) surgical procedures, such as the removal of impacted third molars, which are performed in an oral surgeon's office, a light form of general anesthesia is usually used. With this level, the patient still breathes spontaneously so the airway does not need to be maintained artificially with a breathing tube, although the protective reflexes around the larynx are depressed. A long-acting local anesthetic is often used also. This has the added benefit of keeping the patient free of pain from 6 to 12 hours after the procedure. While longer procedures, from 30 minutes to 4 hours or more, can be performed in a dental office or a dental surgical facility, they are better done in a hospital operating room where the staff and equipment to handle emergencies are available.

The minimum number of dental personnel involved in administering general anesthesia in a dental office are an anesthesiologist, an assistant, and a circulating nurse. The person who administers the anesthetic must have completed a minimum of two years of training in anesthesiology. He or she could be a dentist, a physician anesthesiologist, or a certified registered nurse anesthetist.

Patients who have severe systemic diseases that may or may not limit their activity, as well as patients for whom a dentist or physician determines that general anesthesia should not be administered in a dental office, should always be admitted to a hospital and receive it there. When general anesthesia is administered in a hospital, the dentist performing the dental or surgical procedure does not need to be trained in anesthesiology, as the hospital will supply a dentist, physician anesthesiologist, or certified registered nurse anesthetist.

Emergencies during general anesthesia, although uncommon, are more frequent than they are with conscious sedation. With other methods of pain control available for the dental patient, general anesthesia should not be used unless necessary.

If you are having general anesthesia, you will be evaluated more thoroughly before the procedure than if you were having conscious sedation. The following laboratory tests may be required: urinalysis, complete blood count, and a hematocrit and/or hemoglobin count. Chest radiographs and electrocardiograms usually are taken for persons over the age of 35. Refraining from food and drink for six hours is essential (as it is also for intravenous sedation) to avoid vomiting that could obstruct the airway or infect the lung during the procedure. General anesthesia may be more difficult to perform on obese persons, particularly if they have short, thick necks, or on persons who have significantly decreased cardiac and/or pulmonary function or a history of myasthenia gravis or poliomyelitis, in which the chest muscles have been compromised.

Posttreatment Pain Relief

For the vast majority of dental procedures, nonnarcotic analgesics (aspirin, acetaminophen) or nonsteroidal anti-inflammatory drugs (e.g., ibuprofen) are sufficient to relieve mild to moderate pain. For more severe pain, especially that which can arise after surgical extractions or periodontal or endodontic treatments, narcotic analgesics, which require a prescription, may be necessary. Dentists are licensed to write prescriptions for these medications.

Although effective for pain, narcotics have side effects. They are constipating; can cause nausea, gastrointestinal upset, and drowsiness; and can produce dependence. You should not drive, operate machinery, or drink alcohol while under their influence.

CHAPTER 20

In an Emergency

Many different types of injuries can involve the teeth or skin and bones of the face. Most are the result of automobile, sports, or other accidents. When the injury appears serious or when a considerable amount of pain is involved, people know to seek prompt professional care. There are, however, dental injuries that may not seem as significant but still require immediate dental care. The following pages describe some dental emergencies and what you should do for them before you can reach and/or are treated by your dentist.

PREPARATION

One of the most important things you can do to prepare for a dental emergency is to have the number of your dentist accessible at all times. Post it on your refrigerator, carry it in your wallet, and put it in your address book, along with other emergency telephone numbers (e.g., the fire and police departments, physicians, and hospital). You should also give the number of the dentist to your children, in case they should be injured at school or in your absence. When abroad, in case of an emergency, a listing of U.S.-trained dentists can be obtained from the U.S. consulate in the country in which you are traveling.

TOOTHACHE

Even if the pain from a toothache is bearable, you should never ignore it. It may signal caries, an abscess, periodontal, or endodontic problems. Quick dental attention can remedy the problem and may mean the difference between saving or losing a tooth.

If you have a toothache:

- *Call your dentist and follow instructions.*
- Take, as directed by your dentist, an over-the-counter pain medica-

tion, such as acetaminophen (e.g., Tylenol) or a nonsteroidal anti-inflammatory drug (e.g., ibuprofen) to relieve the pain.

- Do *not* place aspirin or any other medication directly on your tooth or gums.
- Rinse your mouth with warm water to remove debris and food particles.
- Use dental floss to remove food particles trapped between your teeth.
- Avoid very hot, cold, or sweet foods and beverages if they cause discomfort.

PROBLEMS WITH ORTHODONTIC APPLIANCES

For all problems with orthodontic appliances, call your dentist immediately and follow instructions. Until you can visit your dentist or orthodontist, the following may be done:

- For wires that are irritating your lips or cheeks, use beeswax, gauze, or part of a cotton ball to cover the end of the wire. Do not use chewing gum.
- Do not try to pull the orthodontic wire out.
- Remember to take any loose orthodontic appliances or portion(s) of a broken appliance with you to the dentist.

OBJECTS CAUGHT BETWEEN TEETH

If you have something trapped between your teeth, try removing it before you call your dentist. To do so:

- Use dental floss carefully.
- Do not use sharp implements.
- Rinse gently with warm water.
- Brush your teeth.

If you cannot remove what is caught between your teeth, call your dentist.

BLEEDING

The measures listed here should be taken if:

- You bite your tongue or lip and the bleeding does not stop after ten minutes.
- After a tooth extraction, the area begins to bleed. (If you feel the bleeding is significant, you may not want to wait and may instead decide to seek treatment immediately.)

In either of these instances, if the bleeding continues, try to stop the bleeding. To do so:

- Use a clean gauze or cloth and apply direct pressure to the area.
- Continue applying the pressure for five minutes.
- If the bleeding continues, apply pressure for five minutes using a moist tea bag.
- *If the bleeding still continues and you are unable to stop it with direct pressure, call your dentist. If you are unable to reach your dentist, continue applying pressure and go to a hospital emergency room.*

DENTAL INFECTIONS

In general, the faster the onset of swelling and pain, the more serious the infection. Symptoms of dental infections include:

- Pain
- Fever
- Discharge of pus
- Foul odor
- Swelling
- Temperature

Call your dentist if you experience any of the symptoms of a dental infection. If you cannot reach your dentist and your symptoms continue, go to a hospital emergency room.

Infections that need immediate attention may have additional symptoms. They are:

- Difficulty speaking and swallowing
- Swelling of the tongue and under the tongue
- *If you find it difficult to swallow or speak, call your dentist immediately. If you cannot reach your dentist, do not wait. Go directly and without delay to a hospital emergency room.*

KNOCKED OUT (AVULSED) TOOTH

A permanent tooth that has been avulsed or completely knocked out of its socket suffers damage to its nerves, blood supply, and often the bone that supports it. Whether the tooth can be successfully put back (replanted) usually depends on how long it has remained outside the mouth. When a tooth is replanted within 30 minutes of being avulsed, it has a better chance of survival. Teeth that remain out of the mouth longer have much less chance of survival. Therefore, you must act quickly.

If a permanent tooth is knocked out:

- Pick the tooth up by the crown and not the root(s).
- If the tooth is visibly soiled, gently rinse it. If milk is immediately available, use it to rinse the tooth. If milk is not available, clean the tooth by holding it under gently running cold water. Be careful not to scrub or touch the root as this can injure the remaining attached tissue and will reduce the chance of the tooth being successfully replanted.
- Gently reinsert the tooth into its socket. Keep the tooth in place by using pressure from your finger or by biting on a clean cloth or gauze. If replanting is not possible (especially in the case of a young child) or you are concerned the tooth may be swallowed, place it in a container of milk. If you cannot place the tooth in milk and you are not concerned about swallowing it, you may place it under your tongue. If you cannot do any of these, place the tooth in plastic wrap or wet towel.
- *See your dentist immediately. Remember to take the tooth.*

TOOTH FRACTURES

Tooth fractures can involve the crown, the root(s), or both. A fracture of the crown can be confined to the enamel or include the dentin and/or the pulp. Injury to the pulp demands the most involved treatment. Although fractures of the crown may be the most obvious, it is important that you recognize the symptoms of other types of fractures so that you know to seek prompt dental care.

Broken Tooth (Complete Crown Fracture)

If your tooth breaks:

- Gather the broken pieces (if you can) and bring them to your dentist. Sometimes they can be bonded back onto the tooth.
- Rinse your mouth gently with *warm* water to remove dirt or debris from the injured area.
- If your tooth breaks, swelling may occur. Apply ice wrapped in a towel or a cold compress to the face around the area of swelling.
- *Call your dentist and follow instructions.*

Fractures of the Enamel Only

Many times these fractures are not visible and can only be diagnosed by symptoms. Symptoms include:

- Discomfort when chewing
- Discomfort if the fracture has penetrated the enamel completely
- Discomfort if the sharp edges of the fractured enamel touch and irritate your lips and/or tongue

Call your dentist as soon as possible. Even though a fracture involving only the enamel seems small, it can, at times, result in permanent damage to the tooth.

Fractures of Both Enamel and Dentin

Symptoms are:

- Discomfort with chewing
- Sensitivity to changes in temperature
- Loose tooth fragments

Call your dentist immediately. The treatment the dentist provides will depend on the location and severity of the fracture. The dentist may clean and dry the tooth and then place a protective barrier over the exposed dentin to protect the pulp from further irritation. The tooth is usually restored temporarily with composite material. After six to eight weeks the tooth may be restored permanently.

Fractures Involving the Pulp

These fractures require the most immediate attention. You may even be able to see the pulp. The symptoms associated with fractures involving the pulp are generally the most severe and include:

- Discomfort with chewing
- Sensitivity to changes in temperature
- Loose tooth fragments

Call your dentist immediately. Treatment varies, depending on a number of factors, including how much of and how long the pulp has been exposed. Treatments may include pulp capping, pulpotomy, root canal therapy, or extraction.

OTHER TYPES OF INJURIES TO THE TEETH

Some of the different types of injuries a tooth can sustain are described in Box 20.1. Most result from a blow or trauma to the tooth. Although the type injury the tooth experiences determines its treatment and prognosis, none requires special measures on your part. To avoid delay in seeking dental care, it is important that you are able to recognize the symptoms.

DEFINITIONS OF
SOME DENTAL TERMS

The following are definitions of some of the dental terms used in this chapter.

Avulsion. Complete displacement or a tooth knocked from its socket. When this occurs, the nerves and blood supply to the tooth and its connection to the periodontal ligament are severed.

Extrusion. As a result of a blow, a tooth becomes partially pushed out of its socket. When this occurs, the periodontal ligament and the blood supply and nerves to the pulp of the tooth are severed.

Complete Tooth Fracture. A fracture that results in loss of tooth structure.

Incomplete Tooth Fracture. A fracture that results in no loss of tooth structure.

Luxation Injuries. These vary in severity and result from a blow to the tooth. The tooth is moved in, but not displaced from, its socket. This severs some of the fibers of the periodontal ligament and fractures or bruises the wall of the alveolar socket. Types of luxation injuries include:

Concussion. The damage causes the periodontal ligament to hemorrhage and fluid to build up in the pulp. Since the periodontal ligament remains intact, the tooth does not become loose.

Intrusion. This is a severe type of luxation injury, in which the tooth is pushed into the alveolar socket. The socket is fractured, and the pulp and periodontal ligament are damaged. Complications often occur, including death of the pulp, root resorption, and loss of bone support.

Lateral Luxation. This is a severe injury in which the crown is pushed backward and the root of the tooth is displaced toward the front of the mouth.

Subluxation. As with concussion, this injury results in hemorrhage of the periodontal ligament and fluid buildup in the pulp. Unlike concussion, the periodontal ligament ruptures, and the tooth becomes loose.

The trauma to the tooth may result in a change of position (extraction, intrusion, lateral luxation). The direction of change will dictate the type and extent of emergency treatment that is required. The dentist may reposition and splint the tooth. If it is not possible to reposition the tooth, it may be possible to move it orthodontically at a later date. The dentist may need to treat the tooth endodontically or it may need to be extracted. At times, opposing teeth may need to be reduced slightly to prevent further trauma.

Symptoms associated with a change in position due to trauma include:

- Looseness
- A tooth that after trauma appears longer than the other teeth
- Pain when chewing
- Inability to have teeth come together
- Bleeding from the gingival sulcus
- Being partially visible or not visible at all if the tooth is intruded (pushed up)

See your dentist as soon as possible. If you are unable to reach your dentist, go to the hospital emergency room.

Trauma may also result in an injury in which the tooth does not appear to have moved (concussion, subluxation). Although these injuries do not appear to be as great, they can result in symptoms that should be evaluated by your dentist. These symptoms include:

- Pain when chewing
- Sensitivity to tapping
- A feeling of looseness
- Bleeding from gingival sulcus

BONE FRACTURES—FRACTURED JAW

Symptoms of a broken jaw include:

- Pain
- Tenderness over the actual injury or a distance from it

- Difficulty chewing
- A change in the way the teeth and jaws come together
- Facial numbness

If you suspect a broken jaw:

- Do not try to move it.
- Immobilize it by tying a piece of cloth (scarf, towel, neck tie, hand-kerchief, etc.) under the jaw and up over the top of the head.
- If there is swelling, apply ice wrapped in a towel or a cold compress to it.
- *Call your dentist immediately. Your dentist may advise you to go to the hospital emergency room or to an oral and maxillofacial surgeon. If you cannot reach your dentist, go immediately to a hospital emergency room and request that you be seen by an oral and maxillofacial surgeon.*

INJURIES TO THE SOFT TISSUES

Injuries can result in cuts, bruises, and scrapes in and around the mouth. Lacerations may require suturing. Immediate treatment will depend on the seriousness and location of the injury. *Call your dentist immediately, describe the injury, and follow instructions. If you cannot reach your dentist right away, go to the emergency room at a hospital and request an oral surgeon.*

Burns from electric cords are a very serious type injury, but fortunately, very rare. They occur most often to children under the age of two years who suck on the ends or lengths of electric cords that are plugged into walls or extension cord sockets. *Individuals who sustain injuries from electric cords should be brought immediately to a hospital emergency room.*

CHAPTER 21

———

Other Concerns About Your Dental Care

In recent years, dentistry has made the news for a number of controversies, among them the suspected transmission of HIV, the human immune deficiency virus that causes AIDS (acquired immune deficiency syndrome), to patients by a dentist; mercury in amalgam fillings; and water fluoridation. In addition, many patients are concerned about radiation exposure from dental radiographs. This chapter separates the facts from the rumors to give you an accurate understanding of these issues.

DENTAL RADIOGRAPHS (X-RAYS)

Radiographs remain one of the most effective and reliable diagnostic tools in dentistry. They can detect a number of different dental diseases and conditions that cannot be seen visually during an oral examination, among them caries and bone loss from periodontal and pulp diseases. Radiographs can uncover many diseases and abnormalities early in their development when they can be treated more easily and less expensively, painfully, and extensively than they can be if treated later. In many instances, early treatment prevents the loss of a tooth. By comparing dental radiographs taken at different intervals, a dentist is able to monitor the progress of your dental health so that all your treatments can be performed at the appropriate times.

What Is a Radiograph?

Ionizing-radiation is a form of electromagnetic radiation that can penetrate bone and soft tissues. Its energy can also expose photographic films to produce radiographic images for dental and medical diagnostic purposes. More radiation is absorbed by dense tissues (teeth and bone) than by soft tissues (cheeks and gingiva). As a result, after penetrating the hard tissues, fewer x-rays are left to reach the film. The outcome is a lighter image of teeth and bone and a darker one of cheeks and gingiva (gums). Carious lesions and bone loss from periodontal disease appear darker because the loss of calcum allows more rays to pass through them to reach the film.

Because a radiograph portrays a three-dimensional image in two planes, it has limitations. For example, it often can be difficult to determine where in the tooth caries is located. And since soft tissues are radiolucent (penetrable by x-rays), changes in the gingiva, such as inflammation and recession, cannot be seen on a radiograph.

Types of Dental Radiographs

Depending on the treatment proposed and the conditions or diseases suspected, different types of radiographs are made. Intraoral radiographs are taken with the film within the mouth (contained in a cardboard wafer and sometimes attached to a holder); extraoral radiographs are taken from outside the mouth.

The following are common intraoral radiographs:

Bitewing. These films reveal the crowns of several upper and lower teeth. Because the patient holds the film in position in the mouth by biting down on the film wafer, they can only be made if there are opposing teeth. They are used to detect caries between the teeth and under restorations, and bone loss from periodontal disease and to check that metal fillings fit properly.

Periapical. These films show several entire teeth (crowns and roots) and a small amount of the periapical bone (surrounding the root tips). They are used to detect conditions of the root and bone and the structure and eruption of the tooth, such as missing, impacted, and fractured teeth, cysts, tumors, abscesses, as well as bone patterns of some systemic diseases.

Full-Mouth Survey. This is a combination of 14 or more periapical and 4 bitewing films of the back teeth. The precise number of films that will be made depends on the size of the mouth, the position of the teeth, and what technique is used. This series shows all the teeth (crowns and roots) and the alveolar bone surrounding them.

Occlusal. One film can show a complete arch (upper or lower) with the entire structure of the teeth, in addition to the palate, and some of the surrounding periapical area. They are used to locate roots, to reveal extra, unerupted, and impacted teeth, to identify foreign bodies in the jaws or stones in the salivary gland ducts, to visualize the maxillary sinuses, and to determine the extent and nature of fractures of the jaws. They are also recommended when patients are unable, because of pain or muscle spasms, to open their jaws wide enough for periapical radiographs.

The following are extraoral radiographs:

Panoramic. These radiographs take a wide (panoramic) view of all the teeth; the upper and lower jaws, including the temporomandibular joints; and other structures. They are taken to reveal impacted teeth, cysts, fractures, jaws problems, and fragments of roots. They are useful for evaluating general oral health and to detect large bony lesions but do not show caries or bone loss well.

Lateral Skull Radiographs. These radiographs, used for cephalometric analysis in orthodontic treatment, are discussed in Chapter 15.

Computed Tomography (CT). CT scans, better known for their medical applications, are being increasingly used for dental purposes. With CT, a radiographic image passes through a section of the body and is captured by a detector that sends an electrical signal to a computer. The computer analyzes the different densities of the tissue to produce an image.

CT for dentistry is most often used in hospitals to evaluate diseases and injuries to the head and neck for both diagnosis and surgical planning. Because the soft tissues are better seen with CT than with regular radiography, metastases of the lymph nodes are more easily detected with them. Most recently, CT has replaced panoramic radiography to evaluate the jaws (to determine whether sufficient bone is available) before placing osseointegrated implants.

CT of the head usually involves a higher radiation dose than does radiography, which produces a series of plain films of the skull. This higher dosage is generally considered justified because of the greater amount of information that can be gathered.

Magnetic Resonance Imaging (MRI). Soft tissues, and soft tissue tumors, metastases of the lymph nodes, and the disc in the temporomandibular joint are ideally visualized with this modality.

Digital Radiography. In this new twist, the x-rays develop not on film but on a radiation detector and form an electronic image. This is received by a television camera and transmitted to a computer in digital form or stored in the computer memory. The images can be viewed immediately on a video screen or recalled at a later time. Subtraction radiographs (described in Chapter 7), which use digital imaging to subtract an image taken earlier from a later one, are useful new tools for detecting the progression of periodontal disease.

Digital radiography can take pictures from within or outside the mouth. The average dose of radiation absorbed from one intraoral image produced using electronic imaging by video camera has been estimated to be about 80 percent less than the dose received using E-speed film.

Risks and Concerns

It is widely known that large doses of x-radiation can have deleterious effects on tissues. X-rays alter the electrostatic charges and the molecular bonding ability of proteins; this results in damage to normal tissue functioning. Such changes can produce cancer and birth defects.

What is not known is what effects, if any, long-term cumulative exposure to low doses of radiation exposure causes. The amount of x-radiation that is absorbed by the tissues from a radiograph is called the dose. The dose is measured in a unit of measurement called a rem or a sievert.

The dose equivalent involved in a full-mouth dental radiograph of 21 films is 113 millirems. (The amount of radiation a patient receives from dental x-rays is so minute that it must be measured in millirems, which are one-thousandths of a rad or rem.) In contrast, we receive (and tolerate with no untoward effects), on average, 300 millirems per year from radiation to which we are constantly exposed from environmental sources in the earth (e.g., radon gas) and outer space.

Measures That Can Be Taken
to Reduce Radiation Exposure

Because of the uncertainty over the cumulative effects of exposure to low doses of radiation, both governmental and professional dental groups, along with individual dentists, have taken the following steps to reduce the level of exposure to radiation during dental radiographs.

Regulation. Dental radiographic equipment that is manufactured or sold in the United States after 1974 must comply with performance standards set by the federal government. These include specifications for increased filtration and kilovoltage settings. In addition, all radiographic equipment must meet state, county, or city radiation health codes.

Risk Versus Benefit Analysis. Dental radiographs should be made only on recommendation of a dentist and after a clinical examination.

Equipment. Various modifications can be made in the equipment to reduce a patient's exposure to radiation from a dental radiograph. A collimator is a disk in the head of the machine that narrows the x-ray beam so that fewer scatter beyond the area to be filmed. Most states require that the beam of x-radiation be restricted by collimation to no greater than 2.75 inches. Smaller beam collimators that reduce the scatter radiation by between 45 and 95 percent and the dosage delivered to bone marrow by 90 percent are available.

Within the last decade, new machines have become available that produce x-radiation with higher kilovoltage x-ray photons, allowing for shorter periods of exposure. These machines produce fewer lower-energy x-ray photons, which do not have sufficient energy to make an x-ray image but do add to the overall dosage of radiation a patient receives. These constant potential x-ray machines can reduce a patient's radiation exposure by as much as 30 percent.

Filtration also removes the low-energy x-radiation photons. Dental radiographic units are sold with built-in filtration, but additional filters can further reduce radiation by between 25 and 71 percent. Using long cones further reduces radiation to the patient.

Film Speed. D speed and E speed are the two film speeds commercially available for intraoral dental radiographs. E speed is faster, more sensitive, and safer (it reduces exposure to radiation by up to 50 percent). The faster film also reduces the number of retakes needed when either the patient or the machine moves.

Lead Shields. Most states require the use of a lead apron during direct exposure to radiation during dental radiographs for all patients. A lead apron reduces radiation exposure to the chest, abdomen, and gonads by up to 94 percent; the use of a thyroid collar reduces radiation exposure to the thyroid gland by the same amount. Thyroid collars cannot be used for panoramic exposures because they block areas that need to be filmed.

Retaining Your Radiographs. To avoid duplicating radiographs, if you switch dentists, you should ask to have your radiographs sent to your new dentist.

Frequency. After chest radiographs, dental radiographs are the most frequently performed radiographic examinations in the United States. One of the most effective ways to reduce exposure to radiation from dental

---

BOX 21.1

GUIDELINES FOR FREQUENCY OF DENTAL RADIOGRAPHS

The following guidelines for the frequency of administering radiographs are recommended by the Center for Devices and Radiological Health (under the auspices of the U.S. Department of Health and Human Services, Public Health Services of the Food and Drug Administration).

FIRST VISIT—To Assess Dental Diseases and Growth and Development

Children with Primary Teeth. Bitewing radiographs of the back teeth *if* they are in contact with each other

Children with Primary and Permanent Teeth. Periapical / occlusal and bitewing radiographs of the back teeth or panoramic and bitewing radiographs of the back teeth

Patients with Permanent Teeth (until the eruption of their third molars) and Adults with Teeth. Bitewings of the back teeth and selected periapicals; if dental disease is present or there is a history of extensive dental treatment, full-mouth or panoramic radiographs

Patients without Teeth. Occlusal or panoramic radiographs

RECALL VISIT

For Patients with Caries or High-Risk Factors for Caries*

Children with Primary and Primary and Permanent Teeth. Bitewing radiographs of the back teeth every 6 months until no caries is evident

Patients with Permanent Teeth (until the eruption of their third molars). Bitewing radiographs of the back teeth every 6 to 12 months until no caries is evident

Adults with Teeth. Bitewing radiographs of the back teeth every 12 to 18 months

For Patients with No Caries and No High Risk Factors for Caries

Children with Primary Teeth. Bitewing radiographs of the back teeth every 12 to 24 months *if* the teeth are in contact with each other

Children with Both Primary and Primary and Permanent Teeth. Bitewing radiographs of the back teeth every 12 to 24 months

Patients with Permanent Teeth (until the eruption of their third molars). Bitewing radiographs of the back teeth every 18 to 36 months

Adults with Teeth. Bitewing radiographs of the back teeth every 24 to 36 months

For Patients with Periodontal Disease or Past Treatment for It

All Ages with Teeth. Selected periapical and/or bitewing radiographs for places where periodontal disease (other than gingivitis) is evident

To Assess Dental Diseases and Growth and Development

Children with Primary Teeth. Not usually necessary

Children with Both Primary and Primary and Permanent Teeth. Cephalometric or panoramic radiographs

Patients with Permanent Teeth (until the eruption of their third molars). Periapical or panoramic radiographs to evaluate third molars

Adults with Teeth. Not usually necessary

Patients without Teeth. Do not require radiographs at recall visits for five to seven years.

> *If you are at high risk for caries, you may have one or more of the following:
> A past history of high level or recurrent caries
> Restorations of poor quality
> Poor oral hygiene
> Insufficient exposure to fluoride
> Frequent consumption of sucrose
> Extended nursing (from bottle or breast)
> A family history of poor dental health
> Defects of enamel
> Xerostomia (dry mouth)
> Inherited dental abnormalities
> Many restorations
> A history of chemo- or radiation therapy
> A developmental disability

radiographs is by reducing the frequency with which they are made. The schedule (see Box 21.1) recommended for how often they should be taken depends on an individual's age, oral hygiene, history of dental disease, propensity to caries, specific dental problems, and past dental treatment.

MERCURY IN DENTAL AMALGAMS

In its over-150-year history as a material for dental restorations, the mercury content of amalgam has sparked sporadic debates about its safety. The recent allegations about its deleterious effects made by individual dentists and researchers and sensationalized in the media are discussed here.

Reputed Problems

Toxicity. Depending on the dose and duration of exposure, mercury vapors can cause health problems, including irritability, memory loss, depression, tremor, kidney inflammation, and swollen gums. Sudden poisoning, such as that which results from swallowing the metal can produce nausea, vomiting, bloody diarrhea, and kidney failure. The pertinent question in dentistry, however, is, "can these harmful effects result from the mercury vapors released from the amalgam fillings placed by your dentist in your mouth?"

It is estimated that individuals not exposed to the metal in their work receive between 10 and 20 micrograms (per gram of creatine) of the element each day from food, air, and water. A number of studies have concluded that the contribution of mercury in someone with between 8 and 12 tooth surfaces restored with amalgam fillings ranges between 1 and 2 micrograms per day, which is about 10 percent of the normal daily intake. The level necessary to cause the most *minimal* of neurological symptoms is 25 micrograms. This is six times higher than the maximum amount (4 micrograms) of mercury released and absorbed by an individual who has many amalgam restorations.

If mercury vapors from amalgam fillings were to cause neurological problems from toxicity, the group most affected would be dentists and personnel who work in dental offices and are routinely exposed to large amounts released during the placement of amalgam restorations. Indeed, measurements taken between 1975 and 1983 of the urinary levels of mercury in these workers revealed levels well elevated above those in the general population. Of the approximately 30 percent of the dentists who had elevated levels, none experienced difficulties practicing dentistry.

At high dosages, mercury can cause neurological problems. Yet the symptoms many claim are relieved after the removal of their amalgam restorations do not correlate with *any* amount of mercury exposure. For example, some persons have claimed that amalgam can cause cancer, but a higher cancer rate has not been found.

Some individuals have also claimed that multiple sclerosis is connected to amalgam restorations and that their removal has caused a quick reversal of the disease. If amalgam fillings were the cause of the neurological problems associated with the disease, an overnight cure would not be possible. In the process of removing amalgams, anywhere from one-and-a-half to four times the amount of mercury vapor that is present daily in someone with amalgam fillings is released. Therefore if amalgam fillings were to cause or contribute to this ailment, removing them would cause an immediate *exacerbation,* not relief, of the symptoms. Furthermore if mercury from amalgam fillings accumulates over time, then its effects take a while to dissipate; this makes immediate cures of multiple sclerosis on removal of amalgam fillings not possible.

The National Multiple Sclerosis Society has added its support to this reasoning and cautions against the removal of amalgam fillings as a treatment for the disease. It acknowledges that spontaneous remissions and relapses are a characteristic pattern of the disease and that placebo effects can occur. (When placebos, inactive substances or treatments, are given, up to 70 percent of persons can show real, demonstrable improvement because they believe they are receiving an effective treatment.)

Allergies. Allergic reactions to mercury in amalgam fillings are rare. The consensus of a number of studies is that less than 1 percent of the population is hypersensitive, or allergic, to mercury. This leaves over 99 percent of the population who should display no reactions to amalgam fillings.

The symptoms most individuals who are allergic to mercury experience are localized red or whitish, and sometimes ulcerated lesions of the oral mucosa near the fillings. Most of these disappear completely within a few days after the amalgam is removed and replaced with another restorative material. Generalized symptoms like eczema (a skin inflammation characterized by itchy, red blisters on the skin) and urticaria (hives) on the face, legs, and arms are *extremely* rare. Many persons who display these symptoms have a personal or family history of allergies to metal.

Impairment of Kidney Function. Because mercury is excreted via the urine, which is produced and eliminated by the kidneys, these organs are susceptible to dysfunction when the mercury levels of blood and urine are high. From studies of industrial workers, it has been determined that kidney function is not impaired until the urinary mercury levels are approximately 25 times higher than those associated with numerous amalgam fillings.

Swedish studies reported no kidney impairment in persons with amalgam fillings, and they found no differences in liver status, blood cell variables, and some other bodily functions between persons with amalgam fillings and those without them. A study conducted by the American Dental Association also found no statistical association between elevated urinary mercury levels in dentists and kidney dysfunction.

Recommendations

If you experience localized or generalized allergic reactions after having amalgam restorations placed, you should be evaluated by an allergist. If the allergist discovers you are allergic to mercury, you should have your amalgam fillings removed and replaced with another restorative material. If you know you are allergic to mercury or another metal (e.g., if you develop rashes from wearing rings of various metals), you should have a restorative material other than amalgam placed originally to avoid any possible problems.

In the absence of an allergic reaction, you should *not* have your amalgam fillings removed and replaced simply because of what appears to be unsubstantiated fears of ill effects caused by absorbing mercury from the fillings. As explained in Chapter 9, removing an existing filling sacrifices sound and healthy tooth structure.

A decision on which restorative material to choose when having a new filling placed should depend on many factors (discussed in Chapter 6), including aesthetics and personal preference. Although other restorative materials (composite resins, glass ionomers, gold and gold alloys, and porcelains) have been suggested by antiamalgamists as "safer" alternatives to amalgams, none are free of adverse effects.

INFECTION CONTROL

The report of six patients infected with HIV, the virus that causes AIDS, by a dentist in Florida sent shock waves through the dental community and chills up and down the spines of dental patients. As frightening as this is, dental patients should take comfort in the singleness of this event.

There is only one dentist believed to have transmitted HIV to a patient. How the dentist transmitted HIV to his patients remains unknown, even after extensive investigations by the Centers for Disease Control (CDC), which were subsequently analyzed by the U.S. General Accounting Office and other health agencies.

Since the dentist is no longer alive and the practice has been sold and the office remodeled, it seems unlikely that the mystery will be solved. The measures dentists are required to take to prevent the possible spread to or from their patients and themselves and other dental workers of the deadly but fragile HIV, the more virulent hepatitis B virus, and other infections or viruses (including the common cold) are now considered.

Infectious Control Procedures

The Occupational Safety and Health Administration (OSHA) has issued mandatory infection control procedures that all dental offices with one or more employees must follow. The purpose of the OSHA measures is to minimize the risk of the transmission of infectious diseases to employees. In doing so, it is presumed that patients also will be protected. States that administer their own plans must adopt standards that are at least as effective as the federal guidelines. Included among the regulations dentists and staff must follow are:

- The adoption of universal precautions. This means dentists and their assistants should treat all blood and saliva as if it were infectious for HIV and hepatitis B.
- Gloves, face masks, protective clothing, and eyegear must be worn when touching instruments, materials, or surfaces that may be contaminated with blood or saliva.
- Lab jackets must be removed as soon as possible if splashed with blood or saliva or when leaving the work area.
- Gloves must be changed between patients.
- Dental workers must wash their hands before and after treating each patient and after touching with their bare hands objects that are likely to be contaminated.
- Impervious covers, which are removed and replaced between patients, should be placed on surfaces, such as x-ray heads and light switches.
- Contaminated needles and other disposable sharp instruments, such as endodontic files, must be discarded in closable, puncture-resistant, and leakproof containers.
- Waste and contaminated materials must be disposed of in compliance with local, state, and / or federal laws.
- An EPA-registered disinfectant (capable of killing *Mycobacterium tuberculosis,* the organism responsible for tuberculosis) should be used in the treatment room between patients and at the end of the

day on hard surfaces that cannot otherwise be sterilized, such as counter tops.

- Reusable instruments, such as drill bits, hand pieces, and mirrors, should be sterilized between uses with steam under pressure (autoclaved), dry heat, or chemical vapor.
- The sterilization units should be checked at least once a week with a biologic indicator (e.g., a spore test) to verify that the machine is operating properly. Indicators that change color when exposed to heat are not sufficient to do this. When attached to a pack of instruments, these heat-sensitive indicators are useful in that they let the staff know that that pack has been processed through the sterilization machine.

Cross Contamination

Once dentists (or hygienists or dental assistants) don gloves and begin treating you, the only things they should touch are your mouth, the dental instruments, and objects, such as light switches, that have disposable covers on them. If they touch any other object, for example, a light switch that does not have a disposable cover, while or after working on you or another patient, it can easily become contaminated. The germs then can be spread when someone else touches that surface. Although a dentist may comply with the OSHA regulations (e.g., wear gloves), additional measures are needed to avoid the many opportunities throughout the day for inadvertent cross contamination.

FLUORIDE

Fluoride is a form of fluorine, which is the thirteenth most abundant element in the earth's crust. When water flows over rocks containing it, the compounds dissolve so that some soluble fluoride ions are present in all sources of water, including the oceans. Fresh water can contain anywhere from 0.1 to over 12 parts per million of fluoride, some of which exceeds the maximum contaminant level of 4 parts per million that the Environmental Protection Agency considers a risk to health. Most municipalities that supplement their water with fluoride to ensure dental health do so at levels between 0.7 and 1.2 parts per million. Fluoride is also present naturally in some amounts in all foods and beverages; fish and brewed teas contain higher amounts than other foods.

Overwhelming evidence shows that the addition of fluoride to water supplies has been the single most effective measure against dental caries. It also has been shown to be safe. Yet despite fluoride's proven cost-effective anticaries effects and its safe use by millions of Americans and over 250,000,000 persons in more than 30 other countries, the opposition to adding it to drinking water continues.

In 1993, a committee of the National Research Council, part of the National Academy of Sciences (a private organization chartered by Congress to conduct research for the U.S. government), reviewed scientific studies on fluoride. The following is a summary of their conclusions:

- The addition of fluoride to drinking water at the levels of 0.7 to 1.2 parts per million is appropriate.
- A review of over 50 epidemiological studies (of the incidence, distribution, and control of disease in a population) showed no association between exposure to fluoride and an increased risk of cancer in humans.
- At the levels of 0.7 to 1.2 parts per million fluoride does not increase the risk of kidney disease or stomach or digestive disorders.
- At the appropriate levels of 0.7 to 1.2 parts per million fluoride does not increase the risk of birth defects or infertility nor does it have any other adverse effects on human reproduction. The studies conducted on animals that showed an association between fluoride and mutations involved doses 100 times higher than the average to which people are exposed.
- Some studies found a long-term exposure to fluoride increased the risk of hip or vertebral fractures in people over 80 years. Because these studies were not conclusive the National Institutes of Health are undertaking a long-term study on fluoride and hip fractures.

Over the years, other studies have found:

- No evidence of allergic reactions to fluoride at the levels of 0.7 to 1.2 parts per million.

- Fluoride in drinking water does not cause or contribute to heart disease.
- Fluoridated water does not cause or aggravate physical and mental disorders, such as eye diseases, soft tissue degeneration or disease, thyroid dysfunction, or Alzheimer's disease.

There are only two substantiated risks to *excessive* fluoride exposure: fluorosis and overdose.

Fluorosis can result when too much fluoride is ingested during the years of a child's life when tooth enamel is forming. Depending on its severity, it can cause the enamel to darken and become mottled or pitted. Treatments for it are discussed in Chapter 14. Fluorosis occurs in areas of the country, especially in the south, where the water contains amounts of fluoride several times higher than the level added to water supplies for optimum dental health.

It is estimated that very mild to mild fluorosis occurs in between 10 and 15 percent of children who drink fluoridated water from birth. The increasing manufacture of foods and beverages with fluoridated water may be another cause of mild fluorosis. This degree of fluorosis does not cause health problems and usually does not have aesthetic consequences. The teeth are frequently whiter and more attractive than they would be normally, although the change is often detectable only by a dentist.

The increasing popularity of home water filters and use of bottled water poses the opposite problem: too little fluoride. Water filters can remove most of the fluoride in water and bottled water may not contain it. Many persons who obtain their water from these sources may be receiving less than the optimal amount of fluoride to protect them and their children against caries. (See also Chapter 8.)

In excessive amounts fluoride can be toxic. The amount of sodium fluoride necessary to cause death in an adult is estimated to be 5 grams consumed in a single dose. This is over 10,000 times as much as is contained in a glass of water. Extensive research from different sources has consistently shown that water fluoridation at the approved amounts under controlled conditions by public health authorities is safe. When mortality rates of persons in fluoridated communities (with 1 part per million or more of fluoride) were compared with those living in nonfluoridated communities (with less than 0.4 part per million), the data found fluoride to have no effect on death rates.

PART VII

THE FUTURE
OF DENTISTRY

CHAPTER 22

On the Horizon—A Peek into the Not-So-Distant Future of Dental Care

VIRTUAL DENTISTRY

I n 1932 when Aldous Huxley wrote his novel *Brave New World* about what life would be like in the future, he set it hundreds of years ahead, in the twenty-fifth century. When George Orwell wrote *Nineteen Eighty Four* in 1949, his vision of the future also was years away, albeit not as many.

Today, when dental visionaries imagine what the future of dental care will be, the answers in their crystal ball are less than a decade ahead. Dental experts believe that computers will transform your visit to the dentist in the year 2005. The following is a peek at what lies ahead.

While waiting to see the dentist, you ask a trim computer monitor questions about how to care for your teeth or a dental problem you have. The interactive computer is programmed to answer most of the questions you or other patients have.

Once in the dental chair you can either look at the inside of your mouth on an overhead computer monitor or watch a video. Listening to relaxing music or soothing sounds through a small wireless ear piece relaxes you. While treating you, the dentist and hygienist watch another monitor. The dentist uses a monitor that is built into a cabinet in the operatory to access your dental records and information from your doctors and other healthcare professionals and to find out what medications you are taking and whether there are any changes in your health that might influence your dental treatment, as well as to learn about new materials and therapies. To avoid cross contamination, all computers are operated via voice recognition with cordless microphones, which allow the dentist and staff to move about freely.

At each visit, your vital signs and the measurements of your temporomandibular joints and periodontal crevices are electronically recorded.

If you want, you are able to access your dental virtual record on your computer at home. If the dentist wants the opinion of a dental specialist or physician, your records and pertinent information can be transmitted electronically to them. If a lesion in your mouth appears suspicious, the dentist compares it to an image in the computer's database. A computer program using artificial intelligence reviews your radiographs and reports anything out of the ordinary to your dentist. Conventional radiographs have been replaced by digital radiographs, which require less radiation than traditional x-rays and use no hazardous chemicals for developing. Sedation is accomplished without needles via electronic analgesia. After examining you, the dentist, with the aid of the computer, selects the treatment options you have, lets you know how much your insurance carrier will pay for each type of treatment, and sends all forms and x-rays to and from the insurance companies electronically.

If you require an inlay, crown, or fixed prosthesis, you do not have to bite into an unpleasant-tasting material to make the impression. Instead, your dentist takes an optical impression using a computer program. Slender intraoral cameras that take pictures inside the mouth let your dentist know whether you have decay, oral lesions, or fractured teeth. Obtaining the correct shade for a crown or porcelain laminate veneer is no longer left to your dentist's eye, but is done instead by the computer. The dentist also routinely uses computer imaging to alter your smile on a video screen to show you the changes in appearance a specific dental procedure (e.g., bonding, porcelain veneers, or braces) can make. In designing a removable partial denture, the computer evaluates the force on the teeth and calculates the amount of supporting bone and soft tissue; for orthodontic treatment, a computer predicts the growth of the skull and face and projects its effect on orthodontic treatment.

Of course, the use of computers is not the only advance anticipated for dental care in the not-so-distant future. Although innovations in materials, techniques, technologies, and/or trends are being made in all branches of dentistry, the ones mentioned here are those which your dentist is likely to offer you or those which will have a positive impact on your dental health and appearance.

THE FIGHT AGAINST CARIES

Caries Vaccine

For the last 15 years dental researchers have been working on developing a vaccine that passively rather than actively immunizes against caries (tooth decay), and thus eliminates the need for injections. Progress with humans has been slow because of concerns about safety.

Studies have been conducted using cows, chickens, and plants. Pregnant cows that were inoculated with a vaccine made from bacteria that causes caries produced milk that was high in concentrations of caries-fighting antibodies. More research needs to be done to determine whether these antibodies are safe for humans and whether they can be put into a mouthrinse or consumed in milk for effective use and produced in sufficient quantities for widespread use. Vaccinated chickens produced egg yolks that were also rich in caries antibodies. In experiments, rats that were given these chicken egg yolks had lower levels of caries. The most recent and perhaps the most promising research uses plants to generate the caries-fighting antibodies. Plants offer advantages over cows and chickens. The IgG antibodies cows and chickens produce are not specific to the oral cavity. But plants can be engineered to produce IgA antibodies, the main antibodies in the mouth. Transgenic plants also offer the advantage that they can be raised as food crops (i.e., rice, potatoes, cassava, and peppers), and so provide an easy way to confer passive immunity against caries to vast numbers of people around the world.

Replacement Therapy

Another way being studied to fight caries involves using genetic engineering techniques to construct bacteria that have anticaries properties. In one approach, mutated forms of *Streptococcal mutans,* a bacteria that causes caries, are created. These replacement genes lack the ability to form lactic acid, the dominant acid formed by *S. mutans* bacteria, which attacks tooth structure. In another approach, the normally sticky genes that produce enzymes that allow plaque to adhere to the teeth are replaced with genetically engineered genes, which, theoretically, will result in less formation of plaque. Researchers hope these modified bacteria can be introduced into the mouth via chewable tablets.

Toothpastes and Mouthrinses Containing Triclosan

Toothpastes and mouthrinses that contain triclosan, a germicide with antibacterial properties, are being reviewed by the Federal Drug Administration. Clinical studies have shown they are effective in reducing plaque, gingivitis, and calculus that can cause decay and periodontal disease and in maintaining gingival health. They are especially effective when combined with Gantrez, a binding agent, and zinc citrate. Triclosan-containing oral products are available in Europe, Canada, and elsewhere in the world. They are expected to be marketed in the United States within the next three years if not sooner.

Remineralization Products

Researchers are studying different forms of calcium phosphate salts that help the enamel of teeth remineralize during the early stages of decay. In addition to increasing a tooth's resistance to decay, these compounds can reduce a tooth's sensitivity to cold, heat, air pressure, and touch.

The new products containing amorphous calcium phosphate compounds work by crystallizing to form hydroxyapatite, the main mineral in teeth (and bone). The hydroxyapatite disperses over the tooth's surface where dentin has been exposed to fill in the tiny holes that tooth abrasion or gum recession have created. The new remineralization method is effective in the early stages of decay (before a cavity is formed). These compounds may be incorporated into toothpastes, chewing gum, food, and mouthrinses, as well as a professional gel that can be applied by a dentist.

Alternatives to Amalgams

Even though the release of mercury from amalgam fillings has not been shown to have a negative affect on a patient's physical health (see Chapter 21), some organizations and the media have raised enough concerns about them to motivate companies and dental institutions to search for filling materials that have similar properties to amalgam but contain no mercury. The two nonmercury filling materials described here show promise but are not acceptable substitutes at this time.

Gallium alloy is a filling material that was developed almost 30 years ago in a program supported by the American Dental Association. Although it possesses some of the same properties as mercury-containing amalgam (e.g., it is long-lasting and easy for the dentist to handle and place), it is best when used for filling small cavities. Longer and more-detailed clinical studies are needed before it can be considered an appropriate substitute for amalgam fillings.

A more recent innovation is condensable *silver tin alloy,* a new restorative system. This material consists of particles of silver and tin that are treated with a special wetting agent and then pressed and bonded together by a mechanical condensation process. Although this process shows potential, it is still being tested and evaluated and will not be available commercially for several years.

With no acceptable nonmercury alloy filling material available, many people have become more comfortable having their teeth filled with composite resins (although the dentist may still not want to use them for large fillings) and, in some instances, with glass ionomer cement, instead of with amalgam. (Glass ionomer cement, which adheres well to the tooth surface and releases fluoride, is suitable only for filling areas that do not sustain stress.) Better formulations of composite resins have been and will be developed in the coming years. The newer composite resins are more resistant to wear (this should make them more suitable for filling back teeth) and a bit easier for dentists to handle than the earlier formulations were.

PERIODONTAL DISEASE

Periodontal Disease Vaccine

A vaccine that could produce antibodies to fight the bacteria associated with periodontal disease is being researched. It has been tested on monkeys, but its application for humans is many years away.

Growth Factors

Polypeptide growth factors are naturally occurring protein molecules that play a role in the formation and remodeling of many body tissues and in wound healing. Most of the research on them has taken place outside dentistry. However, there have been a number of recent studies on animals that have revealed that when used together, growth factors promote healing and regeneration of periodontal tissues and stimulate bone growth around titanium implants. The two growth factors that have received the most attention for their ability to improve periodontal regeneration are *insulin-like growth factor* and *platelet-derived growth factor.* Growth factors can now be produced in the laboratory using recombinant DNA technology in quantities sufficient that they no longer need to be obtained from human blood. This reduces the possibility of transmitting bloodborne infections, such as hepatitis, HIV, and cytomegalovirus.

Research on growth factors is still in the experimental phase, but even at this early stage, they show promise for periodontal regeneration, especially of the periodontal ligament and bone around teeth and endosseus implants. It may be at least five years before they will be commercially available for patient use.

PEDIATRIC DENTISTRY

In recent years, there have been a number of legislative proposals to restructure the healthcare system in the United States. However the system changes, shortages in healthcare resources (these include dental care) are expected. Pediatric dentists, already experiencing a shortage of care providers, have begun preparing for this future of dwindling dental care services by employing in their practices *risk assessment,* a concept borrowed from pediatric medicine.

With risk assessment, pediatric dentists concentrate their efforts on identifying the individual children who are at risk of developing dental diseases. To do this, they encourage parents to bring children in for their first dental checkups while very young (preferably within the first year of life). The purpose of this first visit is to determine the child's environmental risk for dental disease and to teach parents what they can do to prevent dental disease for their child. To assess a child's environmental risk for dental disease, the dentist asks the parent about the child's use of the bottle, evaluates the level of fluoride in the child's diet, instructs the parents in infant oral hygiene, and may use a caries activity test (explained in Chapter 8) to determine the amount of caries the parent has. Children at higher risk for dental disease are then given more intensive preventive measures, among them dietary guidance, more frequent checkups, and fluoride in different forms. At later visits the dentist instructs children themselves how to care for their teeth and applies sealants to their teeth.

The belt tightening already under way with healthcare has encouraged the growth of Health Maintenance Organizations (HMOs). This method of delivering care is well suited for using risk assessment, followed by the preventive measures explained above. Because dentists who work for a HMO receive a set amount per month for each patient, a pediatric dentist has a financial incentive to keep a child free of dental disease by providing preventive care, such as instruction in oral hygiene and dietary modification and the use of sealants, to avoid performing the more costly procedures (e.g., fillings or crowns) needed to treat dental disease.

TEMPOROMANDIBULAR DISORDERS

Dentists and other healthcare professionals who treat patients with temporomandibular disorders are very positive about the future. Much of this optimism is due to the increased understanding in recent years of the basic mechanisms of pain and of the body's ability to repair itself after injuries and / or adapt to them. In addition, each year new and better medications that can be used for the pain associated with temporomandibular disorders are introduced.

COMPUTERS IN DENTISTRY

A vast system of computer networks has already created an electronic highway that allows information on almost any topic to be exchanged by computer users anywhere, anytime. On the subject of dental health, this electronic information highway, the Internet, is traveled most often by dentists, dental students, and dental auxiliaries. In the coming years, as the Internet expands, more information on dental care and health is expected to be available to the lay person.

To facilitate the exchange of dental knowledge among dental professionals, the American Association of Dental Schools is creating a Dental Information Network (DENTIN) that will be available to the faculty, researchers, students, and administrators of dental schools, as well as to practicing dentists. Among other functions, DENTIN will provide professionals with a forum to conference electronically and discuss their thoughts on various dental subjects, the ability to "talk" via electronic mail, continuing education courses via computer, and the retrieval of dental information electronically. The wealth of information that can be exchanged electronically has the potential to bring the newest and best information on dental materials, technologies, and procedures to all dentist professionals, even those in remote areas. Patients will benefit by having their dentists knowledgeable about state-of-the-art dental practice.

The Internet is also the repository of a growing multimedia library. Its resources include catalogs, journals, textbooks, images, videos, graphics, and sounds. These can be accessed electronically via special navigating software by computer users around the world. Already through the National Library of Medicine's MEDLINE and other databases, anyone with the appropriate computer hardware (personal computer, modem, and printer) and software can access articles on dental care and health published in dental and medical journals.

A number of dental schools, including the Columbia University School of Dental and Oral Surgery, already have sites on the Internet. Through its Internet site Columbia supplies information about its dental school to prospective dental students, details on the dental services and resources it offers patients, telephone numbers, and information to dentists and patients about AIDS and dental care. As advertising proliferates on the Internet, it is becoming difficult for users to distinguish between information that is authoritative and objective and that which is not. Internet users who obtain their electronic information on dental care from a dental school can be assured of its accuracy.

Of particular interest to many lay Internet users are the thousands of discussion groups (e.g., listserves, newsgroups) on a wide variety of subjects, many of them related to health. These groups allow individuals who have similar interests or problems to discuss them, share remedies, and, in the case of a medical or dental problem, to offer emotional support to each other. When subscribers join a listserve, they put their names in a group mailbox and then receive the messages from the other members of that group as electronic mail on their computers. There are many possibilities for newsgroup support groups on dental problems, including temporomandibular disorders and craniofacial abnormalities. Dentists and other dental care professionals may join these and other electronic discussion groups, and answer questions and share their dental expertise.

DENTAL SYMPTOMS

The table below lists some of the many dental problems you may experience, their symptoms, causes, and what you should do about them.

PROBLEM

Dry mouth (xerostomia)

Symptoms. Mouth feels dry and sore; there may be a burning sensation; lips may crack. Dry mouth reduces or eliminates the amount of saliva produced; this can cause caries and periodontal disease and may increase susceptibility to inflammation, sore mouth, and oral yeast infections, as well as produce difficulties eating, swallowing, and speaking.

Possible Causes. Diseases (e.g., Sjögren's syndrome), radiation of the head or neck, and many medications (e.g., appetite suppressants, antianxiety drugs, antiarrhythmics, anticonvulsants, antidepressants, antihistamines, decongestants, muscle relaxants, antihypertensives).

What to Do. See your dentist. Treatments include frequent sips of water, chewing sugarless gum or sucking sugarless candies, the use of artificial saliva substitutes, avoiding drinking alcohol or using mouthrinses that contain alcohol, and switching or reducing dosages of medications (only on the advice and under the care of a physician). The medication pilocarpine hydrochloride, available by prescription, may help in extreme cases. (If you are considering taking it, talk to your dentist or physician, as there are some restrictions on its use.)

PROBLEM

Different types of oral fungal (Candida) infections

Symptoms. Red, sore, inflamed areas and white patches on the oral mucosa and/or tongue; red, crusty lesions at corners of the mouth, sometimes covered with a pseudomembrane. Sometimes there is difficulty swallowing and a painful burning sensation.

Possible Causes. Medications (antibiotics, such as tetracycline and penicillin, tricyclic antidepressants, corticosteroids), systemic diseases (e.g., diabetes, hypothyroidism, HIV infection, Sjögren's syndrome), inhaled steroids for asthma, radiation of the head and neck, some nutritional deficiencies (e.g., iron, folic acid, malnutrition), and suppression of the immune system.

What to Do. See your dentist. Treatments include oral or topical antifungal medications prescribed by a dentist, avoiding mouthrinses containing alcohol, practicing good oral hygiene, and rinsing with water after using oral steroidal inhalants.

PROBLEM

Gingival hyperplasia (swollen gums)

Symptoms. Firm and painless overgrowth of gingival tissues, most often around the outer surfaces of the teeth. This can increase the risk of irritation and inflammation to the gums.

Possible Causes. Medications (some antiepileptic drugs, calcium channel blockers, cyclosporin), periodontal disease.

What to Do. See your dentist. Regularly brush and floss teeth to reduce plaque and have regular professional cleanings to reduce the incidence and severity of the condition. For severe cases, surgery may be needed to reduce excessive overgrowth.

PROBLEM

Gingivitis

Symptoms. Bleeding, swollen, reddened, and sometimes painful gums. There may be blood on the pillow in the morning.

Possible Causes. Accumulation of plaque; chronic irritation from partial dentures and orthodontic bands and appliances; overhanging margins of fillings, crowns, and other restorations; eruption of a tooth; mouth breathing; hormonal fluctuations during menstruation, pregnancy, and oral contraceptive use; and systemic diseases (e.g., HIV infection).

What to Do. Improve oral hygiene. If the condition does not improve, see your dentist. Treatment depends on the type of gingivitis and its cause. Treatments include improving oral hygiene, oral prophylaxis, scaling and root planing, and orthodontic adjustment to correct crowded teeth or incorrect tooth position. Using mouthrinses may be helpful.

PROBLEM

Canker sores (aphthous ulcers)

Symptoms. Painful and sometimes recurring ulcers on the soft tissues of the mouth. If under one centimeter in size, they usually heal in one week; if larger, they take longer to heal.

Possible Causes. Unknown, but they are brought on by stress, trauma, food allergy, and elevated levels of female hormones. Larger, slow-healing ulcers also may accompany HIV infection.

What To Do. Treatments for recurrent canker sores include topical and systemic steroids, antimicrobial mouthrinses (e.g., tetracycline and chlorhexidine gluconate), and application of topical anesthetics.

PROBLEM

Loose teeth

Symptoms. The teeth move around in their sockets and may shift position and stick out. There may be pain with chewing.

Possible Causes. Damage to the periodontal ligament and destruction of the alveolar bone from periodontitis; dental injury; and, in rare instances, tumors in the jaw. Sometimes teeth that need endodontic therapy are loose.

What to Do. See your dentist. Treatments depend on the cause and may include meticulous home hygiene; regular periodontal examinations; professional tooth cleaning; scaling and root planing; endodontic therapy; bite adjustment; and, for more advanced cases, surgery.

PROBLEM

Stained teeth or gums

Possible Causes. Liquid iron supplements, use of tetracycline when teeth were developing, and mouthrinses containing chlorhexidine.

What to Do. If you take iron supplements, drink liquid iron through a straw and then rinse and brush your teeth. Professional cleaning and polishing reduce or eliminate stains from mouthrinses; bleaching, bonding, veneering, or crowns are recommended for deep tetracycline stains.

PROBLEM

Toothache

Symptoms. Pain in or around one or more teeth. Pain may radiate to the ear or jaw.

Possible Causes. Decay, abscess, periodontal disease, problems with the pulp, and injury. Nondental causes include infected sinuses, facial neuralgia, diseases (e.g., diabetes, alcoholism), vitamin deficiencies, herpes zoster (facial shingles), and cluster headaches.

What to Do. If needed, take nonnarcotic analgesics or nonsteroidal anti-inflammatory medications to relieve the pain. Call the dentist and follow instructions. Possible dental treatments include fillings or other restorations, antibiotics to treat infection, endodontic therapy, extractions, and measures to treat periodontal disease. If the cause is not related to a dental problem, the dentist will refer you to a physician.

PROBLEM

Sensitive teeth

Symptoms. The teeth are sensitive when touched or when in contact with hot or cold.

Possible Causes. Vigorous brushing that causes the gums to recede or wears down the enamel and dentin at the neck of the tooth between the crown and root. The sensations of heat, cold, and touch are more easily transmitted to the nerves in the pulp. Extreme sensitivity to temperatures also can indicate injury to the pulp.

What to Do. Home treatments include brushing with a toothpaste marketed for sensitive teeth (these contain strontium chloride and/or potassium nitrate) and applying gel with stannous fluoride to sensitive teeth (these require a prescription written by a dentist). Professional treatments include covering the sensitive tooth structure with glass ionomer cement or composite resin, and endodontic therapy.

PROBLEM

Grinding and clenching teeth (bruxism)

Symptoms. Abnormal tooth wear, especially on the cusps of teeth, broken restorations, fractured tooth cusps, sensitive and/or loose teeth, pain on chewing, headaches, oral infection, temporomandibular disorders (e.g., limited jaw opening, tenderness of the muscles involved in chewing), and inflamed gums.

Possible Causes. Stress, malocclusions, allergies, sleep positioning, defective restorations, and uneven contact between teeth. Genetic predisposition and central nervous system dysfunction are suspected causes.

What to Do. See your dentist. Treatments depend on the cause(s) and include stress reduction therapy (e.g., visual imagery), changing sleep positions, medications (e.g., nonsteroidal anti-inflammatory drugs, limited use of Valium), biofeedback training, physical therapy, soft-food diet, muscle stretching exercises, heat therapy, and use of intraoral appliances.

PROBLEM

Dental infection

Symptoms. Fever; swelling in and around the mouth, between the teeth and the cheeks, or on the roof of the mouth adjacent to the teeth; a tongue that is raised or difficult to move; difficulty speaking, swallowing, and opening the mouth; pain; tenderness; or pus from oral tissues.

Possible Causes. Infections that begin in the teeth and involve the dental pulp (usually a result of caries), periodontal tissues, tonsils, sinuses, and jaws, and then spread to other areas of the head and neck.

What to Do. Call your dentist immediately. If you cannot reach your dentist and the symptoms are worsening or if you have difficulty swallowing or speaking, go immediately to a hospital emergency room and request an oral and maxillofacial surgeon. Treatments include surgically draining the area of pus and administering oral antibiotics. In severe infections, antibiotics may be delivered intravenously.

PROBLEM

Tooth wear (abrasion and erosion)

Symptoms. Tooth surface that is worn away, often on the cusps of the teeth, in grooves or notches at specific sites such as at the neck of the tooth, or where the teeth are exposed when the mouth is open.

Possible Causes. Force from normal chewing; teeth grinding and clenching; fruit and fruit juices containing citric acid (e.g., lemons, oranges); carbonated drinks; vinegar; chewable vitamin C, aspirin, and iron tablets; abrasive toothpastes; repeated vomiting from bulimia or chronic alcoholism; industrial acids; chronic biting of hard objects (e.g., pins, tacks); and inappropriate use of floss, interproximal brushes, and toothbrushes.

What to Do. First, stop the habit or avoid the offending substance that is causing the tooth wear. Other treatments include the application of topical fluorides, soft splints over the teeth, masks to protect the teeth from industrial acid vapors, drinking acid beverages with a straw, good oral hygiene, and excluding coarse food from the diet. If damage is severe, the teeth may need to be restored with bonded composites or crowns.

PROBLEM

Bad breath (halitosis)

Symptoms. Offensive odors emitted from the mouth.

Possible Causes. Oral diseases and problems (e.g., periodontal disease, diseases of the pulp, caries, defective crowns, appliances, prostheses); tongues that have fissures that trap food debris; poor oral hygiene; certain foods (e.g., onions, garlic, spices); dieting; lesions, tumors, or diseases of the nose or sinuses; respiratory diseases (e.g., bronchitis, bronchiectasis, pneumonia); and oral candidiasis. Psychological factors that affect the perception of oral odor include schizophrenia, organic brain syndrome, depression, types of hypochondriacal psychosis, low self-esteem, and difficulties in interpersonal relationships. The following can aggravate bad breath by reducing salivary flow, which results in dry mouth: diseases (e.g., anemia, AIDS, diabetes), stress, radiation of the head or neck, medications (see above and Chapter 10 for a listing), and mouth breathing.

What to Do. First, try improving oral hygiene by brushing the teeth with a fluoride-containing toothpaste, using a fluoridated mouthrinse (only if recommended by a dentist), flossing, cleaning or brushing the tongue with a brush or spoon, and keeping dentures and implants clean. If the bad breath does not improve immediately and dramatically, see your dentist. Treatments depend on the cause and include antifungal medications; dietary modification; improving oral hygiene; therapies for periodontal disease; remedies for dry mouth (see the previous section); recontouring or replacing defective crowns, appliances, or prostheses; endodontic therapy; and extractions. If a psychological or neurological disorder is suspected, the dentist should refer the patient to the appropriate physician.

PROBLEM

Fractured jaw

Symptoms. Pain and tenderness over the injury or nearby, difficulty chewing, a change in the way the teeth bite together, and facial numbness.

Possible Causes. Injury to the jawbone.

What to Do. Do not move the jaw. To prevent it from moving, tie a scarf or other piece of cloth or clothing around the jaw and over the top of the head. For swelling, apply ice wrapped in a towel or a cold compress to the tender area. Call your dentist immediately. If you are unable to reach your dentist, go directly to a hospital emergency room and ask to be seen by an oral and maxillofacial surgeon.

PROBLEM

Salivary gland disorders

Symptoms. Enlargement, tenderness and/or pain of the salivary gland and decrease or increase in the amount of saliva produced.

Possible Causes. Sjögren's syndrome, trauma, salivary gland stones, infections, cysts, tumors, viruses, nutritional disorders, allergy, alcoholic cirrhosis, HIV infection, and injection of iodine-containing compounds.

What to Do. See your dentist. Treatments include antibiotics and surgery.

PROBLEMS

Fluorosis

Symptoms. White or brown defects on the enamel of the permanent teeth. In extreme cases, the enamel can also become mottled and/or pitted.

Possible Causes. Excessive amounts of fluoride during the years the teeth were forming.

What to Do. Most cases of fluorosis are mild and require no treatment. For more severe cases, treatment depends on the severity of the staining. Options include bleaching, bonding, and sometimes crowns. To prevent fluorosis or further staining, see your dentist to be certain that children receive the correct amount of fluoride in their water and diet and from other sources.

PROBLEM

Glossitis (burning tongue)

Symptoms. Pain, sensitivity, and burning sensations in the tongue; the tongue may appear red and may have sores on it.

Possible Causes. May be related to anxiety, stress, depression, and other psychological and emotional factors; candida infections; and geographic tongue (benign migratory glossitis), a type of glossitis.

What to Do. Your physician should rule out anemia, diabetes, and other systemic disorders. Treatment with antifungal medication should be given if the glossitis is caused by a candida infection. Good oral hygiene may help. Occasionally, if no medical or dental cause can be found, psychological counseling may be advised.

PROBLEM

Angular cheilitis

Symptoms. Deep fissures or cracks at the corners of the mouth that can bleed, ulcerate, and develop a crust on them; pain, especially when opening the mouth wide.

Possible Causes. Candida infections, overclosure of the mouth in someone who is without teeth and without dentures or implants, and nutritional deficiency (of vitamin B). Less frequent causes include staphylococcus and streptococcal infections and herpes simplex virus type I.

What to Do. See your dentist. Treatments depend on the cause and can include antifungal and antibiotic medication, vitamins, and construction of dentures for toothless patients.

PROBLEM

Oral Cancer

Symptoms. A flat or slightly raised red and/or white area (which may or may not be painful) that is firm and stippled (dotted) located on the sides of the tongue or the floor of the mouth just behind the lower front teeth. Oral cancer usually occurs in men over the age of 50 who consume tobacco and excessive amounts of alcohol. The sore may hurt when touched.

Possible Causes. Tobacco and excessive amounts of alcohol.

What to Do. See your dentist immediately. Treatments include surgery by an oral and maxillofacial surgeon or a head and neck surgeon, sometimes followed by radiation therapy and chemotherapy.

PROBLEM

Loose dentures

Symptoms. The dentures shift and do not fit securely.

Possible Causes. Resorption of the alveolar bone, shrinkage of the supporting soft tissues, and a retracted tongue.

What to Do. See your dentist or prosthodontist. The denture may need to be relined, rebased, or replaced.

PROBLEM

Loose implants

Symptoms. The implants or the tooth or teeth shift, budge, or move and the implants do not fit securely.

Possible Causes. The implant did not heal properly in the bone, or there is a loose or broken connection between the implant and the teeth or denture.

What to Do. See your dentist. If the implant did not heal properly in the bone, it may need to be removed and allowed to heal before being replaced. If the connection of the tooth or teeth, bridge, or denture to the implant is loose, a screw may need to be replaced.

PROBLEM

Denture sore mouth (stomatitis)

Symptoms. The area in the mouth underneath the dentures becomes inflamed and sore.

Possible Causes. Candida infection, reaction of the tissues to poorly fitting or unclean dentures, systemic disease, vitamin deficiencies, a residue of denture cleaner, irritation from wearing dentures too long, or allergy to dental material (extremely rare).

What to Do. See your prosthodontist. Remedies include cleaning the dentures by using a brush or ultrasonic device or by soaking them in an antifungal solution; relining the dentures with a tissue conditioner; making a new denture; or treatment with an antifungal medication (e.g., amphotericin, miconazole, nystatin), available only by a prescription.

PROBLEM

Temporomandibular disorders

Symptoms. Pain in the face or head; noises (clicking, grating, popping) when the jaw is opened or closed; limited range of jaw movement; sore jaw muscles; headache; temporary or permanent locking of the jaw; pain on yawning, chewing, or opening the mouth; inability to chew correctly; and tooth grinding.

Possible Causes. Injuries to the jaw joint and oral habits (e.g., grinding the teeth, clenching the jaw, biting the fingernails).

What to Do. If symptoms persist, see your dentist for a thorough evaluation. Treatments include soft-food diet, heat and cold therapy, muscle exercise and massage, mouthguards, relaxation therapies, medications (e.g., anti-inflammatories, muscle relaxants, antianxiety drugs, narcotic analgesics, antidepressants), and trigger point injections. In persistent and very painful cases, surgery (arthroscopy, reconstructive open-joint surgery) may be indicated.

GLOSSARY

Definitions for some of the more common dental terms are presented here. Others can be found in separate chapters (for example, Chapter 4 includes definitions of insurance terms, and Chapter 20 a description of some types of dental injuries).

abrasion—tooth wear caused by mechanical forces other than chewing, such as improper tooth brushing or holding objects between the teeth.

abutment—a tooth (or implant) that supports a dental prosthesis.

alveolar bone—the part of the jaw that surrounds the roots of the teeth.

alveolar process—the curving part of the jaw into which the teeth sink or are embedded.

alveolus—the socket in the alveolar bone into which the root of a tooth fits.

amalgam—an alloy of different metals including mercury used as a filling material.

ankylosis—a condition in which two hard tissues that are normally not fused are fused together. When this happens to a tooth and the alveolar bone, the tooth erupts only partially.

anterior disc displacement—see internal derangement.

apical foramen—the opening at the tip of a root where blood vessels and nerves enter the root canal of a tooth.

apicoectomy—removal of the tip of a tooth root.

arthroscopy—a surgical procedure in which an arthroscope is inserted into the temporomandibular joint in order to view the joint.

articular disc—the disc of fibrous tissue within the temporomandibular joint that fits over the condyle or end of the mandible and cushions its movement.

attached gingiva—the gingival tissues that lie over the alveolar process of the jaw and are strongly attached to the bone and underlying teeth.

attrition—the wearing down of tooth structure caused by tooth-to-tooth contact in normal chewing or with bruxing (tooth grinding).

bitewing radiographs—radiographic films that reveal the crowns of several upper and lower teeth as they are biting down.

bleaching—a cosmetic dental procedure that whitens teeth using a bleaching solution.

bonding—a cosmetic dental procedure in which composite resin is applied to a tooth to change its shape and color. Bonding also refers to how fillings, orthodontic appliances, or certain fixed partial dentures are attached to teeth.

bridge—see fixed partial denture.

bruxism—the habitual grinding or clenching of teeth.

calculus—deposits of hardened or calcified plaque on teeth. Also called tartar.

caries—an infectious dental disease that can destroy tooth structure. Commonly called decay.

cariogenic—caries promoting.

cast, diagnostic—a stone or plaster model of the teeth and adjoining structures. Also called study model.

cavity—a hole in a tooth caused by caries.

cementum—hard tissue covering the roots of the teeth.

cephalometric analysis—an analysis of measurements of the skull and jaw taken from lateral skull radiographs that is used to evaluate the shape of the skull and face for orthodontic treatment.

cleft lip—a birth defect in which there are one or more fissures in the upper lip, a result of the failure of the embryonic upper jaw and midline tissues to grow sufficiently and come together during their development.

cleft palate—a birth defect in which the two sides of the palate failed to grow together and fuse. This creates a hole or gap in the middle of the palate (roof of the mouth).

conscious sedation—a level of sedation in which patients are less aware than usual of what is taking place around them but are able to breathe and swallow on their own.

crown—the part of the tooth that is visible and covered with enamel. Also a restoration that replaces the tooth structure lost from the crown of the tooth.

curettage—the cleaning or scraping of the walls of periodontal pockets that is performed for treatment of periodontal disease.

cusp—the pointed portion of the crown of the tooth.

debridement—removing foreign matter or dead tissue remnants.

decay—the common term for caries.

deciduous—a term for primary teeth.

dental assistant—a member of a dental staff who helps the dentist by performing a variety of professional, administrative, and secretarial duties. What duties he or she can perform to assist the dentist at the chair (for example, helping during surgery, taking impressions of teeth) depend on the regulations of the state in which he or she is employed.

dental hygienist—a dental care professional who performs preventive maintenance services, such as scaling and polishing teeth and applying topical fluorides and sealants. In some states he or she is allowed to perform other dental care duties.

dental prosthesis—an artificial device that replaces one or more missing teeth.

dental specialist—a dentist who has received postgraduate training in one of the eight recognized specialties in dentistry.

dentin—hard tissue surrounding the pulp of a tooth and beneath the enamel and cementum.

dentinal tubule—tubules within the dentin of a tooth that are filled with fluid and can transmit a number of stimuli, such as heat and cold from the outside of the tooth to the nerves within the pulp, resulting in pain.

dentition—the arrangement, number, and type of teeth.

denture—a set of artificial teeth that are not fastened permanently in the mouth.

denture base—the part of a denture that fits over the gums and holds the artificial teeth.

digital radiography—a radiographic process in which the images are formed electronically and transmitted in digital form to a computer where they can be viewed immediately on a video screen or stored for later viewing.

discectomy—surgical removal of part or all of the disc within the temporomandibular joint.

dry mouth—see xerostomia.

dry socket—delayed healing of the tooth socket after extraction possibly caused by infection or a problem with the blood clotting.

edentulous—toothless.

enamel—hard outside tissue covering the crown of the tooth.

enamel recontouring—see tooth reshaping.

endodontics—a specialty of dentistry concerned with preventing, diagnosing, and treating diseases and injuries of the dental pulp and the soft tissues and bone surrounding the tip of the root.

endodontist—a dentist who has received additional specialty training in endodontics and restricts his or her practice to diagnosing and treating diseases and injuries of the dental pulp and the soft tissues and bone surrounding the tip of the root.

endosteal implant—a type of dental implant that is surgically placed in the jaw bone.

erosion—wearing down of tooth structure, caused by chemicals (acids).

eruption—when a tooth emerges through the gums.

filling—the common term for a dental restoration.

fixed appliances—orthodontic appliances, commonly known as braces, that are bonded to the teeth to produce different tooth movements to reposition teeth for orthodontic therapy.

fixed partial denture—a fixed dental prosthesis that usually is cemented to abutment teeth to replace one or more missing teeth. Also called a fixed bridge.

fluoride—a mineral that is added to water and given by drops or tablets to harden enamel and reduce caries.

fluorosis—a condition in which the permanent teeth become discolored and pitted from the ingestion of abnormally high levels of fluoride during the time when the teeth are forming.

free gingiva—the small strip of gingival tissues along the margin of the gingiva.

frenum—muscle fibers covered by mucous membranes that attach the lips, tongue, or cheek to other parts of the oral mucosa.

full-mouth radiographs—a combination of 14 or more periapical and 4 bitewing films of the back teeth. This series reveals all the teeth (crowns and roots) and the alveolar bone surrounding them.

functional appliances—orthodontic appliances used either exclusively or before and after treatment with fixed appliances (braces) to change the relationship of the jaws.

general anesthesia—a deep level of sedation in which patients lose consciousness, feel no pain, and have no memory of what is taking place around them. Medical equipment may be needed to assist them in breathing. It is usually reserved for longer surgical dental procedures, such as surgery on the jaw.

general dentist—a dentist who takes care of the general dental needs of patients and refers them to dental specialists when needed.

gingiva—the mucous membranes that cover the roots of the teeth and the surrounding alveolar bone. Commonly called gums.

gingival crevicular fluid—fluid that is released from the gum tissues into the gum pocket.

gingival hyperplasia—an overgrowth of gingival tissues.

gingival sulcus—the space between the free gingiva and the tooth.

gingivectomy—a surgical procedure for the treatment of periodontal disease that removes part of the gum to reduce the depth of the periodontal pocket. It can also be performed for cosmetic purposes, to make the front teeth longer and even up teeth that seem to be of different lengths as a result of the unevenness of their gum margins.

gingivitis—an inflammation of the gingiva.

glossitis—an inflammation of the tongue.

guided tissue regeneration—a procedure during flap surgery for periodontal disease in which a membrane is inserted between the alveolar bone and the bone graft to encourage the gum tissues to grow onto the alveolar bone.

implant, dental—a cylinder or other material that is inserted into the alveolar bone to provide a base to hold artificial teeth.

impacted tooth—a tooth that is prevented from erupting (emerging through the gums) because it is obstructed by another tooth, bone, or soft tissue.

infection control procedures—measures that dentists are required by the Occupational Safety and Health Administration to take to reduce the risk of transmitting infectious diseases to employees.

inlay—a restoration that fits within a prepared cavity in a tooth.

internal derangement—the disc within the temporomandibular joint becomes displaced or slipped, so that it prevents the jaw from fully opening. Also called anterior disc displacement.

interproximal—between the teeth.

intravenous sedation—the introduction of medications intravenously (through the blood stream) to produce varying levels of sedation.

malocclusion—problems in the way in which the teeth of the upper jaw occlude (come together) with the teeth in the lower jaw.

mandible—lower jaw.

mandibular prognathism—a skeletal deformity in which the lower jaw is more developed than the upper jaw and the chin is prominent.

mandibular retrognathism—a skeletal deformity in which the upper jaw appears larger or more developed than the lower jaw, the chin looks receded, and the upper teeth protrude over the lower teeth.

Maryland bridge—a type of fixed partial denture not requiring crowns. Instead the prosthesis is bonded to the natural teeth to secure it.

maxilla—upper jaw.

mouthguards—mouthpieces that fit over the teeth to prevent injury to the teeth and surrounding structures during athletic or other activities or from grinding and to treat temporomandibular disorders.

nightguard bleaching—bleaching teeth by the patient, monitored by the dentist.

nitrous oxide with oxygen—chemicals that are inhaled by the patient to produce a light level of conscious sedation. Often called laughing gas or sweet air.

obstructive sleep apnea—a disorder in which breathing stops for short periods of time during sleep.

occlusal radiograph—a radiograph (x-ray picture) that reveals a complete lower or upper dental arch, the entire structure of the teeth, the palate, and some of the surrounding periapical area on one film.

occlusion—contact between the biting (occlusal) surfaces of the upper and lower teeth.

occlusal—the top or biting surfaces of the molars.

onlay—a restoration that replaces the cusps and biting surface of a tooth.

oral and maxillofacial surgeon—a dental specialist who diagnoses and surgically treats diseases, injuries, and abnormalities of the hard and soft tissues of the neck, face, head, and jaws.

oral mucosa—the pink-red tissues lining the mouth.

oral pathologist—a dental specialist who studies and occasionally diagnoses the causes and effects of diseases of the mouth and surrounding regions.

orthodontics—the specialty of dentistry that deals with malocclusions and problems in the spacing and positioning of teeth.

orthodontist—a dental specialist who limits his or her practice to the diagnosis, prevention, and treatment of malocclusions and problems with spacing and positioning of teeth.

orthognathic surgery—surgery performed to correct facial imbalances caused by abnormalities of the bones of the jaws.

osseointegration—the process by which bone heals around an implant.

overdenture—a dental prosthesis that is supported by natural tooth roots or implants.

palate—the hard and soft tissues of the roof of the mouth.

panoramic radiograph—a "wide-angle" radiograph that includes the upper and lower jaws on one film.

parotid glands—major salivary glands located in front of and below the ears.

partial denture—a removable prosthesis that replaces several missing teeth.

pediatric dentist—a dental specialist who treats the dental needs of children and also may treat the dental needs of adult special patients.

pellicle—a thin nonbacterial film from saliva that covers the teeth.

periapical—the tissues surrounding the tip of the root of a tooth, including the peridontal ligament connective tissue and bone.

periapical radiograph—a film that shows several entire teeth (crowns and roots) and specifically includes a small amount of the periapical bone (surrounding the root tips).

periodontal abscess—an infection in the gum pocket that is capable of destroying both hard and soft tissues.

periodontal disease—a group of infectious diseases that affect the periodontium.

periodontal ligament—tendonlike tissues surrounding the root of the tooth that attach the tooth to the jawbone.

periodontal pocket—a small crevice or space between the tooth and gingiva that is created as a result of the destruction of the collagen tissues by the bacteria present in periodontal disease.

periodontist—a dental specialist whose practice is limited to the detection, diagnosis, prevention, and treatment of periodontal diseases.

periodontitis—the more-advanced stages of periodontal disease that damage the supporting structures of the teeth: the cementum, periodontal ligament, and alveolar bone.

periodontium—the hard and soft structures that support the teeth: the gingiva, alveolar process, cementum, and periodontal ligament.

plaque—the soft, transparent substance composed of bacteria and its toxic byproducts that accumulates on the teeth.

pontic—the artificial tooth on a fixed partial denture.

prophylaxis, oral—a professional cleaning that removes food, beverages, tobacco stains, and tartar from and polishes the teeth above the gumline.

prosthodontist—a dental specialist who replaces missing teeth with a variety of dental prostheses.

public health dentist—a dental specialist who does not treat individuals but instead focuses on preventing and controlling dental diseases and promoting dental health through public programs. He or she often works for a government or an academic medical center.

pulp—loose, soft connective tissue within the tooth that contains blood vessels and nerves.

pulp canal—the space within the root of a tooth. Also called root canal.

pulp chamber—the space within the crown of the tooth that contains pulp tissue.

pulpectomy—a procedure that removes the diseased pulp from within the root canal.

pulpitis—inflammation of the pulp.

pulpotomy—a procedure that removes the diseased pulp from within the crown of the tooth only.

radiograph—an image produced by projecting radiation, as x-rays, on photographic film. Commonly called x-ray.

ranula—a cyst that can develop under the tongue in the floor of the mouth.

rebase—to replace the denture base.

reconstructive open joint surgery—various surgical procedures, in which the temporomandibular joint is exposed, that are used to repair problems with the joint and its surrounding structures.

reline—to resurface the side of the denture that is in contact with the soft tissues of the mouth to make it fit more securely.

removable appliances—removable orthodontic appliances used to effect simple tipping movements of one tooth or a group of teeth.

resorb—dissolve.

restoration—the replacement of lost tooth structure with metal, plastic, or cement materials.

retainer—a removable or fixed device that is used after orthodontic treatment to hold teeth in their new position until the bones and tissues reorganize.

root—the portion of the tooth beneath the gums that is embedded into the alveolus.

root canal—the channel inside the root that contains pulp tissue.

root canal therapy—a procedure in which the diseased pulp is removed from the root canal(s) and pulp chamber, and the area filled in to treat and / or prevent inflammation in the periapical tissues.

root caries—caries that affects the surfaces of the tooth roots.

root planing—a procedure that removes bacteria, calculus, and diseased cementum or dentin from the surface of the tooth roots or in the periodontal pockets.

scaling—professional removal of plaque, tartar, and stains from teeth.

sealants—plastic resin placed on the biting surfaces of molars to prevent bacteria from attacking the enamel and causing caries.

sialadenitis—the formation of stones, or calculi within the ducts of major and minor salivary glands.

sialography—radiography of the salivary ducts and glands after radiopaque dye has been injected into them.

Sjögren's syndrome—an autoimmune disorder mostly affecting older women that is characterized by partial or complete cessation of saliva and tears. It also can be associated with rheumatic disease, such as rheumatic arthritis, lupus, or scleroderma.

stomatitis—inflammation of the membranes in the mouth.

sublingual glands—major salivary glands located in the mucosa on the floor of the mouth.

submandibular glands—walnut-sized major salivary glands located beneath the tongue.

tartar—deposits of hardened or calcified plaque on teeth. Also called calculus.

temporomandibular joint—the joint that connects the lower jaw (mandible) to the base of the skull (temporal bone).

temporomandibular disorders—a variety of problems that affect the temporomandibular joints and/or the muscles involved in chewing.

tooth reshaping—a procedure in which small amounts of enamel are removed from a tooth to reshape it. Also called enamel recontouring.

veneering—a cosmetic dental procedure in which prefabricated veneers of acrylic resin or porcelain are bonded onto a tooth to change its shape and color.

xerostomia—a condition in which the mouth lacks or is deficient in saliva. Also called dry mouth.

x-ray—see radiograph.

APPENDIX 1

Directory of
Some Dental Associations

American Dental Association
211 East Chicago Avenue
Chicago, IL 60611
312-440-2500

Academy of Dentistry for Persons
with Disabilities
211 East Chicago Avenue
Chicago, IL 60611
312-440-2661

Academy of General Dentistry
211 East Chicago Avenue,
Suite 1200
Chicago, IL 60611
312-440-4300

American Association of Endodontics
211 East Chicago Avenue,
Suite 1100
Chicago, IL 60611
312-266-7255

American Association of Oral and
Maxillofacial Surgeons
9700 West Bryn Mar Avenue
Rosemont, IL 60018-5701
1-800-822-6637

American Association of Orthodontics
401 North Lindberg Boulevard
St. Louis, MO 63141-7816
314-993-1700

American Academy of Pediatric
Dentistry
211 East Chicago Avenue,
Suite 1036
Chicago, IL 60611
312-337-2169

American Academy of Periodontology
737 North Michigan Avenue,
Suite 800
Chicago, IL 60611-2615
312-787-5518

American College of Prosthodontics
211 East Chicago Avenue,
Suite 1000
Chicago, IL 60611
312-573-1260

American Association of Public
Health Dentistry
10619 Jousting Lane
Richmond, VA 23235
804-272-8344

APPENDIX 2

Directory of Dental Schools

UNITED STATES

ALABAMA
University of Alabama
School of Dentistry
University Station
Birmingham, AL 35294

CALIFORNIA
University of California, Los Angeles
School of Dentistry
Center for the Health Sciences
Los Angeles, CA 90024-1668

University of California at San Francisco
School of Dentistry
513 Parnassus Avenue, Room S-630
San Francisco, CA 94143-0430

Loma Linda University
School of Dentistry
Loma Linda, CA 92350

University of the Pacific
School of Dentistry
2155 Webster Street
San Francisco, CA 94115

University of Southern California
School of Dentistry
University Park—MC 0641
Los Angeles, CA 90089-0641

COLORADO
University of Colorado
School of Dentistry
4200 East Ninth Ave., Box C-284
Denver, CO 80262

CONNECTICUT
University of Connecticut
School of Dental Medicine
263 Farmington Avenue
Farmington, CT 06030-3915

DISTRICT OF COLUMBIA
Howard University
College of Dentistry
600 W Street, NW
Washington, D.C. 20059-0001

FLORIDA
University of Florida
College of Dentistry
P.O. Box 100405
Gainesville, FL 32610-0405

GEORGIA
Medical College of Georgia
School of Dentistry
120 15th Street, Room AD1119
Augusta, GA 30912-1000

ILLINOIS
University of Illinois at Chicago
College of Dentistry
801 South Paulina Street
Chicago, IL 60612-7211

Northwestern University
Dental School
240 East Huron Street
Chicago, IL 60611-2972

Southern Illinois University
School of Dental Medicine
2800 College Avenue
Alton, IL 62002-4789

INDIANA
Indiana University
School of Dentistry
1121 West Michigan Street
Indianapolis, IN 46202-5186

IOWA
University of Iowa
College of Dentistry
100 Dental Science Building
Iowa City, IA 52242-1010

KENTUCKY
University of Kentucky
College of Dentistry
800 Rose Street
Lexington, KY 40536-0084

University of Louisville
School of Dentistry
501 South Preston
Louisville, KY 40292

LOUISIANA
Louisiana State University
School of Dentistry
1100 Florida Avenue
New Orleans, LA 70119

MARYLAND
University of Maryland at Baltimore
Dental School
666 West Baltimore Street
Baltimore, MD 21201

MASSACHUSETTS
Boston University
School of Graduate Dentistry
100 East Newton Street
Boston, MA 02118

Harvard School of Dental Medicine
188 Longwood Avenue
Boston, MA 02115

Tufts University
School of Dental Medicine
1 Kneeland Street
Boston, MA 02111

MICHIGAN
University of Detroit Mercy
School of Dentistry
2985 East Jefferson Avenue
Detroit, MI 48207-4282

University of Michigan
School of Dentistry
1011 North University Avenue
Ann Arbor, MI 48109-1078

MINNESOTA
University of Minnesota
School of Dentistry
515 Delaware Street, S.E.
15-209 Moos Tower
Minneapolis, MN 55455

MISSISSIPPI
University of Mississippi
School of Dentistry
2500 North State Steet
Jackson, MI 39216-4505

MISSOURI
University of Missouri—Kansas City
School of Dentistry
630 East 25th Street
Kansas City, MO 64108-2784

NEBRASKA
Creighton University
School of Dentistry
2500 California Plaza
Omaha, NE 68178-0240

University of Nebraska Medical
Center
College of Dentistry
40th and Holdrege Streets
Lincoln, NE 68583-0740

NEW JERSEY
University of Medicine and Dentistry
of New Jersey
New Jersey Dental School
110 Bergen Street
Newark, NJ 07103-2400

NEW YORK
Columbia University
School of Dental and Oral Surgery
630 West 168th Street
New York, NY 10032

New York University
College of Dentistry
345 East 24th Street
New York, NY 10010-4099

State University of New York
at Buffalo
School of Dental Medicine
325 Squire Hall, 3435 Main Street
Buffalo, NY 14214-3008

State University of New York at
Stony Brook
School of Dental Medicine

Health Sciences Center
Stony Brook, NY 11794-8700

NORTH CAROLINA
University of North Carolina at
Chapel Hill
School of Dentistry
CB #7450, 104 Brauer Hall
Chapel Hill, NC 27599-7450

OHIO
Ohio State University
College of Dentistry
305 West 12th Avenue
Columbus, OH 43210-1241

Case Western Reserve University
School of Dentistry
10900 Euclid Avenue
Cleveland, OH 44106-4905

OKLAHOMA
University of Oklahoma
College of Dentistry
1001 Stanton L. Young Boulevard
P.O. Box 26901
Oklahoma City, OK 73190-3044

OREGON
Oregon Health Sciences University
School of Dentistry
611 S. W. Campus Drive
Portland, OR 97201

PENNSYLVANIA
University of Pennsylvania
School of Dental Medicine
4001 West Spruce Street
Philadelphia, PA 19104

University of Pittsburgh
School of Dental Medicine
3501 Terrace Street
Pittsburgh, PA 15261-1933

Temple University
School of Dentistry
3223 North Broad Street
Philadelphia, PA 19140-5096

PUERTO RICO
University of Puerto Rico
School of Dentistry
Medical Sciences Campus
P.O. Box 365067
San Juan, PR 00936-5067

SOUTH CAROLINA
Medical University of South Carolina
College of Dental Medicine
171 Ashley Avenue
Charleston, SC 29425-2601

TENNESSEE
Meharry Medical College
School of Dentistry
D. B. Todd Boulevard
Nashville, TN 37208

University of Tennessee
College of Dentistry
875 Union Avenue
Memphis, TN 38163

TEXAS
Baylor College of Dentistry
P.O. Box 660677
Dallas, TX 75246-0677

University of Texas—Health Science
Center at Houston

Dental Branch
P.O. Box 20068
Houston, TX 77225-0068

University of Texas—Health Science
Center at San Antonio
Dental School
7703 Floyd Curl Drive
San Antonio, TX 78284-7906

VIRGINIA
Medical College of Virginia
Virginia Commonwealth University
School of Dentistry
P.O. Box 980566
Richmond, VA 23298-0566

WASHINGTON
University of Washington
School of Dentistry
D322 Health Sciences Building SC-62
Seattle, WA 98195-9950

WEST VIRGINIA
West Virginia University
School of Dentistry
Health Sciences Center North
Medical Center Drive
Morgantown, WV 26506-9400

WISCONSIN
Marquette University
School of Dentistry
604 North 16th Street
Milwaukee, WI 53233-2188

CANADA

ALBERTA
University of Alberta
Faculty of Dentistry
Dentistry Pharmacy Building
Edmonton, Alberta
Canada T6G-2N8

BRITISH COLUMBIA
University of British Columbia
Faculty of Dentistry
350-2194 Health Science Mall
Vancouver, BC
Canada V6T-1W5

MANITOBA
University of Manitoba
Faculty of Dentistry
780 Bannatyne Avenue
Winnipeg, Manitoba
Canada R3E-OW3

NOVA SCOTIA
Dalhousie University
Faculty of Dentistry
5981 University Avenue
Halifax, NS
Canada B3H-3J5

ONTARIO
University of Toronto
Faculty of Dentistry
124 Edward Street
Toronto, Ontario
Canada M5G-1G6

University of Western Ontario
Faculty of Dentistry
London, Ontario
Canada N6A-5C1

QUEBEC
Universite Laval
Faculté de Medicine Dentaire
Sainte-Foy, Quebec
Canada G1K-7P4

McGill University
Faculty of Dentistry
3460 University Street
Montreal, Quebec
Canada H3A-2B2

Université de Montreal
Faculté de Medicine Dentaire
2900 Edouard-Montpe
Montreal, Quebec
Canada H3C-3J7

SASKATCHEWAN
University of Saskatchewan
College of Dentistry
Saskatoon, Saskatchewan
Canada S7N-OWO

APPENDIX 3

Directory of
U.S. Dental Associations

STATE

Alabama Dental Association
836 Washington Street
Montgomery, AL 36104-3839

Alaska Dental Society
3400 Spenard Road, Suite 10
Anchorage, AK 99503-3738

Arizona State Dental Association
4131 North 36th Street
Phoenix, AZ 85018-4761

Arkansas State Dental Association
2501 Crestwood Road, #205
North Little Rock, AR 72116-7613

California Dental Association
Post Office Box 13749
Sacramento, CA 95853-4749

Colorado Dental Association
3690 South Yosemite Street, #100
Denver, CO 80237-1808

Connecticut State Dental Association
62 Russ Street
Hartford, CT 06106-1522

District of Columbia Dental Society
502 C Street North East
Washington, D.C. 20002-5810

Delaware State Dental Society
1925 Lovering Avenue
Wilmington, DE 19806-2157

Florida Dental Association
1111 East Tennessee Street,
Suite 102
Tallahassee, FL 32308-6914

Georgia Dental Association
2801 Buford Highway, North East,
#T-60
Atlanta, GA 30329-2137

Hawaii Dental Association
1000 Bishop Street, Suite 805
Honolulu, HI 96813-4208

Idaho State Dental Association
1220 West Hays Street
Boise, ID 83702-5315

Illinois State Dental Society
1010 South Second Street
Springfield, IL 62704-3005

Indiana Dental Association
Post Office Box 2467
Indianapolis, IN 46206-2467

Iowa Dental Association
505 5th Avenue, Suite 333
Des Moines, IO 50309-2322

Kansas Dental Association
5200 South West Huntoon Street
Topeka, KS 66604-2365

Kentucky Dental Association
1940 Princeton Drive
Louisville, KY 40205-1838

Louisiana Dental Association
320 Third Street, #201
Baton Rouge, LA 70801-1307

Maine Dental Association
Post Office Box 215
Manchester, ME 04351-0215

Maryland State Dental Association
6450 Dobbin Road
Columbia, MD 21045-5824

Massachusetts Dental Society
83 Speen Street
Natick, MA 01760-4125

Michigan Dental Association
230 Washington Square North,
Suite 208
Lansing, MI 48933-1312

Minnesota Dental Association
2236 Marshall Avenue
St. Paul, MN 55104-5758

Mississippi Dental Association
2630 Ridgewood Road
Jackson, MS 39216-4920

Missouri Dental Association
Post Office Box 1707
Jefferson City, MO 65102-1707

Montana Dental Association
Post Office Box 1154
Helena, MT 59624-1154

Nebraska Dental Association
3120 O Street
Lincoln, NE 68510-1533

Nevada Dental Association
6889 West Charleston Boulevard,
Suite B
Las Vegas, NV 89117-1600

New Hampshire Dental Society
Post Office Box 2229
Concord, NH 03302-2229

New Jersey Dental Association
1 Dental Plaza
North Brunswick, NJ 08902-4313

New Mexico Dental Association
3736 Eubank Boulevard Northeast,
#A1
Albuquerque, NM 87111-3556

The Dental Society of the State of
New York
7 Elk Street
Albany, NY 12207-1002

North Carolina Dental Society
Post Office Box 12047
Raleigh, NC 27605-2047

North Dakota Dental Association
Post Office Box 1332
Bismarck, ND 58502-1332

Ohio Dental Association
1370 Dublin Road
Columbus, OH 43215-1009

Oklahoma Dental Association
629 West I 44 Service Road
Oklahoma City, OK 73118-6032

Oregon Dental Association
17898 Southwest McEwan Avenue
Portland, OR 97224-7217

Pennsylvania Dental Association
Post Office Box 3341
Harrisburg, PA 17105-3341

Rhode Island Dental Association
200 Centerville Road
Warwick, RI 02886-0204

South Carolina Dental Association
120 Stonemark Lane
Columbia, SC 29210-3841

South Dakota Dental Association
Post Office Box 1194
Pierre, SD 57501-1194

Tennessee Dental Association
Post Office Box 120188
Nashville, TN 37212-0188

Texas Dental Association
Post Office Box 3358
Austin, TX 78764-3358

Utah Dental Association
1151 East 3900 S Ste B160
Salt Lake City, UT 84124-1216

Vermont State Dental Society
132 Church Street
Burlington, VT 05401-8401

Virginia Dental Association
Post Office Box 6906
Richmond, VA 23230-0906

Panama Canal Dental Society
17410 1st Place Southwest
Seattle, WA 98166-3704

Washington State Dental Association
2033 6th Avenue, Suite 333
Seattle, WA 98121-2526

West Virginia Dental Association
1002 Kanawha Boulevard East
300 Capitol Street
Charleston, WV 25301-2809

Wisconsin Dental Association
111 East Wisconsin Avenue,
Suite 1300
Milwaukee, WI 53202-4807

Wyoming Dental Association
Post Office Box 1123
Cheyenne, WY 82003-1123

TERRITORY

Puerto Rico, Colegio de Cirujanos
Dent
200 Avenue Domenech
San Juan, P R 00918-3507

Virgin Islands Dental Association
Post Office Box 10422
St. Thomas, VI 00801-3422

GOVERNMENT

Air Force Dental Corps
HQ USAF/SGD
110 Luke Avenue Southwest,
Room 400
Bolling AFB DC 20332-5113

Navy Dental Corps
Office of the Secretary
of Defense
The Pentagon #30372
Washington, D.C. 20310-0000

Veterans Affairs
5205 Continental Drive
Rockville, Maryland 20853-1119

Army Dental Corps
Chief, Army Dental Corps

2250 Stanley Road
Fort Samuel Houston, TX 78234-6185

Navy Dental Corps
2603 Oakton Glen Drive
Vienna, VA 22181-5342

INDEX

abrasion, 157–59, 168–69, 397–98
  in adults, 158
  in endodontics, 221–22, 224
  in prosthodontics, 278
abscesses:
  acute apical, 223, 225–26, 228
  emergencies and, 356
  endodontic, 125
  periapical, 88, 232
  periodontal, 125, 228
  in periodontal disease, 112
  toothaches from, 396
  x-rays of, 367
acetaminophen, 200, 325, 349, 354, 357
acquired immune deficiency syndrome (AIDS),
     152, 170, 366, 376, 391
  dentists for people with, 28
  oral problems associated with, 197–98
  xerostomia in, 163
acrylic resins:
  in cosmetic dentistry, 248–49
  in prosthodontics, 282, 284, 286, 289, 293
acute apical abscesses, 223, 225–26, 228
acute apical periodontitis, 225–26
acute necrotizing ulcerative gingivitis (ANUG),
     109–10
acute periapical abscesses, 232
acute pseudomembranous candidiasis, 170
adenoids, 138, 257, 262, 338
adolescents:
  caries in, 150, 153
  dental care for, 149–53
  dental development in, 13
  dentists for, 32, 139
  fluoride supplements for, 143, 150
  periodontal disease in, 110, 112–13, 151
  removal of wisdom teeth from, 152
  sexually transmitted diseases in, 152–153
  sports injuries in, 151
  tobacco and snuff use of, 153
  women as, 180–82
adrenal insufficiency, 207–8
adult periodontitis, 112, 183

adults:
  bruxism in, 156, 164
  caries in, 155, 158–60, 163, 165
  dental aesthetics in, 164–65
  dental care for, 155–65
  dental changes in, 155–59
  dental problems in, 159–65
  fluorides and, 158–59, 380
  halitosis in, 162–63
  illnesses in, 155–56, 160, 163
  oral cancer in, 161–62
  orthodontics for, 165, 256, 258–59
  periodontal disease in, 155–56, 160–62
  re-restorations for, 159–60
  wear and tear in, 156–59
  x-rays for, 163, 371–72
advanced education in general dentistry
     (AEGD), 30
aesthetics:
  in prosthodontics, 276, 278–79, 284,
     288
  see also cosmetic dentistry
age and aging:
  dental changes related to, 155–56
  for eruption of permanent teeth, 16
  for eruption of primary teeth, 15, 132–33
  in extractions, 324–25
  in orthodontics, 259
  and pain, 344
  and periodontal disease, 113, 121
  stains caused by, 68
  TMD and, 303
  see also adolescents; adults; children, 6-
     through 12-year-old; elderly; infants and
     children
alcohol and alcoholism:
  and cosmetic dentistry, 245
  and dental development, 22
  and oral and maxillofacial surgery, 331
  in oral cancer, 161, 400
  periodontal disease from, 110
  and prosthodontics, 285
  in tooth wear, 157–58, 397

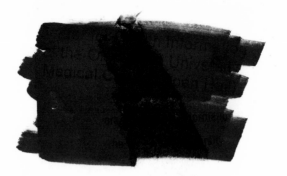